Hot Topics in Acute Care Surgery and Trauma

Series Editors

Federico Coccolini
Pisa, Italy

Raul Coimbra
Riverside, USA

Andrew W. Kirkpatrick
Calgary, Canada

Salomone Di Saverio
Cambridge, UK

Editorial Board

Luca Ansaloni (Cesena, Italy); Zsolt Balogh (Newcastle, Australia); Walt Biffl (Denver, USA); Fausto Catena (Parma, Italy); Kimberly Davis (New Haven, USA); Paula Ferrada (Richmond, USA); Gustavo Fraga (Campinas, Brazil); Rao Ivatury (Richmond, USA); Yoram Kluger (Haifa, Israel); Ari Leppaniemi (Helsinki, Finland); Ron Maier (Seattle, USA); Ernest E. Moore (Fort Collins, USA); Lena Napolitano (Ann Arbor, USA); Andrew Peitzman (Pittsburgh, USA); Patrick Rielly (Philadelphia, USA); Sandro Rizoli (Toronto, Canada); Boris Sakakushev (Plovdiv, Bulgaria); Massimo Sartelli (Macerata, Italy); Thomas Scalea (Baltimore, USA); David Spain (Stanford, USA); Philip Stahel (Denver, USA); Michael Sugrue (Letterkenny, Ireland); George Velmahos (Boston, USA); Dieter Weber (Perth, Australia)

This series covers the most debated issues in acute care and trauma surgery, from perioperative management to organizational and health policy issues.

Since 2011, the founder members of the World Society of Emergency Surgery's (WSES) Acute Care and Trauma Surgeons group, who endorse the series, realized the need to provide more educational tools for young surgeons in training and for general physicians and other specialists new to this discipline: WSES is currently developing a systematic scientific and educational program founded on evidence-based medicine and objective experience. Covering the complex management of acute trauma and non-trauma surgical patients, this series makes a significant contribution to this program and is a valuable resource for both trainees and practitioners in acute care surgery.

More information about this series at http://www.springer.com/series/15718

Joseph M. Galante • Raul Coimbra
Editors

Thoracic Surgery for the Acute Care Surgeon

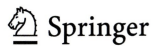

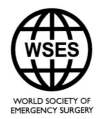

WORLD SOCIETY OF
EMERGENCY SURGERY

Editors
Joseph M. Galante
Davis Medical Centre
University of California, Davis
Sacramento, CA
USA

Raul Coimbra
Riverside University Health System Medical Center
Comparative Effectiveness and Clinical Outcomes Research Center - CECORC
Riverside, CA
USA

Loma Linda University School of Medicine
Loma Linda, CA
USA

ISSN 2520-8284　　　　　　　　ISSN 2520-8292　(electronic)
Hot Topics in Acute Care Surgery and Trauma
ISBN 978-3-030-48492-7　　　　ISBN 978-3-030-48493-4　(eBook)
https://doi.org/10.1007/978-3-030-48493-4

© Springer Nature Switzerland AG 2021
This work is subject to copyright. All rights are reserved by the Publisher, whether the whole or part of the material is concerned, specifically the rights of translation, reprinting, reuse of illustrations, recitation, broadcasting, reproduction on microfilms or in any other physical way, and transmission or information storage and retrieval, electronic adaptation, computer software, or by similar or dissimilar methodology now known or hereafter developed.
The use of general descriptive names, registered names, trademarks, service marks, etc. in this publication does not imply, even in the absence of a specific statement, that such names are exempt from the relevant protective laws and regulations and therefore free for general use.
The publisher, the authors, and the editors are safe to assume that the advice and information in this book are believed to be true and accurate at the date of publication. Neither the publisher nor the authors or the editors give a warranty, expressed or implied, with respect to the material contained herein or for any errors or omissions that may have been made. The publisher remains neutral with regard to jurisdictional claims in published maps and institutional affiliations.

This Springer imprint is published by the registered company Springer Nature Switzerland AG
The registered company address is: Gewerbestrasse 11, 6330 Cham, Switzerland

Series Foreword

Research is fundamentally altering the daily practice of acute care surgery (trauma, surgical critical care, and emergency general surgery) for the betterment of patients around the world. Management for many diseases and conditions is radically different than it was just a few years ago. For this reason, concise up-to-date information is required to inform busy clinicians. Therefore, since 2011 the World Society of Emergency Surgery (WSES), in partnership with the American Association for the Surgery of Trauma (AAST), endorses the development and publication of the "Hot Topics in Acute Care Surgery and Trauma," realizing the need to provide more educational tools for young in-training surgeons and for general physicians and other surgical specialists. These new forthcoming titles have been selected and prepared with this philosophy in mind. The books will cover the basics of pathophysiology and clinical management, framed with the reference that recent advances in the science of resuscitation, surgery, and critical care medicine have the potential to profoundly alter the epidemiology and subsequent outcomes of severe surgical illnesses and trauma.

Federico Coccolini
General Emergency and Trauma Surgery
Ospedale Maurizio Bufalini
Cesena, Italy

Raul Coimbra
Riverside University Health System—Med
Riverside, CA, USA

Andrew W. Kirkpatrick
Department of Surgery and Critical Care Medic
Foothills Medical Centre
Calgary, AB, Canada

Salomone Di Saverio
Department of Surgery (Addenbrooke)
Cambridge University Hospitals NHS Found
Cambridge, UK

Preface

The partnership between the American Association for the Surgery of Trauma (AAST) and the World Society of Emergency Surgery (WSES) centers around emergency surgical care delivered by acute care surgeons (ACS). ACS must be ready to deal with an array of trauma, emergency surgery, and critical care emergencies. They are often called upon day or night, sometimes in austere environments, to care for patients, whom they have never met before, with life-threatening surgical disease. Thoracic-based pathology is one of the more daunting areas faced by ACS making them feel less comfortable treating patients with surgical thoracic diseases due to limited experiences in either training or everyday practice. Unfortunately, thoracic surgical disease, whether a hemothorax or tuberculosis, is common around the world, and diagnosing and treating these patients in a timely fashion is critical if adequate outcomes are to be expected.

This textbook is a "how-to" guide for ACS to treat thoracic trauma and emergencies. The chapters include a focus on pediatrics, low resource environments, trauma and non-trauma conditions, and infectious disease. We have collected the expertise of a cadre of international authors who are members of the AAST and WSES to guide the ACS through the challenges of thoracic emergencies. We hope this textbook will be a valuable tool to improve the care and outcomes of patients with thoracic pathology around the world.

Sacramento, CA   Joseph M. Galante
Riverside, CA   Raul Coimbra

Contents

Low-Resource Environments 1
Marissa A. Boeck, Alain Chichom-Mefire, and Rochelle Dicker

Part I Acute Surgery Thoracic Emergencies

Esophageal Rupture 23
Patrick L. Bosarge and Dennis Y. Kim

Incarcerated Hiatal Hernia 43
Luigi Bonavina and Kenji Inaba

Pulmonary Embolism 53
David Miranda and Joseph Cuschieri

Empyema and Effusions 69
Andreas Hecker, Winfried Padberg, Timothy Browder,
and David A. Spain

Pericarditis and Pericardial Effusions 83
Ho H. Phan, Amanda Phares, Gustavo P. Fraga,
and Lindemberg M. Silveira-Filho

Necrotizing Lung Infections 103
Jill Streams, Jaclyn Clark, Marc de Moya, and Sharon Henry

Incidental Pulmonary Nodule 111
Fabio Ramponi, Cino Bendinelli, Joseph M. Galante,
Luis Godoy, and Anna Xue

Chylothorax 131
Laura Godat, Todd W. Costantini, and Kimberly A. Davis

Part II Trauma

Rib Fractures and Chest Wall Injury 145
Federico Coccolini, Michelle Hamel, Francesco Favi,
and John Mayberry

Pneumothorax and Hemothorax 159
R. Stephen Smith, Erin Vanzant, and Fausto Catena

Pulmonary Contusions and ARDS 169
Emiliano Gamberini, Luca Bissoni, Giovanni Scognamiglio,
and David H. Livingston

Tracheal and Bronchial Injury 191
Preston Miller and Walter L. Biffl

Lung Injury 197
Samuel P. Carmichael II, Yoram Kluger, and J. Wayne Meredith

Cardiac Injury 207
Kristina J. Nicholson, Ravi K. Ghanta, Matthew J. Wall Jr,
and Andrew B. Peitzman

**Blunt Thoracic Aortic Injury in Thoracic Surgery
for the Acute Care Surgeon** 227
Anna Romagnoli, Pedro Teixeira, Viktor Reva, and Joseph DuBose

Thoracic Vascular Trauma 243
Paul T. Albini, Megan L. Brenner, and Raul Coimbra

Diaphragm 253
Stefan W. Leichtle and Michel B. Aboutanos

Part III Special Considerations

Acute Care Pediatric Thoracic Surgical Conditions 263
Julia Grabowski and L. R. Scherer III

Surgical Consideration of Bacteria, Fungi, and Parasites 291
Massimo Sartelli

Travel and Transport 299
Allison Berndtson and Jay Doucet

Low-Resource Environments

Marissa A. Boeck, Alain Chichom-Mefire, and Rochelle Dicker

Epidemiology and Global Disparities

Thoracic pathologies requiring emergent invasive procedures are diverse and multifactorial, spanning from communicable to non-communicable, with a large proportion due to injuries. Although consistent and reliable data are lacking in many low- and middle-income countries (LMICs), various studies provide a glimpse of the thoracic surgery burden and case volume, as well as limitations and potential solutions. A 7-day prospective, observational cohort study of over 11,000 patients in nearly 250 hospitals across 25 African countries showed 1.3% of patients underwent a thoracic procedure, either for lung, gut, or other pathologies [1]. This is comparable to Rwanda's 1.76% of surgical cases being performed for thoracic diagnoses [2]. Data suggest that the number of people actually undergoing surgery pales in comparison to those who likely require it: It is estimated that as few as 10% of people who need thoracic surgical procedures actually undergo the procedure [3]. When comparing pathologies between low- and high-income countries, the main difference is the burden of infectious, inflammatory, and traumatic relative to malignant causes, with the former pathologies being more prevalent in low-resource settings [2, 4–7]. This likely reflects a real disparity, as well as that malignant chest conditions are likely underdiagnosed in LMICs. A 9-year case series from a national

M. A. Boeck
Department of Surgery, Zuckerberg San Francisco General Hospital, University of California San Francisco, San Francisco, CA, USA

A. Chichom-Mefire (✉)
Faculty of Health Sciences, University of Buea and Regional Hospital Limbe, Buea, Cameroon

R. Dicker
Department of Surgery, University of California Los Angeles, Los Angeles, CA, USA
e-mail: RDicker@mednet.ucla.edu

cardiothoracic center in Ghana revealed corrosive esophageal strictures as the most common thoracic pathology, followed by a mixture of malignant and infectious esophageal and pulmonary processes [8]. Additional disease processes more common in LMICs include pericardial effusion and constrictive pericarditis frequently secondary to tuberculosis, prior cardiac surgery, radiation, or trauma [9].

Nearly one-third of the world's population is infected by tuberculosis, leading to over one million deaths and nine million new cases annually, a large proportion of which occur in low-resource settings [10]. Proper medical treatment has an 85–90% success rate; however, those who are not cured frequently have multidrug-resistant or extensively drug-resistant forms, the social impact of which can be enormous. Surgery for tuberculosis is usually reserved for diagnosis, such as pleural drainage and exploration of solitary pulmonary nodules and mediastinal lesions. It is also used for definitive treatment in those with adequate pulmonary and physiologic reserve who fail medical therapy beyond 4 to 6 months and have focal lesions and/or drug resistance, or persistent bronchopleural fistula, tension pneumothorax, massive hemoptysis, empyema-causing sepsis, destroyed lung, or fibrothorax [10, 11].

Based on its direct relation to improved health outcomes, the Lancet Commission on Global Surgery considers 40 surgical, anesthetic, and obstetric (SAO) providers per 100,000 population as the minimum needed, noting that over 70% of the world's population lives in countries with surgical workforce densities below this target [12]. Those trained in cardiothoracic surgery are even more scarce [3, 13]. This leads to many general surgical, as well as non-surgical, providers encountering, and perhaps managing, a wide variety of thoracic pathologies. Frequently, these interactions occur at sites that are remote and have limited access to modern diagnostic and therapeutic instruments, and present referral challenges to higher levels of care. Referral challenges can be due to the acuity of the problem (the patient is too ill to travel), financing, or patient willingness to travel, among others. Factors contributing to a lack of access to thoracic surgical care include limited provider training and experience, and unavailability of surgical equipment for thoracic cases [2]. This chapter is to assist providers in LMICs who may encounter patients with thoracic issues requiring invasive procedures. The goal is to facilitate the rapid diagnosis and treatment of the most common thoracic problems seen in LMICs, as well as how to manage certain pitfalls and challenges should they occur. Supplemental material on management principles for specific pathologies can be found in other chapters of this textbook.

Diagnosis

As in any clinical scenario, one must first start with a thorough history and physical examination to arrive at the proper diagnosis. This is even more essential when advanced diagnostic modalities are unavailable. If possible, adjuncts such as laboratory tests and imaging should be used to further refine the diagnosis, with a frequent need for the clinician to be able to perform, interpret, and apply the exam findings in the absence of formal technicians and specialists. However, the power of the patient's story and exam findings cannot be understated.

History

Whenever possible, take a detailed history from the patient, family members, and/or pre-hospital care providers, including a history of present illness (HPI) and review of systems, past medical and surgical, allergies, current medications, and social and family history. In the HPI, items pertinent to thoracic diagnoses include shortness of breath, cough, chest pain, or dysphagia or odynophagia, elucidating quality, frequency, duration, and modifying or alleviating factors. It is important to know if the patient suffered a blunt or penetrating injury to the thorax, ingested a caustic substance or foreign body, or has a history of intra- or extra-thoracic malignancy or prior pulmonary infections. For infectious pathologies, elucidate if the patient has experienced fevers, chills, or received prior antibiotics or invasive treatments. Determine if the patient smokes, and if so, the quantity and duration. If the patient has a known malignancy, elicit prior pathologic diagnoses, surgeries, and treatment regimens.

Physical Exam

Observe the patient and determine if she or he passes the "eye-ball" test; that is, whether she or he looks reasonably well or ill. If presenting in extremis or as the result of a traumatic injury, follow the primary survey (ABCDEs) of management to address the most critical items first, including Airway, Breathing, Circulation, Disability, and Exposure. Evaluate whether the patient is speaking in full sentences, can only emit a few words before needing another breath, or is unable to phonate. Assess the mouth for foreign bodies, blood or emesis, or severe facial or neck trauma that may compromise the patient's ability to move air to maintain oxygenation and ventilation. Determine if the patient has a normal breathing pattern, or if there is accessory muscle use or diaphoresis, which indicate increased work of breathing and potential impending respiratory failure. Notice if you can hear a patient's breathing without auscultating, which usually takes the form of expiratory wheezing from lower airway obstruction, inspiratory stridor in those with upper airway obstruction, or inspiratory white noise, similar to radio static, in patients with chronic bronchitis or asthma [14]. Observe the chest wall for asymmetric expansion, which in a non-intubated patient suggests pneumonia or pleural effusion on the side with less movement, or right mainstem intubation with decreased movement on the left [14]. Assess the patient's coloring, especially around the lips, with blue hues suggesting hypoxia. Note the heart and respiratory rates and, if available, the blood pressure, oxygen saturation, and temperature. Evaluate the patient's mental status using the Glasgow Coma Scale, with a score of eight or lower suggesting a need for intubation and mechanical ventilation to protect the airway. And finally, remove all of the patient's clothing to avoid missing any injuries or physical exam findings, and cover her or him with a blanket to prevent hypothermia.

Follow the standard physical exam steps of inspect, auscultate, percuss, and palpate, with certain steps expedited for unstable patients. Perform these assessments anteriorly, laterally, and posteriorly on the thorax. When inspecting, look for external signs of trauma or pathology, including abrasions, lacerations, bullet holes, or flail chest, defined as two or more adjacent ribs broken in two or more places with paradoxical chest wall motion on respiration [15]. Always examine both axillae as injuries in these regions have the potential to affect the thorax, as well as down to the costal margin circumferentially, keeping in mind these areas can have both thoracic and abdominal injuries. Assess for jugular venous distention, which can be a sign of fluid overload, obstructive shock, or increased intrathoracic pressure, either due to heart failure, pulmonary embolism, cardiac tamponade, or tension pneumothorax. On auscultation assess for vocal resonance, breath sounds, and adventitious sounds. Decreased heart or lung sounds, crackles, rubs, wheezes, stridor, or rhonchi that may indicate fluid, atelectasis, pulmonary edema, bronchoconstriction, or consolidation in varying degrees. Abnormal vocal resonance can take the form of egophony, where the patient's voice has a nasal quality assessed by the patient saying "EE" and the sound transforming into "AH," bronchophony, where the voice is much louder than normal, or pectoriloquy, where the patient's words are intelligible, all of which can suggest consolidation in the appropriate clinical setting, or if diminished can suggest the presence of fluid [14]. Percuss bilaterally and assess for differences, with areas of hyperresonance that may indicate a pneumothorax versus dullness, which correlates with fluid or consolidation. Palpate for areas of tenderness that suggests fracture or inflammation, and crepitus that indicates air outside the aerodigestive tract.

Labs

If available, send a full set of labs including basic metabolic panel, complete blood count, and coagulation profile. If active tuberculosis is suspected, sputum cultures aided by nucleic acid amplification tests like GeneExpert should be sent in conjunction with imaging. Latent tuberculosis relies more on tuberculin skin and blood tests [16]. If the etiology of a pleural effusion is unknown and laboratory capabilities are available, send the fluid for gram stain, cell count, glucose, lactate dehydrogenase, and protein, with the latter two items determining if the effusion is transudative or exudative based on Light's criteria. A small case series out of Nepal showed fluids high in protein were associated with tuberculosis, parapneumonic and malignant effusions, yet only tuberculosis and malignant effusions had high lymphocyte counts, while those of parapneumonic effusions had predominantly neutrophils. An adenosine deaminase level above 60 U/L was both sensitive and specific for tuberculosis (90–100%, 89–100%, respectively) [17]. If there is concern for infection or malignancy, the fluid or tissue should be sent for gram stain, cell count, and culture (aerobic, anaerobic, fungal, and acid-fast bacilli) or cytology, respectively.

Imaging

The World Health Organization (WHO) estimates potentially two-thirds of the world's population do not have access to basic diagnostic imaging. Yet, it is generally thought around 20–30% of global medical diagnoses require more than clinical evaluations to confirm the underlying pathology, specifically with up to 60% of chest problems and injuries requiring further investigations [18].

Chest Radiography

Conventional radiography is one of the most widely used tests for diagnosing thoracic pathology, especially in low-resource settings. Created in 1895, it is considered safe with approximately 0.20 mGy delivered per exam versus 8–10 mGy per routine computed tomography chest study. These can be performed upright, supine, or decubitus, with posteroanterior (PA) and lateral or portable anteroposterior (AP) views. If looking for a pneumothorax or free fluid, upright chest can facilitate diagnosis by air rising to the apex of the thoracic cavity or fluid collecting at the base, respectively. Appropriate radiographic technique is confirmed by assessing for adequate inspiration, defined as seeing the right hemidiaphragm apex below the tenth posterior rib, motion, assessed by confirming a clear cardiac margin, pulmonary vessels, and diaphragm, penetration, with the ideal being faint visualization of the thoracic spine intervertebral disk spaces, and rotation, confirmed by superimposition of vertical lines drawn between the clavicular heads anteriorly and spinous processes posteriorly. Consolidation consistent with pneumonia will appear as an opacity, potentially with air bronchograms. Solitary pulmonary nodules consistent with neoplasm may appear similarly, requiring further elucidation with history, physical, and additional imaging. Pneumothorax can be identified by a non-dependent lucency along the chest wall medially displacing the visceral pleura on an upright film, or with a "deep sulcus" sign, hyperlucent upper abdomen, or "double diaphragm" sign with the patient supine. Although a clinical diagnosis, if radiography is done in the setting of a presumed tension pneumothorax, you may see hyperlucency, lung medialization, and diaphragmatic depression ipsilaterally, and contralateral mediastinal shift [19].

Tuberculosis is radiographically called "the great imitator" and has three main appearances on chest X-ray. Primary tuberculosis from a first exposure can look like a homogenous consolidation, pleural effusion, lymphadenopathy, or calcified caseating granuloma (Ghon focus). Reactivation tuberculosis frequently has linear opacities and nodules, cavities, and patchy heterogeneous consolidation specifically in the superior segments of the lower lobes and apical and posterior segments of the upper lobes. Finally, military tuberculosis has numerous, subcentimeter nodules throughout both lungs and thickened interlobular septa [16]. Radiographs also allow for the diagnosis of cardiac and vascular pathology, including a widened mediastinum potentially indicating an aortic dissection or rupture [15].

It is useful to read chest radiography in a standard fashion, following the pneumonic DRSABCDE. D is for details of the patient and study, R is for RIPE, standing for Rotation, Inspiration, Picture, and Exposure penetration of the study, and S is for soft tissue and bones, assessing for fractures and subcutaneous air. A stands for airway and mediastinum, assessing the trachea and carina for shift or adequate endotracheal tube placement within 2 to 4 cm of the carina, and mediastinal width. B is for breathing, evaluating the lung fields for pneumothorax, fluid, or consolidation. C refers to cardiac or circulation, which includes heart size and borders and aortic knob. D is for diaphragm, checking for elevation, blunting of costophrenic angles, and air under the diaphragm. E stands for everything else, which includes assessing for foreign bodies, tubes, or subcutaneous air [15].

Ultrasound

Since the World Health Organization's 1985 report on the potential advantages of ultrasound use in developing countries, its application has been on the rise given its relatively low cost, ease of use and interpretation with minimal training, portability, and battery power supply. A recent literature review found sub-Saharan Africa as the most common LMIC geographic area of use [20]. Possible examinations include vascular, cardiac, abdominal, obstetric, traumatic, and musculoskeletal, with studies showing ultrasound findings changing the initial care plan anywhere from 17 to nearly 70% of the time [21].

Pulmonary Exam

Multiple symptoms and potential diagnoses can be further evaluated with ultrasound, including respiratory failure, dyspnea, undifferentiated shock, pleural effusion, pneumothorax, consolidation, diaphragm function, volume status, lung or pleural masses, or thoracic trauma. The exam is typically done with a linear or curvilinear probe oriented to the head or the patient's right side in the longitudinal plane. Set the optimum depth and gain, and examine each hemithorax in multiple rib interspaces at the midclavicular line, midaxillary line, and posteriorly [22]. The following diagnoses have these characteristic sonographic findings:

Pneumothorax

Normal lung should have a "trail of ants" or hyperechoic pleura, which indicates lung sliding and is 100% sensitive to exclude pneumothorax at the location imaged. There should also be A-lines with normally aerated lung, which are hyperechoic lines appearing within the lung parenchyma that are a perpendicular artifact of the ultrasound beam reflecting off the pleura. A lack lung sliding plus or minus A-lines is concerning for a pneumothorax. False positives include a prior history of pleurodesis, severe acute respiratory distress syndrome, severe emphysema, opposing mainstem intubation, and apnea [22, 23].

Pulmonary Edema/Consolidation

As mentioned above, normal lung has A-lines. In the presence of intraparenchymal fluid, B-lines will appear, which are vertical lines that look like spotlights radiating from the probe downward. Specific criteria include that they: (1) extend across the entire image from the pleura downward, (2) move with lung sliding, and (3) eliminate A-lines. The quantity of B-lines correlates with the volume of fluid in the lungs, with a single B-line potentially being a normal finding, especially in a dependent lung zone [23]. Consolidation versus atelectasis can be assessed by the presence of mobile air bronchograms, which indicate a patent bronchus [22].

Pleural Effusion

It can be helpful to position the patient either upright or with the affected side down, to allow fluid to collect in the dependent portion of the thorax and facilitate identification. Using the curvilinear probe oriented parallel to the spine and toward the patient's head in the posterior axillary line, locate the diaphragm and either the liver on the right or spleen and kidney on the left. Look for the "spine sign," which is a refraction artifact of fluid in the pleural space that allows visualization of the spine above the diaphragm, as the normal presence of air does not allow this [22].

Cardiac Function

Heart function can be assessed with ultrasound to help elucidate the cause of undifferentiated shock, the pericardial space, left and right ventricular size and function, left atrial size, volume responsiveness, severe valve dysfunction, and cardiopulmonary symptoms. There are five positions for a basic sonographic cardiac exam, which include the parasternal long-axis, parasternal short-axis, apical four-chamber, subcostal four-chamber, and subcostal inferior vena cava [22]. Details regarding each are outside the scope of this chapter.

Extended Focused Assessment with Sonography in Trauma (eFAST)

The standard Focused Assessment with Sonography in Trauma (FAST) exam includes four views that examine the right upper quadrant, left upper quadrant, subxiphoid, and suprapubic region for free fluid, which appears jet black and collects in the most dependent areas. It is most useful for unstable, blunt trauma patients, where it has 100% sensitivity and specificity when performed by a trained surgeon [24]. FAST can also be useful for penetrating injury to the "cardiac box" (between the nipples laterally and from the sternal notch to the xiphoid) to assess the pericardium for fluid, as well as in multicavity penetrating injury to examine both the thorax and abdomen to determine which cavity to explore first [25]. The extension (eFAST) includes looking anteriorly at both hemithoraces for pneumothorax, with ultrasound having increased sensitivity over chest X-ray (86–98% vs. 28–75%, respectively). Although operator-dependent, studies have shown a low 5% error rate after completing ten FAST exams, with a leveling off of the learning curve after 30 exams [21].

Computed Tomography

Although more sensitive and specific than the above imaging modalities for a broad range of pathologies, reliable access to computer tomography (CT) in low-resource settings is scarce. Although 70% of countries responding to a World Health Organization assessment ($n = 121$) reported at least one CT unit per million population, only 14% of low-income countries met this bar versus 100% of high-income countries [26]. CT is most frequently found at higher-level and private facilities, usually in urban settings. When available, these images are useful in specifying the presence or absence of thoracic pathology, and can help further elucidate if a procedure is warranted.

Diagnostic Modality Pitfalls

Even if the technologies exist, there are numerous challenges for appropriate use and maintenance. Out-of-service periods for radiography machines are common, either due to a lack of trained technicians or replacement parts and software, or limited electricity or battery power. A group examining 24 years of inventory data from 16 countries in the Americas, Africa, and Southeast Asia found nearly 40% of equipment in LMICs was out of service, with X-ray machines topping the list at 47%. The state of the equipment depends not only on its presence but also on health technology management, training, and resources and infrastructure, which frequently do not accompany equipment implementation [27]. CT or digital X-ray machines usually require intermittent or permanent high-speed internet access, with authorized representatives from the manufacturer needed to install and maintain the equipment, which can be costly and are associated with delays due to company representative travel [16]. Hospitals may run out of blood draw supplies and laboratories may lack reagents to run tests, or the test duration may make the results irrelevant for acute problems. Most healthcare systems in LMICs require payment prior to study performance, which frequently is outside of a patient's financial means. Many hospitals and clinics rely on radiography machines external to their facilities, necessitating patient transport as well as stability to undergo the usually unmonitored travel and study duration.

Management

Pain

Chest pathology can cause significant pain with profound effects on a patient's ability to maintain adequate oxygenation and ventilation. Multiple modalities exist to optimize a patient's ability to sustain their respiratory capacity without mechanical interventions, the latter of which are frequently lacking in low-resource settings. Opioids are critical for adequate post-operative analgesia for moderate to severe pain; however, 50% of the world's population living in the poorest countries receive under 1% of the morphine-equivalent opioids distributed [28]. Oral, parenteral, and intramuscular forms of tramadol, paracetamol, and other nonsteroidal anti-inflammatory drugs (NSAIDs) exist in many low-resource settings, as well as injectable and topical local anesthetics (e.g. xylocaine), all of which should be used in a multimodal pain regimen [29]. While spinal anesthesia is fairly accessible, access to other forms of regional anesthesia is limited, with epidurals only done by trained anesthetists and paraspinal analgesia not routinely performed. Ketamine is commonly used in the pediatric population, [30] with studies in adults as either an intravenous infusions or subcutaneous injections showing promise [31].

Anesthesia

Thoracic surgery frequently necessitates single lung ventilation, achieved with either a bronchial blocker or a double-lumen endotracheal tube and fiberoptic scope. Yet these items are often absent in many facilities, not to mention a lack of trained anesthesiologists as well. Work arounds for a lack of supplies include double lung ventilation with low tidal volumes, blind placement of double-lumen tubes with subsequent auscultation and observation of chest rise to assess proper placement, and endobronchial intubation or fogarty catheter insertion into the non-operative side [30].

Blood Transfusion

There is a persistent lack of safe blood products in low-resource settings, [32] as exhibited by 80% of the world's population having access to only 20% of the world's blood supply [33]. However, chest pathology and its required interventions, especially for trauma, frequently require blood transfusions. These challenges can potentially be solved by autologous blood transfusions. Techniques for autologous blood transfusion include a predeposited donation, perioperative or periprocedural salvage, and acute normovolemic hemodilution. Predeposited donations are for planned operations, with visits starting 4–5 weeks before surgery with one unit collected per week. Normovolemic hemodilution occurs immediately preoperatively for patients predicted to lose 20% or more of blood volume during the operation. One to 1.5 l are removed while replacing the volume with crystalloid or colloid, and the collected blood is anticoagulated and reinfused during the procedure as needed [34]. Periprocedural blood salvage can involve anything from simple, inexpensive sterile bottles to advanced cell washing devices. If a Pleurovac with a standard collecting device or a Cell Saver is not available, one group describes using a large bore chest drain connected to a sterile glass container, usually containing a solution to prevent clotting (e.g. citrate-phosphate-dextrose-adenine), and a funnel created from several layers of sterile gauze. The collected blood is then re-infused once the bottle is full using a standard blood infusion set with a filter [35]. Others have described using a simple, sterile, disposable bag with heparin added prior to transfusion [36]. Autologous transfusion has been studied in multiple settings, from both the thoracic and peritoneal cavities, showing equivalent or better patient outcomes than allogenic transfusions [34, 37].

Tube Thoracostomy

Indications
If the patient is found to have a pneumothorax, hemothorax, or pleural effusion compromising their respiratory status, insertion of a chest tube is warranted. If there is concern for a tension pneumothorax, exhibited by decreased breath sounds, JVD,

hypotension, pneumothorax with tracheal deviation on chest radiography, and/or low oxygen saturation, the patient should undergo immediate needle decompression with a 14-gauge angiocath in the anterior axillary line at the fourth or fifth intercostal space. A rush of air with immediate improvement in the patient's vitals will confirm the diagnosis. A subsequent formal tube thoracostomy will then need to be performed. If the patient has a sucking chest wound, a gauze dressing taped on three sides should immediately be applied over the wound, which allows air to escape while preventing subsequent re-entry into the thoracic cavity.

Procedure

A standard tube thoracostomy is best completed with the patient in the supine or lateral decubitus position with the normal lung side down, and arm raised above the head to open the rib spaces. The recommended insertion point irrespective of the underlying pathology is in the fourth or fifth interspace in the mid-axillary line. On men, this corresponds with the nipple, and in women just superior to the inframammary fold. Essential supplies are listed in Table 1. The procedure should be performed under sterile conditions using local anesthesia. A skin incision is made with a scalpel, large enough to accommodate one finger for subsequent investigation of the pleural space, and a clamp is used to bluntly dissect the soft tissue toward the pleural space in a posterior direction to facilitate subsequent tube placement. Always dissect *over* the rib, since the neurovascular bundle with the intercostal artery, nerve, and vein lie underneath and can be inadvertently injured, causing difficult-to-control hemorrhage. Once the soft tissue and muscle have been dissected and you have reached the rib, close the clamp and in a controlled fashion with two hands "pop" into the pleural space. A rush of air or fluid will confirm entry in the proper space. Open the clamp parallel to the ribs to create an opening large enough for your finger and the subsequent tube. Insert a finger and feel for lung, as well as any loculations, which can be bluntly released. It can help to place a clamp at the tip of the chest tube to facilitate insertion into the pleural cavity. Once the tip has entered the pleural cavity, remove the clamp and thread the tube into a posterior apical position. The external end of the chest tube should be

Table 1 Tube thoracostomy supplies	Hat, mask, eye protection, sterile gown, and gloves
	Sterile prep (e.g. Chlorhexidine, betadine)
	Sterile drape/towels
	Local anesthetic (e.g. lidocaine, bupivacaine)
	Sterile syringe and needle
	Sterile scalpel
	1–2 large sterile clamps (e.g. Kelly)
	Sterile chest tube
	Sterile, non-absorbable suture (e.g. 0 silk)
	Sterile dressing and tape (e.g. Vaseline impregnated + gauze)
	Drainage container (e.g. Pleurovac)
	± suction

attached to a drainage container below the level of the patient for removal of fluid via gravity or with a water seal that allows for removal of air without re-entry into the pleural cavity.

In the absence of a formal chest tube, you can use a pigtail catheter (e.g. 8–14 French) or central venous catheter (e.g. 16 gauge) placed via a percutaneous, Seldinger technique, [38] or a urinary catheter of sufficient size. We recommend against the use of thoracostomy tubes with trocars due to the high incidence of iatrogenic injuries during placement. In the absence of a formal Pleurovac device, you can use a sterile urine drainage bag system placed below the level of the patient's chest for gravity drainage, [38] with intermittent applied suction based on machine availability and triage based on patient stability. Occasionally, a chest tube will remain clamped between interval suction episodes, requiring close patient monitoring given the risk for decompensation due to tension pneumothorax. If a water seal is needed for pneumothorax evacuation, a bottle can be half filled with water and the external end of the thoracostomy tube placed below the surface (Fig. 1). Although attachment of the drainage container to suction facilitates more rapid removal of air or fluid and apposition of the visceral to parietal pleura, this modality is not essential.

Management

Chest tube management includes tracking daily drainage output and quality, performing a physical exam to assess for improvement, assessing for the presence of an air leak in the water seal chamber, indicated by air bubbles, and, if available, subsequent imaging to assess for resolution of the underlying pathology. For pneumothorax, once the lung is stably re-expanded, the chest tube is changed from suction to

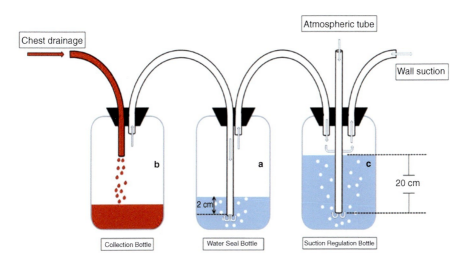

Fig. 1 Example of improvised simple water seal system used for the management of a chest tube. (Reprinted/adapted by permission from: Springer Nature, Fundamentals of General Surgery by Francesco Palazzo COPYRIGHT 2018)

water seal (if not done previously), and if no evidence of lung collapse, the chest tube is removed. For a pleural effusion, hemothorax, empyema, or post-operatively, removal can be considered once the fluid is serous to serosanguinous and is draining under 150–200 ml per 24-h period.

Chest tube removal requires scissors or a scalpel and an occlusive dressing. The suture securing the chest tube is cut, and the patient is instructed to exhale, sometimes best accomplished by asking them to hum. The chest tube is removed in one swift motion and the occlusive dressing secured in place to prevent re-entry of air into the pleural cavity. This dressing should be left in place for 72 h to allow apposition of the underlying tissues.

Pitfalls and Challenges

Complications of tube thoracostomy insertion include entry into the abdominal cavity with possible associated injury, injury to the lung, intercostal neurovascular bundle, or heart with varying degrees of blood loss, improper insertion (e.g. subcutaneous, fissure), adhesions with inability to insert the chest tube, and infections.

Many pneumothoraces or pleural effusions are chronic in nature due to a lack of access to care. Upon evacuation, these patients are at risk for developing re-expansion pulmonary edema. Prevalence in the literature ranges from 0.3 to 32.5% with higher numbers associated with pneumothoraces, although clinically significant cases are likely less than 1%. Patients at highest risk include those who are younger, have lung collapse over 1 week or need three or more liters of fluid removed, or have large pneumothoraces. Upon initial re-expansion, a patient may experience pain as well as coughing, tachypnea, dyspnea, hypoxia, tachycardia, or hemodynamic instability anywhere from 1 to 24 h after the procedure [39]. For pleural effusions, it can be helpful to temporarily clamp the drainage catheter to stop the removal of fluid, and allow the patient and lung to adjust. We usually recommend draining fluid in 1-l increments to avoid re-expansion sequelae. Should the latter occur, the treatment is mainly supportive, including supplementary oxygen as well as diuresis to facilitate intraparenchymal fluid removal.

Thoracotomy

Indications

Reasons to perform a thoracotomy include lung resection or palliation for either a mass or tuberculosis, washout, and decortication, penetrating thoracic trauma with evidence of injury, traumatic diaphragm or bronchus rupture, cardiac tamponade, esophageal injury, and resuscitation for a witnessed traumatic cardiac arrest.

Procedure

For an elective procedure, the standard position is a posterolateral thoracotomy done over the fifth intercostal space, corresponding to the lung fissure. The patient is positioned in the lateral decubitus position with the operative side up, and the bed is flexed to open the rib spaces. Important landmarks are identified, including the tip of the scapula, the costal margin, and the xiphoid, the incision is planned and marked, and the patient sterilely prepped and draped. The incision typically extends from 3 cm posterior to the scapula tip halfway between the scapula and spinous process to the anterior axillary line. The skin is incised, and the soft tissue, Scarpa's fascia, and the latissimus dorsi muscle are divided. You will encounter the auscultatory triangle, bordered by the trapezius, serratus anterior, and scapula. Sparing of the serratus anterior by freeing it from the surrounding soft tissue and rotating it forward preserves shoulder motion and shortens recovery time. To facilitate rib spreading, the muscle can be detached from the sixth, seventh, and eighth ribs. The intercostal muscle is then divided from the top of the sixth rib, taking care to avoid injuring the neurovascular bundle on the underside of the fifth rib. This is continued as close to the costochondral junction anteriorly and transverse processes of the vertebral body posteriorly to maximize rib spreading [40]. Once adequate rib spreading is achieved, the Finochietto rib spreader is inserted and slowly opened. Note any areas of tension that require additional muscle release to avoid an iatrogenic rib fracture.

Resuscitative thoracotomies in the setting of trauma are performed in the anterolateral position on the left side in the fourth or fifth intercostal space with the patient in the supine position and sterilely prepped. An incision is made with a scalpel from the sternum laterally to the bed and carried down to the rib through the subcutaneous tissue and musculature. Entry into the pleura is done bluntly with a clamp or finger, and completed with Metzenbaum scissors to avoid injury to the underlying lung. The Finochietto rib spreader is inserted with the handle toward the bed and opened. Cardiac massage is performed by a sterile assistant, while the proceduralist divides the inferior pulmonary ligament, taking care not to continue too far superiorly and injure the inferior pulmonary vein. The spine is identified posteriorly, with the aorta lying just anterior to this. The aorta is circumferentially bluntly dissected with a finger or large clamp and cross-clamped or occluded with direct pressure. Cardiac massage with the adjunct of intracardiac epinephrine and volume resuscitation is continued until the return of systemic circulation or a determination of death. If pulmonary hemorrhage is the cause of shock, a large clamp can be applied to the lung hilum temporarily, followed by tractotomy via stapling, and intermittent clamp removal to identify and control the bleeding via suture ligation. In low-resource settings, a resuscitative thoracotomy is rarely indicated as necessary items both to perform the procedure and for subsequent management are frequently lacking, including surgical trays outside of the operating theater, blood products for resuscitation, mechanical ventilation, and an intensive care unit.

Management

Post-operative management of the patient depends on the underlying pathology. Recommendations for chest tubes and pain control can be found in the preceding sections.

Pitfalls and Challenges

The main difficulties with performing a thoracotomy include suboptimal patient positioning, lack of necessary surgical tools, and inadvertent injury to underlying structures, including the lung, heart, and vasculature. Whenever possible, ensure the patient is appropriately positioned prior to incision as outlined above. If an underlying structure is injured during incision, the appropriate repair should be undertaken.

Pericardial Drainage and Pericardiectomy

Indications

Pericardial drainage is required if a significant amount of fluid accumulates between the visceral and parietal layers impairing cardiac function, leading to tamponade physiology. This fluid can be exudative, sanguineous, chylous, or transudative, and develop acutely, subacutely, or chronically. Inflammation of the pericardium causing scarring and fibrosis that eventually prevents expansion and constricts the heart's ability to fill necessitates removal. The most common cause of both of a pericardial effusion and constrictive pericarditis in LMICs is tuberculosis [41].

Procedure

For pericardiectomy, you can enter the chest via a median sternotomy, left anterolateral thoracotomy, the Harrington approach ("U" incision with the base at the left sternal border), and the Churchill (bilateral thoracotomy), with the latter two being mainly historical. A dissection limited to the anterior surface between the left and right phrenic nerves laterally, and from the great vessels cranially to the diaphragm, and inferior vena cava caudally leads to significant functional improvement. However, some still argue that a radical or total pericardiectomy provides better results [9].

Pericardial drainage can be performed either via percutaneous pericardiocentesis under echocardiographic or fluoroscopic guidance by a trained operator, or surgically via a pericardial window, with the latter being the gold standard [42]. The ideal entry site for echo-guided drainage is at the site of maximal fluid and where the effusion is closest to the transducer. Fluoroscopic-guided drainage is commonly performed via a subxiphoid approach, advancing a needle to the left shoulder at a 30° angle to the skin while alternating aspirating for fluid and injecting small amounts of dilute contrast from an attached syringe. Once in the proper position, a guidewire is introduced, followed by dilation, and pigtail catheter placement for further fluid removal [43].

Surgical drainage, allowing decompression into the pleural or peritoneal cavities, can be performed via an anterior thoracotomy or subxiphoid approach, thoracoscopy, or transdiaphragmatic during a laparotomy. The portion of pericardium excised should be enough to prevent recurrence [44].

Management

For pericarditis, patients should receive NSAIDs, colchicine, and/or steroids, with judicious use of diuretics given the likely decreased cardiac output [41]. If a pericardial drain is placed, it is recommended to keep until draining less than 30 ml over 24 h in order to maximize visceral and parietal pericardial adherence [42].

Pitfalls and Challenges

Complications of pericardiocentesis include myocardial or coronary vessel laceration or perforation, air embolism, arrhythmias, pneumothorax or hemothorax, or entry into the peritoneal cavity with potential injury to abdominal viscera [42].

Tracheostomy and Cricothyroidotomy

Indications

Tracheostomies are mainly performed for patients in need of prolonged chronic mechanical ventilatory support, which may be impractical in low-resource settings with limited mechanical ventilators and intensive care units. Optimal timing continues to be debated, with reasonable criteria being intubation for 1–2 weeks without an expected improvement or a need for enhanced pulmonary toilet and decreased sedation. Benefits include patient comfort, secure airway, improved oral hygiene, and pulmonary toilet, decreased risks of vocal cord injury, subglottic stenosis, and sinusitis, and phonation with fenestrated devices. Cricothyroidotomies are an emergent method of securing the airway when translaryngeal intubation is not possible [40].

Procedure

In preparation for the procedure, a tracheostomy appliance is selected. Most come in a variety of sizes (adult range Jackson 4–10), variable lengths, cuffed versus uncuffed, and fenestrated versus non-fenestrated [45]. Typically, size six or greater are initially chosen to allow for maximal pulmonary toilet and bronchoscopy. Cuffed appliances are needed when the patient requires mechanical ventilatory support. If unavailable, a traditional endotracheal tube can be used with length modifications as appropriate.

Open tracheostomy is performed with the patient in the supine position, and the neck extended, making sure to identify the anatomic landmarks of the sternal notch and cricoid and thyroid cartilages. The ideal entry location is at the second or third tracheal ring, which is usually 1 to 2 cm above the sternal notch. A 2- to 3-cm transverse skin incision is made, dividing the subcutaneous tissues and platysma transversely, cutting the anterior superficial cervical fascia longitudinally, and splitting the strap muscles bluntly. The thyroid gland is typically seen and can either be elevated superiorly or the thyroid isthmus can be divided to enhance visualization. Traction sutures with monofilament permanent suture (e.g. 2-0 Prolene) are placed around the second and third tracheal rings laterally, both to elevate the trachea and to secure the airway in the immediate post-operative period should the appliance become dislodged. The pretracheal fascia is incised, and a horizontal cut is made in the space between the second and third tracheal rings, with subsequent division of the third ring bilaterally creating a flap. The opening is enlarged by dilation, and the endotracheal tube is slowly retracted by the anesthesia team until the tube is above the tracheostomy site. The tracheostomy tube is then laterally inserted through the tracheal opening, and subsequently rotated into the correct position, with cuff inflation and mechanical ventilation attached. The tracheostomy appliance is sutured to the skin with non-absorbable sutures in four quadrants. Proper placement is confirmed by physical exam, auscultation, end tidal CO_2, ventilator settings, and bronchoscopy, both to confirm appropriate placement and to remove accumulated secretions or blood [40].

Cricothyroidotomy starts with the patient in the supine position with a shoulder roll to facilitate neck extension, and the neck sterilely prepped and draped. The cricothyroid membrane is identified, and either a vertical midline or horizontal incision is made, and the soft tissue is bluntly dissected until reaching the cricothyroid membrane. A horizontal incision is made in the membrane, with subsequent dilation and placement of a small endotracheal tube or tracheostomy tube. Position is confirmed by exam, auscultation, and end tidal CO_2, and the tube is secured in place. Due to a higher rate of subglottic stenosis, if continued ventilatory support is required, the cricothyroidotomy is converted to a standard tracheostomy within 2–3 days [40].

Management

Tracheostomy tube care involves daily examination and cleaning externally and internally, with methods to reduce any areas of appliance pressure that can lead to skin erosion and ulcers, suctioning of the tube, and inner cannula cleaning. Cuff deflation should occur when the patient no longer needs mechanical ventilation and there is no concern for aspiration. If the tube becomes dislodged within 7 days of creation, it should be replaced with the same size tube or a size smaller. If this is not possible, the patient should undergo orotracheal intubation. The initial tube should be replaced within 3–7 days after initial insertion for an adult, and sutures should be removed with tracheal ties maintained [46].

For decannulation, an evaluation is done to ensure that the reasons for the tracheostomy tube have adequately resolved. Additionally, the patient needs to tolerate cap trials with an uncuffed tube, have an adequate mental status for airway protection without evidence of gross aspiration, and have a strong cough. The tube may require exchange and/or downsizing to facilitate capping and ensure the placement of an uncuffed tube. After tube removal, clean and cover the site with a dry gauze dressing, which should be changed daily. The patient should apply digital pressure over the site when talking or coughing to reduce air leak [46].

Pitfalls and Challenges

The main risks of both procedures include bleeding and infection. Tracheostomy issues can include fistulas, between the trachea and esophagus or trachea and innominate artery, tracheal stenosis secondary to granulation tissue, tracheomalacia, infection or hemorrhage from the stoma, and swallowing dysfunction. A frequent challenge in low-resource settings is a lack of mechanical ventilators. If this is the case, patients will require continuous bag-mask ventilation by staff and family members, either until they recover or a mechanical ventilator becomes available. This lack of supplies is frequently linked to a lack of space or existence of intensive care units. As already mentioned, tracheostomy appliances may not be readily available, which can be substituted with a standard endotracheal tube.

Conclusion

Many contributors to the global burden of disease reside in the thoracic cavity. Of the top ten causes of mortality in low-income countries in the 2017 Global Burden of Disease Study, at least three have thoracic manifestations warranting intervention, including respiratory infections and tuberculosis, neoplasms, and HIV/AIDS [47]. In the face of this burden, and with a severe shortage of both specialist and general surgical providers in low-resource settings, it is critical that all medical providers be trained in the basic diagnosis and safe management of emergent thoracic pathology. Healthcare facilities must be outfitted with the minimum necessary components to provide this care, including basic diagnostic imaging modalities and supplies to perform the previously described procedures. In this way, patients can receive the care they need irrespective of where they live.

References

1. Biccard BM, Madiba TE, Kluyts H-L, Munlemvo DM, Madzimbamuto FD, Basenero A, et al. Perioperative patient outcomes in the African Surgical Outcomes Study: a 7-day prospective observational cohort study. Lancet. 2018;391(10130):1589–98. https://doi.org/10.1016/S0140-6736(18)30001-1.
2. Ramirez AG, Nuradin N, Byiringiro F, Ntakiyiruta G, Giles AE, Riviello R. General thoracic surgery in Rwanda: an assessment of surgical volume and of workforce and material resource deficits. World J Surg. 2019;43(1):36–43. https://doi.org/10.1007/s00268-018-4771-y.
3. Linegar A, van Zyl G, Smit F, Goldstraw P. Pleuro-pulmonary disease in Central South Africa: a thoracic surgical deficiency. S Afr Med J. 2010;100(8):510–2.
4. N'Dong FO, Mbamendame S, Offobo SN, Kaba MM, Mbourou JB, Diané C. Cardio-thoracic surgical experience in Gabon. Cardiovasc Diagn Ther. 2016;6:S74–S7.
5. Iddriss A, Padayatchi N, Reddy D, Reddi A. Pulmonary resection for extensively drug resistant tuberculosis in Kwazulu-Natal, South Africa. Ann Thorac Surg. 2012;94(2):381–6. https://doi.org/10.1016/j.athoracsur.2012.03.072.
6. Mefire AC, Pagbe JJ, Fokou M, Nguimbous JF, Guifo ML, Bahebeck J. Analysis of epidemiology, lesions, treatment and outcome of 354 consecutive cases of blunt and penetrating trauma to the chest in an African setting. S Afr J Surg. 2010;48(3):90–3.
7. Somocurcio JG, Sotomayor A, Shin S, Portilla S, Valcarcel M, Guerra D, et al. Surgery for patients with drug-resistant tuberculosis: report of 121 cases receiving community-based treatment in Lima, Peru. Thorax. 2007;62(5):416–21. https://doi.org/10.1136/thx.2005.051961.
8. Tettey M, Tamatey M, Edwin F. Cardiothoracic surgical experience in Ghana. Cardiovasc Diagn Ther. 2016;6:S64–73.

9. Tettey M, Sereboe L, Aniteye E, Edwin F, Kotei D, Tamatey M, et al. Surgical management of constrictive pericarditis. Ghana Med J. 2007;41(4):190–3.
10. Dewan RK, Pezzella AT. Surgical aspects of pulmonary tuberculosis: an update. Asian Cardiovasc Thorac Ann. 2016;24(8):835–46. https://doi.org/10.1177/0218492316661958.
11. Molnar TF. Tuberculosis: mother of thoracic surgery then and now, past and prospectives: a review. J Thorac Dis. 2018;10:S2628–S42.
12. Meara JG, Leather AJM, Hagander L, Alkire BC, Alonso N, Ameh EA, et al. Global surgery 2030: evidence and solutions for achieving health, welfare, and economic development. Lancet. 2015;386(9993):569–624. https://doi.org/10.1016/S0140-6736(15)60160-X.
13. Linegar A, Smit F, Goldstraw P, van Zyl G. Fifty years of thoracic surgical research in South Africa. S Afr Med J. 2009;99(8):592–5.
14. McGee S. Evidence-based physical diagnosis. 4th ed. Amsterdam: Elsevier; 2018.
15. ATLS Advanced trauma life support student course manual. 10th ed. Chicago: American College of Surgeons; 2018.
16. Radiology in global health: strategies, implementation, and applications. Cham: Springer; 2019.
17. Dhital KR, Acharya R, Bhandari R, Kharel P, Giri KP, Tamrakar R. Clinical profile of patients with pleural effusion admitted to KMCTH. Kathmandu Univ Med J (KUMJ). 2009;7(28):438–44.
18. WHO. Essential diagnostic imaging. Geneva: Department of Essential Health Technologies; 2011.
19. Fundamentals of diagnostic radiology. Philadelphia: Wolters Kluwer/Lippincott Williams & Wilkins Health; 2012.
20. Becker DM, Tafoya CA, Becker SL, Kruger GH, Tafoya MJ, Becker TK. The use of portable ultrasound devices in low- and middle-income countries: a systematic review of the literature. Tropical Med Int Health. 2016;21(3):294–311. https://doi.org/10.1111/tmi.12657.
21. Sippel S, Muruganandan K, Levine A, Shah S. Review article: use of ultrasound in the developing world. Int J Emerg Med. 2011;4:72. https://doi.org/10.1186/1865-1380-4-72.
22. AIUM. Practice parameter for the performance of point-of-care ultrasound examinations. J Ultrasound Med. 2019;38(4):833–49. https://doi.org/10.1002/jum.14972.
23. Doerschug KC, Schmidt GA. Intensive care ultrasound: III. Lung and pleural ultrasound for the Intensivist. Ann Am Thorac Soc. 2013;10(6):708–12. https://doi.org/10.1513/AnnalsATS.201308-288OT.
24. Ferrada P, Stassen N. Bedside ultrasound for surgeons. In: Butler KL, Harisinghani M, editors. Acute care surgery: imaging essentials for rapid diagnosis. New York: McGraw-Hill; 2015.
25. Matsushima K, Clark D, Frankel HL. Surgeon performed ultrasound in acute care surgery. In: Moore EE, Feliciano DV, Mattox KL, editors. Trauma. 8th ed. New York: McGraw-Hill; 2017.
26. WHO. Global atlas of medical devices. Geneva: WHO; 2017.
27. Perry L, Malkin R. Effectiveness of medical equipment donations to improve health systems: how much medical equipment is broken in the developing world? Med Biol Eng Comput. 2011;49(7):719–22. https://doi.org/10.1007/s11517-011-0786-3.
28. Bhadelia A, De Lima L, Arreola-Ornelas H, Kwete XJ, Rodriguez NM, Knaul FM. Solving the global crisis in access to pain relief: lessons from country actions. Am J Public Health. 2018;109(1):58–60. https://doi.org/10.2105/AJPH.2018.304769.
29. Size M, Soyannwo OA, Justins DM. Pain management in developing countries. Anaesthesia. 2007;62(Suppl 1):38–43. https://doi.org/10.1111/j.1365-2044.2007.05296.x.
30. Parab SY, Myatra SN. Thoracic anesthesia in the developing world. In: Slinger P, editor. Principles and practice of anesthesia for thoracic surgery. Cham: Springer; 2019. p. 699–716.
31. Tuchscherer J, McKay WP, Twagirumugabe T. Low-dose subcutaneous ketamine for postoperative pain management in Rwanda: a dose-finding study. Can J Anesth. 2017;64(9):928–34. https://doi.org/10.1007/s12630-017-0914-0.
32. Blood safety and availability. Geneva: World Health Organization. 2019. https://www.who.int/en/news-room/fact-sheets/detail/blood-safety-and-availability. Accessed 25 Aug 2019.

33. Roberts DJ, Field S, Delaney M, Bates I. Problems and approaches for blood transfusion in the developing countries. Hematol Oncol Clin North Am. 2016;30(2):477–95. https://doi.org/10.1016/j.hoc.2015.11.011.
34. Osaro E, Charles AT. The challenges of meeting the blood transfusion requirements in Sub-Saharan Africa: the need for the development of alternatives to allogenic blood. J Blood Med. 2011;2:7–21. https://doi.org/10.2147/JBM.S17194.
35. Baldan M, Giannou CP, Rizzardi G, Irmay F, Sasin V. Autotransfusion from haemothorax after penetrating chest trauma: a simple, life-saving procedure. Trop Dr. 2006;36(1):21–2. https://doi.org/10.1258/004947506775598725.
36. Kothari R, Pandey N, Sharma D. A simple device for whole blood autotransfusion in cases of hemoperitoneum and hemothorax. Asian J Surg. 2019;42(4):586–7. https://doi.org/10.1016/j.asjsur.2019.01.018.
37. Rhee P, Inaba K, Pandit V, Khalil M, Siboni S, Vercruysse G, et al. Early autologous fresh whole blood transfusion leads to less allogeneic transfusions and is safe. J Trauma Acute Care Surg. 2015;78(4):729–34. https://doi.org/10.1097/ta.0000000000000599.
38. Singh K, Loo S, Bellomo R. Pleural drainage using central venous catheters. Crit Care. 2003;7(6):R191. https://doi.org/10.1186/cc2393.
39. Meeker JW, Jaeger AL, Tillis WP. An uncommon complication of a common clinical scenario: exploring reexpansion pulmonary edema with a case report and literature review. J Community Hosp Intern Med Perspect. 2016;6(3):32257. https://doi.org/10.3402/jchimp.v6.32257.
40. Sugarbaker DJ, Bueno R, Colson YL, Jaklitsch MT, Krasna MJ, Mentzer SJ, et al. Adult chest surgery. 2nd ed. New York: McGraw-Hill; 2014.
41. Yacoub M, Mahajan K. Constrictive-effusive pericarditis. Treasure Island: StatPearls Publishing; 2019.
42. Imazio M, Adler Y. Management of pericardial effusion. Eur Heart J. 2012;34(16):1186–97. https://doi.org/10.1093/eurheartj/ehs372.
43. Adler Y, Charron P, Imazio M, Badano L, Barón-Esquivias G, Bogaert J, et al. 2015 ESC guidelines for the diagnosis and management of pericardial diseases: the task force for the Diagnosis and Management of Pericardial Diseases of the European Society of Cardiology (ESC) endorsed by: The European Association for Cardio-Thoracic Surgery (EACTS). Eur Heart J. 2015;36(42):2921–64. https://doi.org/10.1093/eurheartj/ehv318.
44. Feins EN, Walker JD. Chapter 57: Pericardial disease. In: Cohn LH, Adams DH, editors. Cardiac surgery in the adult. 5th ed. New York: McGraw-Hill; 2018.
45. Tracheostomy. Medtronic. 2019. https://www.medtronic.com/covidien/en-us/products/tracheostomy.html. Accessed 7 July 2019.
46. Mitchell RB, Hussey HM, Setzen G, Jacobs IN, Nussenbaum B, Dawson C, et al. Clinical consensus statement:tracheostomy care. Otolaryngol Head Neck Surg. 2013;148(1):6–20. https://doi.org/10.1177/0194599812460376.
47. Institute for Health Metrics and Evaluation (IHME). GBD compare data visualization. Seattle: IHME, University of Washington. 2018. http://vizhub.healthdata.org/gbd-compare. Accessed 7 July 2019.

Part I
Acute Surgery Thoracic Emergencies

Esophageal Rupture

Patrick L. Bosarge and Dennis Y. Kim

Introduction

Although likely underreported, the incidence of esophageal rupture has been estimated at 3–6 persons per one million per year, which makes this a rare condition [1]. Overall, esophageal perforation occurs most frequently in the thoracic cavity (approximately 70%), followed by both cervical esophageal perforations (approximately 15%) and perforations into the abdominal cavity (approximately 15%) [2, 3]. Most perforations of the esophagus are iatrogenic in nature due to instrumentation performed for diagnostic and therapeutic reasons of the upper gastrointestinal tract or for cardiac evaluation and treatment. Spontaneous perforations, known as Boerhaave's Syndrome, account for approximately 15% of patients with esophageal rupture [4]. Other causes of rupture include external trauma, internal trauma from ingestion of foreign body or caustic agent, and malignancy. This chapter will focus on the management of patients with esophageal rupture secondary to causes other than external trauma.

Etiology

The esophagus is a thin-walled tubular structure that lacks a serosal layer making it vulnerable to rupture or perforation. Once perforation occurs, only loosely organized connective tissue impedes the passage of esophageal contents (food substances, saliva, refluxed gastric contents, etc.) into the mediastinum or adjacent

P. L. Bosarge
University of Arizona College of Medicine—Phoenix, Phoenix, AZ, USA
e-mail: bosarge@email.arizona.edu

D. Y. Kim (✉)
Harbor-UCLA Medical Center, David Geffen School of Medicine at UCLA, Torrance, CA, USA

© Springer Nature Switzerland AG 2021
J. M. Galante, R. Coimbra (eds.), *Thoracic Surgery for the Acute Care Surgeon*, Hot Topics in Acute Care Surgery and Trauma,
https://doi.org/10.1007/978-3-030-48493-4_2

thoracic cavities. Thus, dissemination of infectious and inflammatory agents causes sepsis from mediastinitis and/or pleural contamination that may progress to sepsis, multiple organ failure, and death if left unabated. Mortality rates for esophageal perforation vary depending on the etiology of the perforation and the timing from rupture to presentation. Postemetic perforation has a high reported mortality, which may be as high as 89% [5]. Iatrogenic instrumental perforation has a lower reported mortality most likely because providers have a higher index of suspicion related to the procedural complications. Iatrogenic perforation mortality varies from 5 to 26% [6, 7]. Mortality rates also vary according to the time interval between rupture and treatment with increasing mortality occurring with further delay in therapy.

Despite the potential for iatrogenic esophageal rupture during instrumentation, upper endoscopy and transesophageal echocardiography are quite safe with a reported rupture rate between 1 in 2500 and 11,000 [8, 9]. Overall, most perforations that occur with instrumentation are due to blind insertions or to therapeutic procedures such as dilations. There is a tendency to discover iatrogenic perforations earlier, particularly when the cause is associated with endoscopy. These ruptures tend to be smaller in size than Boerhaave's Syndrome [4]. This may account for the improved mortality that has been witnessed over the past 40 years.

First described in 1724 by Dr. Herman Boerhaave, spontaneous rupture of the esophagus, now associated with the eponym Boerhaave's Syndrome, is not a spontaneous occurrence, but rather esophageal rupture that is caused by a rapid increase of intraesophageal pressure due to vomiting. Frequently, patients with this condition will have a preceding history of overindulgence in both food and alcohol prior to the emesis that subsequently causes rupture. Diagnosis of Boerhaave's syndrome can be difficult as symptomatology can vary significantly. Additionally, delay in presentation for medical care is common for these patients.

Presentation

Presentation of esophageal rupture can vary considerably. This is partially due to the degree of mediastinal contamination and partially due to where the rupture occurs within the esophagus. The location of perforation also varies depending on what is the cause. Spontaneous rupture typically occurs just above the diaphragm and affects the posterior lateral wall of the esophagus. These perforations tend to be longitudinal in nature and more commonly occur on the left versus right side. Instrumental perforations are common in the pharynx and distal esophagus. These perforations tend to be smaller in size and frequently less contamination occurs due to the patient's n.p.o. status.

The classically described presentation of Boerhaave's syndrome is that of a middle-aged male with a recent history of overindulgence in food and alcohol. Although symptoms can vary for patients presenting with spontaneous rupture, some will experience chest pain and subcutaneous emphysema after a recent bout of emesis. This is termed Mackler's triad and is present in approximately 50% of cases.

The typical symptoms that occur following esophageal perforation tend to be related to the location of the perforation. Pain is common and occurs in the lower anterior chest or upper abdomen. Patients may also endorse episodes of vomiting. Subcutaneous emphysema may be present as well. Other symptoms that may be present include neck pain and dysphagia if upper esophageal perforation has occurred. Hematemesis, shoulder pain, and back pain may also indicate esophageal perforation. Perforation due to instrumentation is frequently diagnosed in a more expeditious manner related to symptoms that may develop in the setting of a recent upper gastrointestinal manipulation.

Diagnosis

Physical Examination

Findings on physical examination after esophageal rupture may include tachycardia and tachypnea. Subcutaneous emphysema, abdominal rigidity, and tachypnea are commonly referred to as Anderson triad, which indicates a likely distal esophageal rupture into the abdominal cavity. Fever may be present in some patients. Shock may also be a finding which is more common in delayed presentations. Pneumothorax can occur in as many as 20% of cases associated with spontaneous esophageal rupture. Laboratory analysis should be obtained when esophageal rupture is suspected. Leukocytosis is commonplace for all esophageal perforations. Frequently, metabolic acidosis and lactic acidemia are common with esophageal perforation, particularly if presentation is delayed.

Imaging

Imaging is required for diagnosis of esophageal rupture (Fig. 1).

Plain Radiographs
Patients suspected of having esophageal perforation should have a posteroanterior and lateral chest radiograph and upright abdominal radiograph performed on an urgent basis. Findings on the chest radiographs of pleural effusion (particularly on the left), pneumothorax, pneumomediastinum, and subcutaneous emphysema should raise suspicion for esophageal perforation. Additionally, the upright abdominal radiograph may demonstrate subdiaphragmatic air if the esophagus has perforated into the abdominal cavity.

Contrasted Esophagography
Initially, contrasted esophagography following plain radiography may be performed to look for extravasation of contrast to confirm esophageal rupture. Water-soluble contrast esophagography can aid in determining the location and the extent of the rupture. If water-soluble contrasted esophagography does not demonstrate

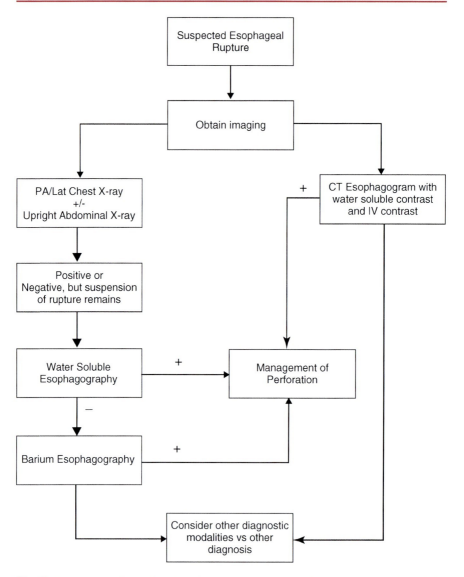

Fig. 1 Diagnostic radiography algorithm for suspected esophageal rupture. (Created by Dr. Patrick Bosarge)

esophageal rupture, and the patient is considered to have a high likelihood of perforation, then thin barium-contrasted esophagography should be obtained. Water-soluble contrast is preferred prior to barium due to the barium causing intense mediastinitis if esophageal perforation exists. One study demonstrated a 22% false-negative rate in diagnosing esophageal perforation using water-soluble contrast, which was then confirmed with barium-contrasted studies in patients who were suspected to have a strong likelihood of rupture [10].

Computerized Tomography

In the situation where contrast esophagography is equivocal or where it is not practical due to endotracheal intubation or inability to swallow, computerized tomography (CT) of the chest is appropriate. Water-soluble oral contrast can be administered 20 min prior to scanning via nasoenteric tube placed in the esophagus to demonstrate extravasation. Intravenous contrast is usually administered to delineate the esophageal wall. Additional clues to perforation which can be seen on CT include extraluminal mediastinal or abdominal gas, pleural or mediastinal fluid, and pneumomediastinum or pneumothorax. Sensitivity and specificity of CT chest for esophageal perforation has been reported as high as 77.7% and 94.3%, respectively [11].

Endoscopy

Esophagogastroduodenoscopy (EGD) is not recommended as the primary mode of diagnosis when acute esophageal rupture is suspected. Endoscopy carries the risk of increasing the size of the original perforation as well as forcing additional insufflated air through the perforation and into the mediastinum and/or pleural cavity. If endoscopy is to be used for diagnostic purposes, it should be noted that endoscopy has poor sensitivity in the cervical esophagus. EGD is appropriate for planning purposes, especially when advanced endoscopic management of esophageal rupture is to be performed.

Thoracentesis

Although rarely needed for diagnosis, aspiration of pleural fluid may reveal acidic pH with elevated amylase content. Purulent and/or malodorous fluid and possibly the presence of food particles in the pleural aspirate can help to confirm the diagnosis of esophageal rupture.

Management

Initial Management

Resuscitative efforts should occur concurrently with the diagnostic workup in patients with suspected esophageal rupture. A definitive airway should be established in patients who are unable to manage their secretions due to an obstruction, as may be seen in the setting of a periesophageal abscess, as well as in patients who present with septic shock and multiple organ dysfunction. Prior to establishing definitive source control, minimally invasive procedures, such as chest tube thoracostomy, may be performed for both diagnostic/confirmatory purposes or as a therapeutic adjunct, particularly in patients with a moderate-sized pleural effusion or associated pneumothorax. Early administration of crystalloids and broad-spectrum antibiotics is critical in patients presenting with sepsis or the systemic inflammatory response syndrome (SIRS). In addition to coverage of gram-positive, gram-negative, aerobic, and anaerobic bacteria, consideration should be given to the administration of an antifungal agent [12].

Key principles in the management of esophageal rupture include:

1. Source control
2. Minimizing further contamination
3. Re-establishing esophageal continuity
4. Establishing distal enteral access

The decision to proceed to surgery should consider several key factors including:

- Etiology (iatrogenic or spontaneous)
- Location (cervical, intrathoracic, or abdominal) and size of defect (Fig. 2)
- Time from rupture to diagnosis
- Presence or absence of sepsis
- Presence of esophageal pathology at site of rupture (malignancy, stricture, obstruction)
- Underlying medical conditions or comorbidities
- Surgeon experience and judgment
- Availability of advanced endoscopic and interventional radiologic resources

Although operative intervention was traditionally considered the gold-standard management strategy for esophageal rupture, contemporary management of this condition requires a multidisciplinary, and often staged, approach, which incorporates both advanced endoscopic and minimally invasive surgical techniques [13]. However, in resource limited environments, an open approach may be the most appropriate.

Nonoperative and Hybrid Approaches to Management

Conservative or nonoperative management of esophageal rupture was first described by Cameron in 1979 and consisted of bowel rest, nasogastric decompression, as well as parenteral antibiotics and nutritional support [12]. Careful patient selection is critical for success (Table 1). Patients considered for a trial of nonoperative management require close follow-up, ongoing supportive care, and monitoring for clinical deterioration. Operative intervention should be considered for those patients who manifest signs of worsening sepsis or fail to improve.

A truly nonoperative or conservative approach to management of esophageal rupture is uncommon as most patients will require some combination of source control (percutaneous, endoscopic, thoracoscopic/laparoscopic), diversion or exclusion, and access for enteral nutrition. One exception may be in patients with an

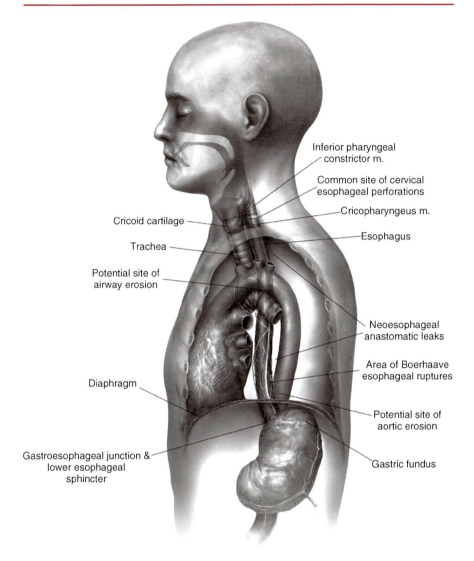

Fig. 2 Common sites of esophageal rupture. (Dickinson, K. J., & Blackmon, S. H. (2015). Endoscopic Techniques for the Management of Esophageal Perforation. *Operative Techniques in Thoracic and Cardiovascular Surgery, 20*(3), 251–278. https://doi.org/10.1053/j.optechstcvs.2016.01.001; permission from Elsevier RightsLink License for re-use in a book/textbook)

iatrogenic cervical perforation in whom conservative or nonoperative management may be employed if there is no evidence of sepsis or descending necrotizing mediastinitis. This multidisciplinary hybrid approach to management is best performed at high-volume centers or esophageal centers of excellence using established treatment algorithms (Fig. 3).

Table 1 Criteria for nonoperative management of esophageal rupture

Early diagnosis (if late, then perforation should be well circumscribed)
Minimal symptoms
Absence of sepsis
Hemodynamically stable
Contained leak or rupture[a]
Minimal pleural soilage
Iatrogenic perforations

aContained rupture is defined as minimum contrast extravasation at the site of perforation or the presence of pneumomediastinum or pneumoperitoneum in the absence of contrast extravasation

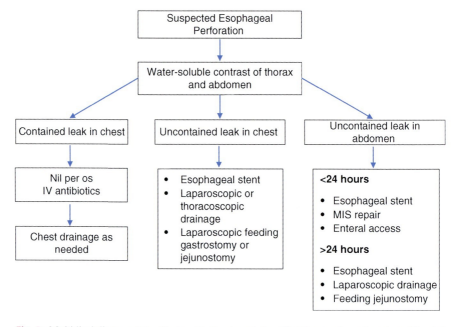

Fig. 3 Multidisciplinary minimally invasive treatment algorithm for esophageal rupture. (Created by Dr. Dennis Kim)

Endoscopic Management

Several endoscopic options exist for the management of esophageal rupture. These include endoscopic stenting and endoscopic defect closure using clips, sutures, and vacuum-assisted closure (VAC) devices [14].

Endoscopic Stenting

Stenting of esophageal rupture may be performed using self-expandable partially or fully covered stents. Although originally used as a palliative adjunct in patients with advanced esophageal cancers, stents have emerged as a valuable adjunct in the management of esophageal rupture. Several variables should be taken into account when considering placement of an esophageal stent including location, the presence of underlying esophageal disease processes, and patient comorbidities. In general, stents are not recommended for cervical esophageal rupture as they are not well-tolerated. Intrathoracic esophageal ruptures or perforations that are contained to the mediastinum are ideal scenarios for the off-label use of stents. Stents placed across the gastroesophageal junction are associated with a high rate of reflux. Consideration should be given to placement of a gastric tube to decompress the stomach and insertion of a jejunostomy or gastrojejunostomy tube (Fig. 4).

While stents may be effective in excluding or diverting flow away from the site of esophageal rupture, source control in the form of mediastinal and/or pleural drainage and debridement are mandatory, especially in patients with evidence of mediastinitis or pleural fluid collections. Stent migration is common, particularly when they are placed in the absence of a stricture or esophageal malignancy.

Endoscopic Clipping and Suturing

Endoscopic closure of esophageal ruptures may be performed using clips or suture techniques, particularly for defects ≤1 cm. Two types of endoscopic clips are commonly employed: through the scope clips (TTSCs) and over the scope clips (OTSCs) (Fig. 5). The size of the defect and operator experience are the two variables that should be considered when deciding upon the type of clip to be employed. In general, TTSCs are better suited for smaller defects in which mucosal apposition only is required. Larger, full-thickness defects as is seen with esophageal rupture are better managed using OTSCs. Placement of an esophageal stent may be required as an adjunct to endoscopic clipping.

Following placement of an overtube, endoscopic suturing can be performed using a suturing device (Overstitch, Apollo Endosurgery, Austin, TX). A dual-channel endoscope in inserted, and the defect can be closed in an interrupted or continuous fashion with the aid of a tissue helix which can be deployed to grasp the esophageal mucosa [14].

Endoscopic VAC

Endoscopic VAC may be used effectively to promote granulation and expedite healing of an esophageal rupture, particularly in stable patients who present with more chronic perforations or postoperative leaks [15]. Endoscopic positioning of a small porous sponge secured to a nasogastric tube into the esophageal defect may improve local blood flow, decrease edema, and minimize spillage of secretions. The sponge should be fashioned such that it is smaller than the esophageal defect and the nasogastric tube may be placed on continuous suction. Repeat exchanges are required and should be performed every 48–72 h [12].

Operative Management

Surgical intervention should be undertaken in any patient who does not meet initial nonoperative management criteria and in those patients initially selected for conservative management who subsequently fail to improve or

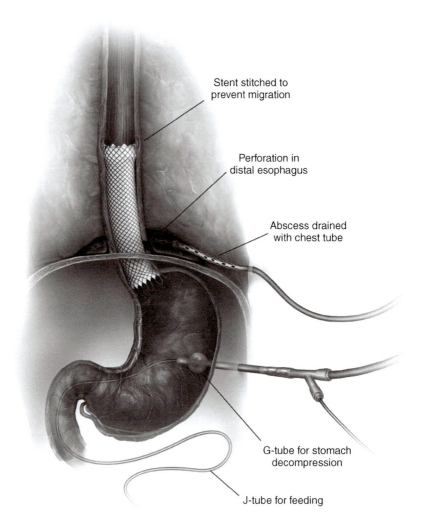

Fig. 4 Deployment of an esophageal stent and distal enteral access. (Dickinson, K. J., & Blackmon, S. H. (2015). Endoscopic Techniques for the Management of Esophageal Perforation. *Operative Techniques in Thoracic and Cardiovascular Surgery, 20*(3), 251–278. https://doi.org/10.1053/j.optechstcvs.2016.01.001; permission from Elsevier RightsLink License for re-use in a book/textbook)

deteriorate clinically. Familiarity with both minimally invasive and open surgical approaches is mandatory for the acute care surgeon managing esophageal emergencies.

Surgical Approach

Access and operative approach to esophageal rupture is guided by the anatomic location of injury. Broadly, the esophagus may be divided into four anatomic areas or locations (Table 2).

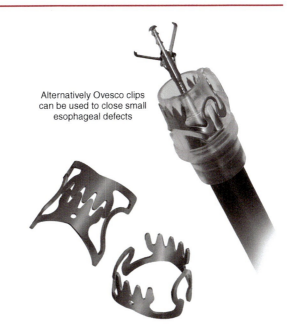

Fig. 5 Endoscopic closure of esophageal perforation using Through the Scope Clips (TTSCs) or Over the Scope Clips (OTSCs). (Dickinson, K. J., & Blackmon, S. H. (2015). Endoscopic Techniques for the Management of Esophageal Perforation. *Operative Techniques in Thoracic and Cardiovascular Surgery, 20*(3), 251–278. https://doi.org/10.1053/j.optechstcvs.2016.01.001; permission from Elsevier RightsLink License for re-use in a book/textbook)

Table 2 Surgical access and incision based on location of esophageal rupture

Location	Incision	Key points
Cervical	Left oblique neck, anterior to SCM	Cervical esophagus at cricopharyngeus is a common location for endoscopic iatrogenic injuries
Proximal 2/3	Right posterolateral thoracotomy	Fourth, fifth, sixth, or seventh intercostal space (depending on exact site of rupture)
Distal 1/3	Left posterolateral thoracotomy	Most common location Seventh or eighth intercostal space
Abdominal	Midline laparotomy or thoracoabdominal	Thoracoabdominal approach used for ruptures that extend across the GE junction

Key tenets of surgical therapy for esophageal rupture include:

- Aggressive debridement of all infected, devitalized, and necrotic tissue
- Irrigation and wide drainage of the mediastinum and pleural spaces
- Decortication in those patients with empyema or trapped lung
- Primary repair, whenever feasible
- Establishment of distal enteral access
  - Several options exist including percutaneous endoscopic gastrostomy (PEG), with or without a jejunostomy extension (PEG-J). In cases where concerns arise over the integrity of the esophageal repair and endoscopic placement of a PEG via the traditional pull or Ponsky method, laparoscopic-assisted, open, or push gastrostomy placement are all viable options. A simpler, short-term option is placement of a nasogastric or nasojejunal tube, particularly in cases where prolonged enteral access is not required.

Management of Intrathoracic Esophageal Rupture

The decision to proceed with a minimally invasive versus open approach is based on several factors: illness severity, degree of contamination, timing of presentation, and surgeon preference.

Video-Assisted Thoracoscopic Surgery (VATS)

Similar to patients undergoing thoracotomy, patients deemed candidates for a VATS should be prepped and positioned in the standard fashion ensuring adequate protection of all bony prominences and placement of an axillary roll to prevent brachial plexus injury (Fig. 6). Insertion of a double-lumen tube and single lung ventilation are critical for adequate surgical exposure. Various port site locations may be used, and the use of a working port for the insertion of open instruments is essential in those patients requiring decortication and aggressive debridement of devitalized tissue and infected fluid collections (Fig. 7). Placement of two large bore chest tubes is important to ensure adequate drainage postoperatively.

Mediastinal drainage may also be accomplished via a mediastinal incision at the sternal notch. Blunt dissection of the paratracheal space, irrigation, and placement of drains is another minimally invasive option in patients with disease limited to the mediastinum.

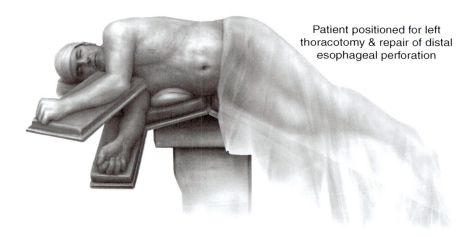

Fig. 6 Patient positioning for both minimally invasive and open approaches to the chest. (Sancheti, M. S., & Fernandez, F. G. (2015). Surgical Management of Esophageal Perforation. *Operative Techniques in Thoracic and Cardiovascular Surgery* 20(3), 234–250. https://doi.org/10.1053/j.optechstcvs.2016.02.002; permission from Elsevier RightsLink License for re-use in a book/textbook)

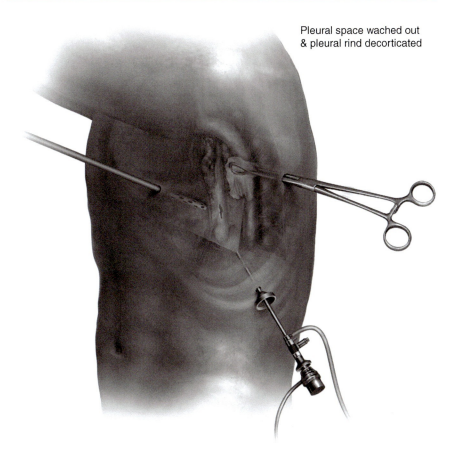

Fig. 7 Video-assisted thoracoscopic surgery (VATS) with demonstration of a working port. (Sancheti, M. S., & Fernandez, F. G. (2015). Surgical Management of Esophageal Perforation. *Operative Techniques in Thoracic and Cardiovascular Surgery*, 20(3), 234–250. https://doi.org/10.1053/j.optechstcvs.2016.02.002; permission from Elsevier RightsLink License for re-use in a book/ textbook)

Thoracotomy

For patients in whom a thoracotomy is required, consideration should be given to placement of a thoracic epidural. The location of the thoracotomy incision is dictated by the site of esophageal rupture. For cases in which exposure is limited, a 1 cm segment of posterior aspect of the inferior rib may be resected. Exposure of the esophagus begins by mobilizing the inferior pulmonary ligament and reflecting the lung anteriorly. The bulging mediastinum may be incised sharply, and the esophagus mobilized and encircled with a Penrose drain (Fig. 8). Careful guided placement of a nasogastric or orogastric tube may assist with identification and mobilization of the esophagus.

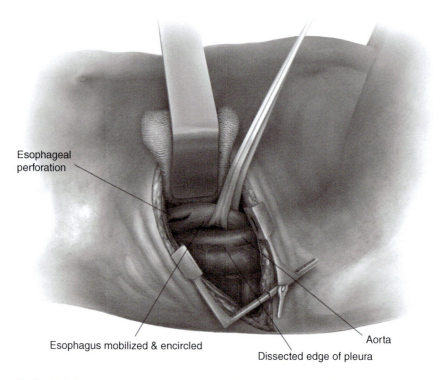

Fig. 8 Mobilization and encircling of the distal esophagus with a Penrose drain. Operative Techniques in Thoracic and Cardiovascular Surgery, 20(3), 234–250. https://doi.org/10.1053/j.optechstcvs.2016.02.002; permission from Elsevier RightsLink License for re-use in a book/textbook)

Primary Repair

Primary repair remains the most common and preferred surgical approach to the management of esophageal rupture. Following initial debridement and removal of devitalized tissue, extension of the myotomy may be required to fully delineate the extent of esophageal mucosal injury (Figs. 9 and 10a). Repair should be performed in two layers: interrupted sutures using an absorbable suture for the mucosal layer followed by interrupted suture repair of the muscular layer with a nonabsorbable suture (Fig. 10b). If concerns for luminal narrowing and potential stricture are present, consideration may be given to repair over a dilator or bougie (32–38 French). Upon completion of the esophageal repair, an air leak test may be performed by inserting a nasogastric tube and positioning it above the repair followed by occlusion of the esophagus distal to the repair, submersion of the esophagus in sterile water or saline, and insufflation to assess for any bubbles.

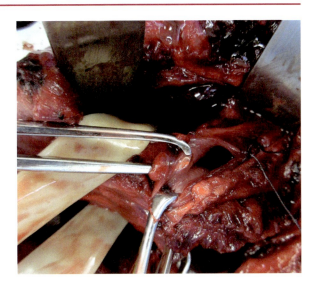

Fig. 9 Mobilization, encircling, and extension of proximal cervical esophageal injury. (Created by Dr. Dennis Kim)

Buttressed Repair with Autologous Tissue
- Neck—Sternocleidomastoid muscle or pectoralis muscle
- Thorax—Pleural, pericardial fat, intercostal muscle
- The decision to use an intercostal flap must be made preoperatively (Fig. 11).
- Abdomen—Gastric fundus, preceded by mobilization of the short gastric arteries or omentum

Exclusion
- Uncommonly performed. May be considered as a damage control technique in unstable patients with significant contamination.
- May be used in patients who present late or in extremis.
- Distal esophageal remnant stapled off, proximal diversion, gastrostomy.

Resection
- Esophagectomy is reserved for the patients in whom an underlying esophageal malignancy has been documented (malignant perforations). Patients with severe esophageal strictures or extensive tissue damage may also be considered for esophagectomy.

At the conclusion of the case, ensure adequate drainage with two large bore chest tubes. Concerns for contralateral hemithorax contamination can be managed transmediastinally or via a separate chest tube thoracostomy.

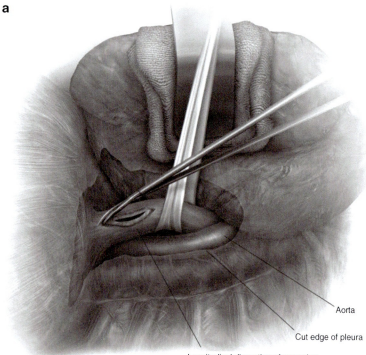

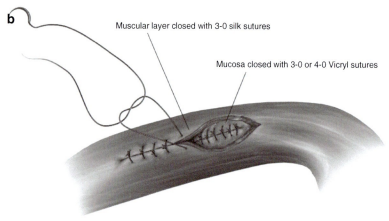

Fig. 10 (**a**) Extension of the esophageal myotomy to expose the full extent of the esophageal mucosal defect. (Sancheti, M. S., & Fernandez, F. G. (2015). Surgical Management of Esophageal Perforation. *Operative Techniques in Thoracic and Cardiovascular Surgery, 20*(3), 234–250. https://doi.org/10.1053/j.optechstcvs.2016.02.002; permission from Elsevier RightsLink License for re-use in a book/textbook). (**b**) Closure of the mucosa using interrupted absorbable suture followed by closure of the esophageal muscular layer. (Sancheti, M. S., & Fernandez, F. G. (2015). Surgical Management of Esophageal Perforation. *Operative Techniques in Thoracic and Cardiovascular Surgery, 20*(3), 234–250. https://doi.org/10.1053/j.optechstcvs.2016.02.002; permission from Elsevier RightsLink License for re-use in a book/textbook)

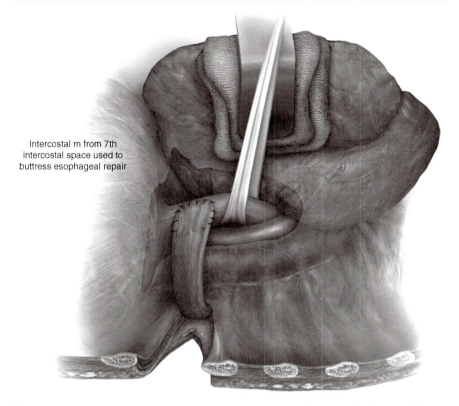

Fig. 11 Use of an intercostal muscle flap to buttress a primary esophageal repair. (Sancheti, M. S., & Fernandez, F. G. (2015). Surgical Management of Esophageal Perforation. *Operative Techniques in Thoracic and Cardiovascular Surgery,* *20*(3), 234–250. https://doi.org/10.1053/j.optechstcvs.2016.02.002; permission from Elsevier RightsLink License for re-use in a book/textbook)

Postoperative Management

Postoperatively, patients with esophageal rupture should be admitted to the intensive care unit for ongoing invasive hemodynamic monitoring and resuscitation.

Sepsis

Broad spectrum antibiotic and antifungal therapy should be continued for a minimum of 7 days. Tissue and fluid culture specimens should be examined, and antimicrobial therapy narrowed, as deemed appropriate. Patients who continue to manifest symptoms and signs of sepsis should undergo imaging to rule out ongoing or recurrent leak and to assess for the size of previously drained collections or the development of new fluid collections or abscesses.

Nutrition

Following esophageal stent placement, contrast esophagogram is usually performed within 24–48 h to confirm exclusion of the rupture. Resumption of oral intake may occur in the absence of a leak. Patients who have undergone an operative repair, postoperative enteral nutrition should be initiated via distal enteral access. Consideration should be given to early parenteral nutrition in those patients without established enteral access in whom a delay to resumption of oral intake is suspected.

Drains and Wound Care
Chest tubes should remain in place until outputs are minimal in patients with pleural effusions and air leaks are resolved in patients with pneumothorax or those who have undergone decortication complicated by an air leak.

Stent Migration
Stent migration is a common complication, particularly in patients in whom a fully covered stent has been deployed. The vast majority of patients will require multiple procedures postinitial stent placement. Duration of stent therapy for esophageal rupture should be limited to 4 weeks. Patients who require a longer duration of stent therapy may require scheduled stent exchange or replacement.

Complications and Outcomes

Leak
Following operative repair, a leak is the most commonly encountered complication in patients with esophageal rupture. Confirmation of a leak is made via contrast esophagogram. In the absence of severe sepsis, conservative management with antibiotics and NPO status should be continued. For leaks that do not respond to these measures, endoscopic strategies may be considered. Uncontrolled leaks and those associated with severe sepsis or shock may require re-operation with employment of damage control techniques as outlined above.

Stricture/Stenosis
Stricture following primary repair of esophageal rupture usually occurs as a late complication. The initial management strategy includes endoscopic serial bougie dilation. The need for re-operative intervention should be made on an individualized basis, specifically among patients who do not respond to endoscopic dilational therapies.

Mortality
Mortality following esophageal rupture continues to remain high. Recent studies demonstrate a mortality rate of up to 18%. Delays in diagnosis are associated with a two-fold increase in death.

Conclusions

Despite significant advances in the diagnostic and therapeutic modalities available to manage esophageal rupture, this condition continues to be associated with significant morbidity and mortality. A high index of suspicion combined with an expeditious workup and timely intervention are paramount to successful outcomes. Emerging endoscopic technologies, combined with minimally invasive techniques, may be successfully employed in properly selected patients in centers with available resources and expertise. Understanding the indications and approaches to operative repair of esophageal rupture is essential for acute care surgeons.

References

1. Soreide JA, et al. Esophageal perforation: clinical patterns and outcomes from a patient cohort of Western Norway. Dig Surg. 2012;29(6):494–502.
2. Sdralis EIK, et al. Epidemiology, diagnosis, and management of esophageal perforations: systematic review. Dis Esophagus. 2017;30(8):1–6.
3. Abbas G, et al. Contemporaneous management of esophageal perforation. Surgery. 2009;146(4):749–55; discussion 755–6.
4. Bufkin BL, Miller JI Jr, Mansour KA. Esophageal perforation: emphasis on management. Ann Thorac Surg. 1996;61(5):1447–51; discussion 1451–2.
5. Derbes VJ, Mitchell RE Jr. Rupture of the esophagus. Surgery. 1956;39(5):865–88.
6. Reeder LB, DeFilippi VJ, Ferguson MK. Current results of therapy for esophageal perforation. Am J Surg. 1995;169(6):615–7.
7. Kiernan PD, et al. Thoracic esophageal perforations. South Med J. 2003;96(2):158–63.
8. Quine MA, et al. Prospective audit of perforation rates following upper gastrointestinal endoscopy in two regions of England. Br J Surg. 1995;82(4):530–3.
9. Sieg A, Hachmoeller-Eisenbach U, Eisenbach T. Prospective evaluation of complications in outpatient GI endoscopy: a survey among German gastroenterologists. Gastrointest Endosc. 2001;53(6):620–7.
10. Buecker A, et al. Esophageal perforation: comparison of use of aqueous and barium-containing contrast media. Radiology. 1997;202(3):683–6.
11. Suarez-Poveda T, et al. Diagnostic performance of CT esophagography in patients with suspected esophageal rupture. Emerg Radiol. 2014;21(5):505–10.
12. Pauli EM, Marks JM. Esophageal perforation. In: Fischer's mastery of surgery, vol. 7. Philadelphia: Wolter Kluwer; 2019.
13. Amudhan A, et al. Management of esophageal perforation: experience from a tertiary center in India. Dig Surg. 2009;26(4):322–8.
14. Dickinson KJ, et al. Utility of endoscopic therapy in the management of Boerhaave syndrome. Endosc Int Open. 2016;4(11):E1146–50.
15. Sudarshan M, et al. Management of esophageal perforation in the endoscopic era: is operative repair still relevant? Surgery. 2016;160(4):1104–10.

Incarcerated Hiatal Hernia

Luigi Bonavina and Kenji Inaba

Introduction

Primary paraesophageal hernia (PEH) is a distinct anatomical and clinical entity that leads to incarceration and volvulus of the stomach in the chest. Because of the volume of herniated abdominal contents, significant hiatal defect, and frail crura, the optimal repair requires correction of both axial and radial tension vectors.

Hiatal hernias are heterogeneous anatomical and clinical entities generally classified into four subtypes. Sliding hernia (type I) results from upward migration of the esophagogastric junction into the mediastinum. Paraesophageal hernia (type II) occurs as a result of an anterior defect in the diaphragmatic hiatus leading to upward dislocation of the gastric fundus alongside the cardia. Progressive enlargement of the hiatus and the hernia sac leads to a mixed paraesophageal and sliding hernia (type III). The latter can evolve into the final disease stage characterized by complete intrathoracic "upside-down" stomach with a variable degree of rotation along longitudinal (organo-axial volvulus) or transverse (meso-axial volvulus) gastric axis. To complete the continuum of disease spectrum, even the transverse colon, small bowel, and other abdominal contents can migrate into the hernia sac (type IV hernia) [1, 2] (Table 1). Paraesophageal hernia (PEH) is estimated to account for about 15% of all hiatal hernias, with type III being the most and type II the least common. Progressive deterioration of the phrenoesophageal ligament may explain the higher incidence of type III PEH in the elderly. Anatomic changes involve thinning of the upper layer of

L. Bonavina (✉)
Department of General and Foregut Surgery, IRCCS Policlinico San Donato, University of Milano, Milan, Italy
e-mail: luigi.bonavina@unimi.it

K. Inaba
Department of Surgery, University of Southern California, Los Angeles, CA, USA
e-mail: Kenji.inaba@med.usc.edu

Table 1 Classification and characteristics of hiatal hernias

Hernia type	EGJ location	Hernia contents	Rx size	Rotation	Major complications
I (sliding)	Intrathoracic	Fundus	1–5 cm	None	Reflux esophagitis, Barrett's esophagus
II (true PEH)	Intra-abdominal	Fundus	1–5 cm	None or organoaxial	Obstruction, strangulation, perforation, bleeding
III (mixed)	Intrathoracic	Fundus+body	>50% of stomach	Organoaxial and mesoaxial	Obstruction, strangulation, perforation, bleeding
IV (mixed +other contents)	Intrathoracic	Fundus + body + other	>50% of stomach +colon / small bowel	Organoaxial and mesoaxial	Obstruction, strangulation, perforation, bleeding

EGJ esophago-gastric junction, *PEH* paraesophageal hernia

the ligament (extension of the endothoracic fascia) and loss of elasticity of the distal layer (extension of the transversalis fascia). Because of continuous cranial stretching from challenges of intra-abdominal pressure, the esophagogastric junction moves extraperitoneally into the thorax through the widened hiatus along with a portion of the lesser curvature of the stomach and forms part of the wall of the hernia sac.

Consequently, the lower esophageal sphincter lies outside the abdominal cavity and is unaffected by its environmental pressures [3]. As the size of the hernia increases, the greater curvature will roll up along the left side of the esophagogastric junction into the posterior mediastinum; the stomach becomes incarcerated above the diaphragm, and a 180° rotation occurs causing an organo-axial or, less commonly, a meso-axial volvulus (Fig. 1). At this stage of the natural history of the disease, mechanical complications may occur secondary to congestion of the gastric mucosa, impairment of pulmonary and cardiac function, and closed-loop gastric outlet obstruction. An incarcerated hiatal hernia may also complicate previously failed antireflux repairs and may occur following esophagectomy and gastric conduit reconstruction.

Clinical Presentation

Up to 50% of patients with PEH are asymptomatic or complain of mild non-specific symptoms. Typical symptoms include postprandial distress, chest discomfort, epigastric fullness, nausea, dyspnea, palpitations, fatigue, regurgitation, retching, and hematemesis [4]. Chronic anemia secondary to occult bleeding and cardiorespiratory impairment secondary to compression of cardiac cavities or lung parenchyma

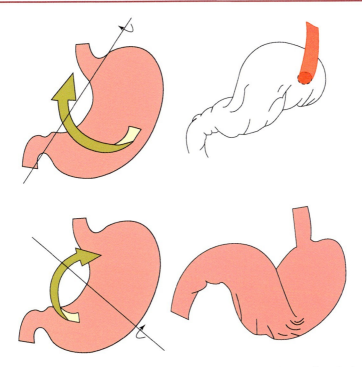

Fig. 1 Organo-axial and meso-axial rotation axes of the intrathoracic gastric volvulus.[From: *GENERAL SURGERY. PRINCIPLES AND INTERNATIONAL PRACTICE, Bland KI et al. (Eds), volume 1, 2nd Edition, Chapter 39, page 432. Springer-Verlag London Limited, 2009]*

are associated with PEH. Acute symptoms mimicking myocardial infarction can develop as a consequence of volvulus with complete gastric outflow obstruction. In as many as 30% of patients, the clinical presentation of a massive and incarcerated intrathoracic stomach may be urgent or emergent [5]. Acute distress with epigastric/chest pain and distension, retching and inability to vomit, and difficulty passing a nasogastric tube (Borchardt triad) can occur as a result of complete obstruction, strangulation, or perforation of the intrathoracic stomach.

Recurrent hernias and para-conduit hiatal hernias following esophagectomy can have a similar clinical presentation. The incidence of para-conduit hernia is 7–10%, and one-third of patients present acutely with hiatal incarceration of the transverse colon or small bowel [6, 7].

Diagnosis and Preoperative Work-up

A PEH is often suspected on an incidental chest X-ray abnormality, most commonly a single or double retrocardiac air-fluid level. In a significant number of elderly female patients, kyphoscoliosis is a common radiological finding. The barium swallow study confirms the diagnosis of incarcerated hiatal hernia with 30–100%

intrathoracic stomach. Computed tomography scan of the chest and abdomen helps to define the anatomical defect, can detect concomitant herniated viscera, and is useful in planning the operative approach. Upper gastrointestinal endoscopy is mandatory to look for esophageal mucosal abnormalities. A type III hernia is identified on retroversion of the scope by noting a gastric pouch lined with rugal folds above the crura impression, with the gastroesophageal junction entering about midway up the side of the pouch. Erosions of the gastric mucosa at the level of the crura impression, known as Cameron's ulcers, are present in about 10% of patients and may cause occult or overt bleeding. In some circumstances, because of the rotation of the stomach, it may be challenging to explore the antropyloric region. Esophageal function studies are usually not necessary in patients considered for elective surgery when symptoms are related to gastric outlet obstruction and distension of the intrathoracic stomach. However, if dysphagia is also present, high-resolution esophageal manometry should be performed to rule out achalasia. Since many of these patients are elderly and frail, a cardiac work up, including cardiovascular magnetic resonance, may be helpful for decision-making before planning elective surgery [8]. For patients presenting emergently with or without signs of sepsis, the CT scan is the single most important diagnostic test to detect early signs of gastric ischemia, perforation, or gangrene of the intrathoracic stomach.

Surgical Treatment

The generally accepted recommendations have been that any medically fit patient should undergo surgical correction of PEH, irrespective of symptoms or age. There is a 30% risk of developing life-threatening complications and a significantly increased risk of mortality with emergent surgery compared to elective repair [9–11]. Some authors advocate a watchful waiting strategy in asymptomatic or minimally symptomatic patients based on the fact that the burden of an emergency operation is not as severe as it was in the past [12]. The traditional approach for repair of PEH has consisted of left thoracotomy or laparotomy. The minimally invasive laparoscopic procedure has quickly gained wide acceptance over the past two decades. The main advantages of the laparoscopic repair include less postoperative discomfort, earlier mobilization, reduced perioperative morbidity, and shorter hospital stay and convalescence. It is imperative that the laparoscopic repair follows the same surgical principles adopted in the traditional operation, that is, complete tension-free reduction of the distal esophagus in the abdominal cavity *en bloc* with the hernia sac, and proper approximation of the crura. However, several areas of controversy persist. These include the recognition and management of a shortened esophagus, and the role of fundoplication, anterior gastropexy, relaxing diaphragmatic incisions, and mesh [13, 14]. In patients presenting acutely, decompression by nasogastric tube or endoscopy and aggressive resuscitation with repletion of intravascular volume are mandatory in preparation for semi-elective surgical therapy. The initial approach of choice is laparoscopy in centers where expertise in advanced minimally invasive surgery is available. However, in unstable patients presenting

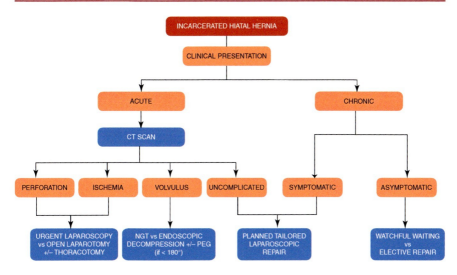

Fig. 2 Management algorithm for incarcerated hiatal hernia

with sepsis and frank signs of ischemia or perforation, laparotomy is recommended as the initial approach, and the chest should also be prepared and draped [15]. Figure 2 shows the proposed management algorithm in patients with incarcerated hiatal hernia.

Technique of Laparoscopic Repair

The patient is placed in the dorsal lithotomy position with reverse Trendelenburg as needed. The surgeon is between the patient's legs. Pneumoperitoneum is induced with the Veress needle placed in the umbilicus or the left hypochondrium, and then maintained at an average pressure of 13 mmHg. The 30-degree-angled scope is inserted through a midline port placed about 15 cm below the xiphoid process. Extended transmediastinal dissection with complete sac excision is mandatory to release axial tension and to reduce at least 3 cm of distal esophagus into the abdomen [16]. By gently pulling the gastric fundus in the caudal direction with atraumatic graspers, dissection of peritoneum off the free edge of the left crus starts at 2 o' clock. Blunt and sharp dissection, with hemostasis provided by ultrasonic shears, is used to expose the entire hernia sac through a relatively avascular plane. The dissection continues anteriorly toward the right crus. The redundant hernia sac that remains attached to the anterior aspect of the esophagogastric junction can be used for retraction. The lesser omentum is then opened and the right crus identified. The dissection continues posteriorly where a large lipoma is usually identified and resected to allow creation of a retroesophageal window. Working through the window from the right side helps to recognize and preserve the posterior vagus nerve, and to complete the dissection of the left crus and the posterior fundus. At this point, the distal esophagus can be safely encircled with a soft silicon drain. The mediastinal cavity is inspected for hemostasis and further blunt/sharp dissection is performed to ensure that an adequate length of the esophagus has been reduced into the abdomen without tension. Occasionally, a staple-wedge Collis gastroplasty may be deemed necessary to further release axial tension [17]. The standard posterior crural repair is performed using interrupted stitches of 2-0 prolene. In patients with oval-shaped hiatus, the left lateral defect can be approximated with an onlay biosynthetic mesh (Phasix) fixed to the crura with a few stitches can be used to reinforce the suture crural repair. To facilitate crura approximation with less radial tension, the pneumoperitoneum pressure should be reduced to 8 mmHg [18] (Figs. 3 and 4). Alternative maneuvers are creating a left pneumothorax through a pleurotomy or performing a right crus relaxing incision [13]. A fundoplication should be routinely added in these patients to prevent gastroesophageal reflux. We prefer a Toupet fundoplication which encompasses the posterior 270° of the distal esophagus. The first two stitches fix the apex of the gastric fundus to the left and the right crura,

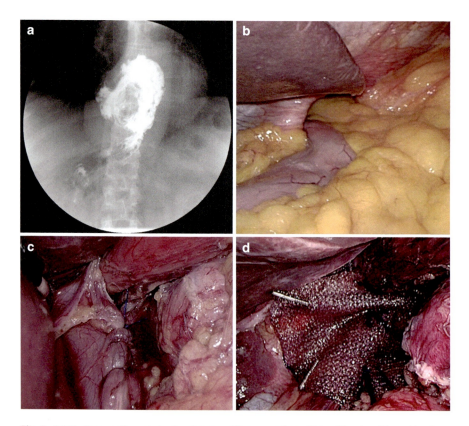

Fig. 3 (**a**) Barium swallow study showing type III paraesophageal hiatal hernia with upside-down intrathoracic stomach; (**b**) Laparoscopic view of large paraesophageal hernia with oval-shaped hiatal defect; (**c**) Posterior crural repair with interrupted permanent sutures; (**d**) Onlay crura augmentation with bio-synthetic Phasix mesh

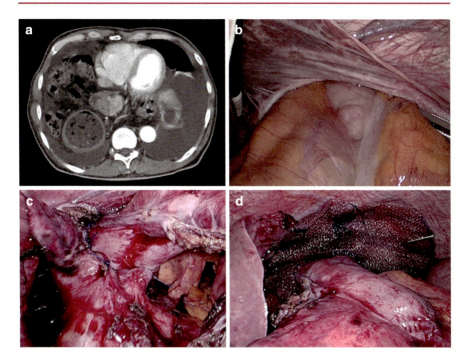

Fig. 4 (**a**) CT scan showing postesophagectomy para-conduit hiatal hernia containing transverse colon; (**b**) laparoscopic view of massive trans-hiatal colon herniation; (**c**) after reduction of the colon, the right side of the gastric conduit is fixed to the right crus with interrupted stitches; (**d**) a bio-synthetic mesh is applied onlay after suture repair of the left diaphragmatic defect

respectively, and additional sutures are placed between the gastric wall and each side of the esophagus [18]. An anterior gastropexy can be added to the repair when the reduced stomach is prone to torsion. A vacuum drain is placed in the mediastinum and a penrose drain under the left liver. All patients undergo a gastrografin swallow study on postoperative day 1, and a clear liquid diet is started. Most patients are discharged home on postoperative day 2 or 3.

Management of Acute Presentations

Decompression of the intrathoracic stomach by nasogastric tube or endoscopy should be a priority in stable patients. After appropriate resuscitation, an endoscopy may be performed on-table in the operating room even in critically-ill and frail patients, when there are doubts about viability of the stomach. Endoscopic unfolding of the volvulus by a J or alpha loop maneuver and repositioning of the stomach with or without percutaneous gastrostomy has been described as an effective strategy in high-risk surgical patients [19, 20]. However, this technique requires a skilled endoscopist and carries a risk of perforation, recurrence is frequent, and a semi-elective surgical repair is warranted in selected individuals. In stable patients, acute clinical presentations of PEH may be dealt with laparoscopy even in patients requiring wedge/sleeve gastric resections or segmental bowel resections. However, emergent situations in critically ill patients with sepsis and evidence of severe gastric ischemia or perforation do require an open approach [21]. Only an anterior gastropexy with or without percutaneous endoscopic gastrostomy should be considered in such circumstances to decrease the incidence of recurrences. Damage control with total gastrectomy and exclusion-diversion is necessary only in the occasional patient presenting with gastric gangrene.

Conclusions

Incarcerated hiatal hernia may be a life-threatening condition, and surgery is the mainstay of treatment. Elective laparoscopic approach for PEH is safe and effective, with a low risk of conversion to open and low complication and mortality rates. Emergency presentations, recurrences, and para-conduit hernias following esophagectomy can often be dealt with laparoscopy but pose more technical challenges. The long-term durability of hiatal repair remains a critical issue that requires further research.

References

1. Skinner D, Belsey R. Management of esophageal disease. Philadelphia: Saunders; 1988.
2. Kahrilas PJ, Kim HC, Pandolfino JE. Approaches to the diagnosis and grading of hiatal hernia. Best Pract Res Clin Gastrenterol. 2008;22:601–16.
3. DeMeester T, Bonavina L. Paraesophageal hiatal hernia. In: Nyhus L, Condon R, editors. Hernia. Philadelphia: Lippincott; 1989. p. 684–93.
4. Wo J, Branum J, Hunter J, et al. Clinical features of type III (mixed) paraesophageal hernia. Am J Gastroenterol. 1996;91:914–6.
5. Hill LD. Incarcerated paraesophageal hernia. A surgical emergency. Am J Surg. 1973;126:286–91.
6. Matthews J, Bhanderi S, Mitchell H, et al. Diaphragmatic herniation following esophagogastric resectional surgery: an increasing problem with minimally invasive techniques? Surg Endosc. 2016;30:5419–27.
7. Brenkman HJF, Parry K, Noble F, et al. Hiatal hernia after esophagectomy for cancer. Ann Thorac Surg. 2017;103:1055–62.
8. Milito P, Lombardi M, Asti E, et al. Influence of large hiatus hernia on cardiac volumes. A prospective observational cohort study by cardiovascular magnetic resonance. Int J Cardiol. 2018;268:241–4.
9. Sihvo EI, Salo JA, Rasanen JV, Rantanen TK. Fatal complications of adult paraesophageal hernia: a population-based study. J Thorac Cardiovasc Surg. 2009;137:419–24.
10. Schlottmann F, Strassle PD, Allaix ME, Patti MG. Paraesophageal hernia repair in the USA: trends of utilization stratified by surgical volume and consequent impact on perioperative outcomes. J Gastrointest Surg. 2017;21:1199–205.
11. Sorial RK, Ali M, Kaneva P, et al. Modern era surgical outcomes of elective and emergent giant paraesophageal hernia repair at a high-volume referral center. Surg Endosc. 2019; https://doi.org/10.1007/s00464-019-06764-4. Epub ahead of print.

12. Stylopoulos N, Gazelle G, Rattner D. Paraesophageal hernias:operation or observation? Ann Surg. 2002;236:492–500.
13. Bradley DD, Louie BE, Farivar AS, et al. Assessment and reduction of diaphragmatic tension during hiatal hernia repair. Surg Endosc. 2015;29:796–804.
14. Tam V, Winger DG, Nason KS. A systematic review and meta-analysis of mesh versus suture cruroplasty in laparoscopic large hiatal hernia repair. Am J Surg. 2016;211:226–38.
15. Bawahab M, Mitchell P, Church N, Debru E. Management of acute paraesophageal hernia. Surg Endosc. 2009;23:255–9.
16. Edye M, Salky B, Posner A, Fierer A. Sac excision is essential to adequate laparoscopic repair of paraesophageal hernia. Surg Endosc. 1998;12:1259–63.
17. Terry ML, Vernon A, Hunter JG. Stapled-wedge Collis gastroplasty for the shortened esophagus. Am J Surg. 2004;188:195–9.
18. Asti E, Lovece A, Bonavina L, et al. Laparoscopic management of large hiatus hernia: five-year cohort study and comparison of mesh-augmented versus standard crura repair. Surg Endosc. 2016;30:5404–9.
19. Tsang TK, Walker R, Yu DJ. Endoscopic reduction of gastric volvulus: the alpha-loop maneuver. Gastrointest Endosc. 1995;42:244–8.
20. Kercher KW, Matthews BD, Ponsky JL, et al. Minimally invasive management of paraesophageal herniation in the high-risk surgical patient. Am J Surg. 2001;182:510–4.
21. Light D, Links D, Griffin M. The threatened stomach: management of the acute gastric volvulus. Surg Endosc. 2016;30:1847–52.

Pulmonary Embolism

David Miranda and Joseph Cuschieri

Introduction

Pulmonary embolism (PE) is a common cause of significant morbidity and mortality. In fact, rates of pulmonary embolism have been estimated to affect greater than 1 out of every 1000 adults annually [1]. The majority of pulmonary embolisms originate from the deep venous system of the pelvis and thighs. As a result, factors associated with deep venous thrombosis (DVT) of the lower extremities increase the risk of PE. Among these factors are prolonged bed rest, congestive heart failure, recent myocardial infarction, malignancy, shock, hypercoagulable states, trauma, and major surgery. Although there has been considerable progress in clinical management and a decreasing incidence of the disease, the severity of PE has been increasing due to simultaneous enhanced survival of patients at greatest risk for PE including advanced malignancy, multisystem severe trauma, and complex major surgery [1, 2]. Although prevention is key to mitigating the disease, appropriate diagnosis when a PE occurs is essential to providing the right treatment to the correct patient without the associated complications of PE treatment in the wrong patient.

Pathophysiology

Acute pulmonary artery obstruction due to embolism or primary thrombosis results in obstructive pathophysiology (Fig. 1). In a minority of patients, pulmonary infarction occurs as small thrombi lodge in distal subsegmental vessels causing pleuritic

D. Miranda
Surgical Critical Care Fellow, University of Washington, Washington, DC, USA
e-mail: Dwmirand@uw.edu

J. Cuschieri (✉)
University of Washington, Washington, DC, USA
e-mail: Jcuschie@uw.edu

© Springer Nature Switzerland AG 2021
J. M. Galante, R. Coimbra (eds.), *Thoracic Surgery for the Acute Care Surgeon*,
Hot Topics in Acute Care Surgery and Trauma,
https://doi.org/10.1007/978-3-030-48493-4_4

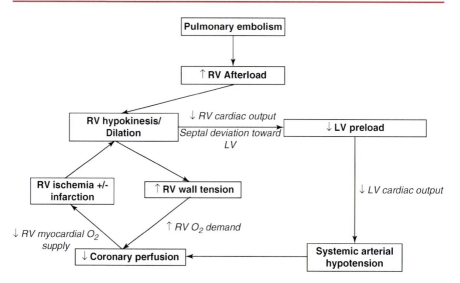

Fig. 1 Pathophysiology of hemodynamic compromises following pulmonary embolism

chest pain and hemoptysis. This is further aggravated by an intense local inflammatory response. As the embolus and subsequent inflammation alters perfusion to otherwise ventilated lung units, dead space physiology occurs. Inflammation also precipitates surfactant dysfunction, atelectasis, and compensatory pulmonary vascular changes where high flow pulmonary perfusion is directed to areas affected by bronchospasm and edema combining to cause functional intrapulmonary shunting. Ultimately, poor V/Q matching occurs and hypoxia can ensue. Patients may develop severe dyspnea, oppressive substernal chest pain, hypotension, and acute cor pulmonale.

Classification

Acute pulmonary embolism represents a spectrum of clinical disease. As a result, pulmonary embolism is categorized into different subgroups that are directly related to the severity of clinical illness. Appropriate categorization is essential to providing appropriate level of care and treatment decisions. Although previous categorizations relied on overall clot burden, the correlation of clot burden and clinical outcome is poorly correlated. As a result, more accurate predictive classifications have been developed that more closely reflect the patient's underlying physiologic and hemodynamic response [3–5].

Currently, the classification systems incorporate validated risk scores, biomarkers, and the patient's hemodynamic status. Three categories of acute pulmonary embolism have been developed—nonmassive (low-risk), submassive (intermediate-risk), and massive (high-risk) (Table 1). Nonmassive pulmonary embolism is not associated with any hemodynamic instability, and more specifically demonstrates no evidence of right ventricular strain, elevation of troponin, or elevation of B-type

Table 1 Mortality risk stratification of pulmonary embolism

PE risk stratification				
Early mortality risk	Shock or hypotension	PESI ≥ 86 or sPESI ≥ 1	Signs of RV dysfunction on an imaging test	Cardiac laboratory biomarkers
High	+	+	+	+
Intermediate-high	–	+	+	+
Intermediate-low	–	+	Either one or none positive	
Low	–	–	Assessment optional: If assessed, both negative	

natriuretic peptide. Submassive pulmonary embolism is not associated with hemodynamic instability but does demonstrate some evidence of cardiac dysfunction as demonstrated by evidence of right ventricular dysfunction by either CT or ECHO, or has elevated biomarkers including B-type natriuretic peptide and/or troponin. Massive pulmonary embolism is associated with hemodynamic instability and shock that is not attributed to a different cause. Thus, the current consensus classification system divides pulmonary embolism into three categories not based on clot size but based on the level of physiologic or clinical deterioration resulting from the embolus.

Diagnosis

Clinical Decision Rules

Several scoring systems have been developed to aid in the diagnosis of pulmonary embolism. Each scoring system should be applied to individual patients appropriately and with caution since clinical suspicion plays a critical role in the actual diagnosis of patients that have suffered from a pulmonary embolism. Three scoring systems are routinely used, the Pulmonary Embolism Rule-Out Criteria (PERC) has been applied in the outpatient and emergency room setting, while the Wells Score and Geneva Score have been applied to hospitalized patients (Tables 2, 3, and 4).

PERC

The PERC scoring system (Table 2) was initially described in 2004. The eight PERC criteria are (1) age greater than or equal to 50; (2) heart rate greater than 100/min; (3) pulse oximetry oxygen saturation less than 95%; (4) unilateral leg swelling; (5) hemoptysis; (6) recent surgery or trauma; (7) prior PE or DVT; and (8) exogenous estrogen use. When none of these factors are present, a pulmonary embolism is unlikely with a sensitivity of 97%, specificity of 22%, and a false-negative rate of under 1% [6]. However, if the clinician suspicion is high, then appropriate laboratory and imaging studies should still be performed.

Table 2 Pulmonary embolism rule-out criteria (PERC)

	Age < 50 years
	Pulse <100/min
	SaO_2 > 94% on room air
	No hemoptysis
	No exogenous estrogen
	No previous DVT or PE
	No surgery or trauma within prior 4 weeks
	No unilateral leg swelling

Table 3 Wells Score

Cancer	1
Heart rate > 100	1.5
DVT or PE history	1.5
Hemoptysis	1
Symptoms of DVT	3
Immobilization > 3 days or surgery < 4 weeks	1.5
No better alternative dx	3
PE risk	≤4 points: PE unlikely ≥4 points: PE likely

Table 4 Geneva Score

Age > 65 years	1
Cancer (active or cured ≤ 1 1 year)	2
Heart rate	75–95 bpm = 3 > 95 bpm = 5
DVT or PE history	1.5
Hemoptysis	1
Unilateral lower limb pain	3
Surgery or lower limb fracture ≤ 1 month	2
Pain on lower limb deep venous palpation and unilateral edema	4
PE probability	≤4 points = low 4–10 points = intermediate 11 points = high

Wells Score

The classic Wells score (Table 3) was initially described in 1998 [7]. Since then, modifications including different cutoffs and corresponding probability levels or alternate weightings of the score items have been proposed, leading to a modified Wells score and a simplified version. The seven Wells criteria are (1) signs of DVT; (2) alternative diagnosis less likely than PE; (3) heart rate greater than 100/min; (f) immobilization for greater than or equal to 3 days/surgery in past 4 weeks; (5) prior DVT or PE; (6) hemoptysis; and (7) active malignancy/palliative situation. In the simplified version, if one or less of these factors is present, then a pulmonary embolism is unlikely.

Geneva Score

The original Geneva score was initially described in 2001. Since then, modifications have been developed to further refine and simplify the scoring in both the Revised Geneva Score and Simplified Geneva Score. Although accurate, it is less dependent on the provider assessment than the Wells score. The nine Geneva criteria are (1) age greater than 65; (2) prior DVT or PE; (3) surgery or fracture within a month; (4) active malignancy; (5) unilateral lower limb pain; (6) hemoptysis; (7) heart rate between 75 and 95/min; (8) heart rate greater than or equal to 95/min; and (9) pain on deep palpation of the lower limb with unilateral edema (Table 4). In the simplified version, if a score of 4 or less is present, then a pulmonary embolism is unlikely [8].

D-Dimer

D-Dimer is a sensitive marker for pulmonary embolism and can exclude PE without need for further testing in patients with low clinic probability. D-dimer levels greater than 500 ng/ml may suggest the presence of PE. However, since D-dimer increases with age, the false-positive rate in older individuals increases. Thus, the threshold for a positive D-dimer should be calculated as the patient's age multiplied by 10 ng/ml for patients older than 50 years. When used in combination with the Wells score in patients with a low clinical suspicion, further testing can be safely withheld. Although the use of D-dimer is useful in the outpatient setting, it appears less useful in the inpatient setting and patients with either a history of previous venous thromboembolic events, trauma, or malignancy [9].

Diagnostic Imaging

Venous Duplex

The presence of a proximal deep venous thrombosis (DVT) in a patient with a suspected PE is highly predictive of a PE and thus warrants treatment. As a result, Doppler and B-mode ultrasonography may be used to demonstrate the presence of a DVT. However, a negative result does not exclude PE and requires further investigation [10].

Chest Radiography

Chest X-ray is not specific for pulmonary embolism, but is important in ruling out other diseases. Traditional radiographic findings, including Westermark's sign (focal peripheral hyperlucency) and Hampton's hump (wedge-shaped consolidation), are neither specific nor sensitive for pulmonary embolism.

Radionucleotide (V/Q) Scan

Historically, V/Q scanning was the most common means of diagnosis of pulmonary embolism, but it is no longer the most sensitive or specific study. The study is based on the presumption that an embolic obstruction of the pulmonary vasculature will produce a perfusion defect without a change in ventilation. However, prior to the rapid emergence of CT, the PIOPED study demonstrated a specificity of only 10% [11]. As a result, the clinical probability plays a critical role in the interpretation of this study.

Pulmonary Angiogram

Although angiography continues to be referred to as the "gold standard" for diagnosis with a sensitivity of 63–100% and a specificity of 55–96%, the increasing accuracy of CT has limited the need for this invasive test. Although this study is limited by the invasive nature, it does allow for potential interventions to be undertaken during the angiography (Fig. 2). As a result, in rare instances in patients with suspected massive PE that may require catheter-directed interventions, this may be considered an option for both diagnosis and therapy.

CT Scan

Computed tomography pulmonary angiography has good diagnostic accuracy for pulmonary embolism and has become widely available (Fig. 3). The test is relatively easy to perform, and as a result has become the major means of diagnostic

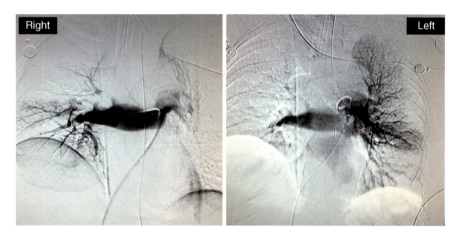

Fig. 2 Catheter-directed pulmonary embolectomy. On right, initial pulmonary angiogram demonstrating clot burden in right and left pulmonary system, in particular to blood flow to right upper lobe and left lung. On left, pulmonary angiogram demonstrating good perfusion to left lung following embolectomy

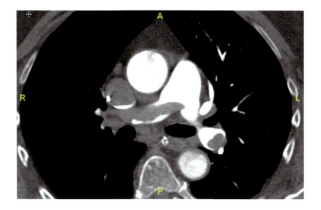

Fig. 3 CT PE demonstrating clot burden throughout pulmonary circulation, with obstruction of right main pulmonary outflow tract

imaging for pulmonary embolism. However, similar to angiography, it exposes patients to ionizing radiation and contrast media that may be contraindicated in patients with severe renal impairment [12].

MRI

Magnetic resonance imaging angiography offers a noninvasive examination of the pulmonary vasculature without the need for ionic contrast. However, the accuracy of MRI in establishing the diagnosis of PE is poor, with nearly 19% of cases being inconclusive [12].

V/Q Single-Photon Emission Computed Tomography

Ventilation/perfusion single-photon emission computed tomography is an emerging technique that results in considerably less radiation exposure than CT angio with PE protocol (CTPE)and avoids the need for intravenous contrast. The diagnostic accuracy of PE in terms of sensitivity and specificity is similar to CTPE. However, the precise role of this modality has not been sufficiently validated for use in routine clinical practice.

Cardiac/Hemodynamic Evaluation

Troponin

Circulating troponin aids in evaluation of evidence of cardiac ischemia. Circulating levels of both troponin I and troponin T are associated with early and late morbidity and mortality following an acute PE. Elevation of troponin I of a level of greater than 0.1 ng/ml implies evidence cardiac ischemia and is consistent with a submassive PE [13].

Natriuretic Peptides

Elevated natriuretic peptides are associated with increased early morbidity and mortality following an acute pulmonary embolism. Both brain natriuretic peptide (BNP) and N-terminal pro-BNP if elevated have been associated with a 9.51- and 5.74-fold increased risk of early mortality, respectively. A BNP value of greater than 100 pg/ml or NT-proBNP greater than 900 pg/ml is suggestive of a submassive pulmonary embolism [14].

Electrocardiogram

Obtaining an EKG helps in differentiating between acute myocardial infarction, pericarditis, and pulmonary embolism. Signs of acute right ventricular overload due to acute pulmonary artery obstruction include sinus tachycardia, rightward shift of the axis, right bundle branch block, and an $S_I Q_{III} T_{III}$ pattern. However, lack of these finding does not rule out a less significant pulmonary embolism.

CT

Dilation of the right ventricle determined by CT is associated with increase in hospital and mortality within 3 months. Although the determination of right ventricular dilation by CT varies, a right ventricle diameter divided by left ventricle diameter of greater than 0.9 is the typical value demonstrating right ventricular dysfunction and suggestive of a submassive PE. The degree of clot burden, however, as demonstrated by CT has not been shown to be prognostic for early or late-term outcome.

ECHO

Transesophageal echocardiography (TEE) usually reveals indirect evidence of pulmonary embolism with acute dilation of the right ventricle and elevated pulmonary artery pressures. Transthoracic echocardiography and TEE can identify clot in the main PA and proximal right PA, but the proximal left PA is often obscured. The primary benefit of TEE is to rule out segmental wall motion defects that might suggest acute infarction, tamponade, and to define whether there is clot proximal enough to warrant an attempt at catheter-directed or surgical removal. Evidence of right ventricular dysfunction by echocardiography following an acute PE is associated with a 2.53-fold increase in early mortality [15].

Prognostication

One of the reasons diagnosing PE into specific classifications is for prognosis. As VTE and PE began to be more associated with hospitalized patients, a formal strategy to predict and prevent development of PE was launched and Various Risk

Assessment Models (RAMs) have been developed to quantitatively predict risk. The Padua Prediction Score and IMPROVE RAM were the first widely used models that were valid in medical patients [16, 17]. However, a more encompassing tool emerged that was also valid among surgical populations—The CAPRINI RAM. This is currently the most robust and used prediction model having been validated in 250,000 patients and 100 clinical trials. The model works via a series of short scoring surveys for both the patient and the healthcare provider. It is dynamic in that it can be used for re-evaluation over the clinical course of a patient's illness and provide new scores and updated treatment options [18].

The pulmonary embolism severity index (PESI) was developed as a clinical prediction tool for 30-day mortality [19]. The PESI consists of 11 clinical variables that can be assessed at the time of diagnosis (Table 5). The PESI does not rely on any imaging or laboratory studies, but several studies have demonstrated increased predictive value with incorporation of laboratory values, specifically troponin and BNP. The benefit of this prediction model is to aid in initial management of patients and to determine which patients are best treated solely with anticoagulation and potential limited hospitalization. This index has been demonstrated to be reliable and reproducible for prognostication of patients with acute PE.

Management

The principle behind PE treatment is to reduce or remove clot burden in order to prevent hemodynamically significant strain on the heart and improve pulmonary gas exchange. The treatment options for PE occupy a spectrum of increasingly invasive options from medical and systemic treatments, to more invasive and targeted approaches up to and including circulatory assist treatments.

Table 5 Pulmonary Embolism Severity Index (PESI) and Simplified Pulmonary Embolism Severity Index

	PESI	Simplified PESI
Age	Age in years = # points	>80 years = 1 point
Cancer	30	1
Heart rate ≥ 110	20	1
Chronic heart failure	10	1
Chronic pulmonary disease	10	
Systolic blood pressure < 100 mmHg	30	1
Arterial oxyhemoglobin saturation < 90%	20	1
Altered mental status	60	–
Temperature < 36 °C	20	–
Respiratory rate > 30 breaths per minute = 20	20	–
Male sex = 10	10	–
30-day mortality risk	≤65 points: Very low 66–85 points: Low 86–105 points: Moderate 106–125 points: High >125: Very high	0 points = low ≥1 = very high

Medical Therapy

Anticoagulation

Early therapeutic anticoagulation has been demonstrated conclusively to reduce recurrence and improve mortality in acute PE [20]. For this reason, in patients with relatively low bleeding risk, systemic anticoagulation should be empirically started in all patients with high clinical suspicion of PE even before diagnosis is confirmed. And, systemic anticoagulation should remain a foundation of treatment even when additional interventional treatments are considered [21]. The particular choice of anticoagulant used depends on clinical factors such as hepatic and renal function, but in general when more advanced treatments are sought for intermediate- and high-risk PE, the flexibility of unfractionated heparin drip is the preferred choice for interventional radiology and surgical teams. For low-risk PEs, and for outpatient management of clinically stable intermediate- and high-risk PEs after advanced treatment, the Direct Oral Anticoagulants (DOACs) are now a first-line treatment along with low-molecular-weight heparin [5, 22]. Duration of treatment in PE mirrors that of DVT and accounts for provoking events and risk factors for bleeding. Specifically, patients with a first episode of low-risk or intermediate-risk PE should receive anticoagulation for at least 3 months. If there were transient provoking factors (i.e. major surgery, immobility >3 days, hormone therapy that was subsequently stopped) within the past 3 months, the duration should not be extended. If, there are sustained provoking factors, anticoagulation therapy may be increased up to 6–12 months on a case-by-case basis, although there continues to be no high-level evidence for specific duration recommendations longer than 6 months [23]. Additionally, patients that do not have evidence of provoking factors should undergo workup for hypercoagulable state that may require lifelong therapy.

Thrombolysis

Systemic thrombolysis is given with the intent of clot dissolution, restoration of pulmonary perfusion and subsequent V/Q matching, and relief of right ventricular afterload. It has been shown that decreased right ventrical (RV) afterload and treating with systemic thrombolytics compared to heparin alone improve outcomes such as hemodynamic collapse when administered in intermediate- and high-risk PE [24, 25]. However, significant complications at prohibitively high rates in the form of intracranial hemorrhage have been conclusively demonstrated, and now systemic thrombolytics are cautiously administered to a narrow group of patients [26]. This group may include patients in cardiac arrest from known PE, patients with right heart thrombus, and patients with high-risk PE and low risk of bleeding. In fact, for patients with massive PE and no contraindications, systemic thrombolysis is considered first-line therapy based mainly on meta-analysis data that found a reduction in recurrent PE or death from 19.0% without treatment to 9.4% with thrombolytic [27]. There is currently not significant high-quality data regarding use of systemic thrombolytics in submassive PE specifically with regard to which outcomes would improve or how that should tip the risk/benefit analysis given the known high complication rates [28].

Inhaled Nitric Oxide

The intended use of inhaled nitric oxide is to harness its property of selective vasodilation only to pulmonary vasculature adjacent to airways participating in inhalation of the gas, thereby reducing RV afterload and strain without causing systemic hypotension. There have been several studies including a randomized control trial demonstrating improved hemodynamics and reduced RV strain; however, the data has not yet been conclusive enough to drive use of nitric oxide into current guidelines [29, 30].

Catheter-Directed Therapy

Catheter-Directed Thrombolysis

Thrombolysis with a continuous infusion of low-dose thrombolytic via a catheter in the pulmonary artery attempts to achieve the advantages of systemic thrombolysis without the distant bleeding risks. There have been a few prominent prospective trials assessing the benefits of this technology, and they have demonstrated better RV-to-left ventrical (LV) ratio reduction compared to heparin alone as well as improved hemodynamics without significant incidence of catastrophic bleeding events [31, 32]. These studies were done in patients with predominantly high-risk PE and underscore the relative safety and efficacy of the technology. However, there is still not good data about which intermediate-risk PE patients would benefit nor do these studies address the challenges of expertise availability and rapid mobilization of high resource interventions compared to lower-resource intravenous systemic thrombolytics. For now, the indicated population appears to be high-risk PE patients with relative contraindications to systemic thrombolysis and intermediate-risk PE patients with signs of impending clinical deterioration [33].

Catheter-Directed Embolectomy

Percutaneous embolectomy is an approach without any significant supportive data which may be an option for patients who have a contraindication or failure of thrombolysis, do not have a cardiothoracic surgeon available for surgical embolectomy, and do have interventionalists and expertise to offer catheter-directed embolectomy. As there are potentially a sizeable number of patients with intermediate- and high-risk PE who may fit this scenario, additional research is warranted. Nevertheless, when patients with contraindication to thrombolysis do not have the option of surgical embolectomy, it is reasonable to consider this approach [33].

Surgery

The indication for surgical pulmonary embolectomy is a patient with intermediate- to high-risk PE who has an absolute contraindication to thrombolysis or is failing thrombolysis. A majority of consensus guidelines support this role for surgical embolectomy even in the presence of pre-operative thrombolysis [4, 5, 21].

Observational studies have found that while mortality used to be high for this surgery, it is beginning to come down into the single-digit percent range. And while there has never been a randomized control trial comparing systemic thrombolysis to surgical embolectomy, both have shown improved RV function and hemodynamics while thrombolysis is associated with more bleeding [34, 35]. Given the challenging decision making around endovascular and surgical treatment in these critically ill patients, it is important to rapidly involve a structured, expert-led, multi-disciplinary Pulmonary Embolism Response Team (PERT) to make these decisions (PERT flow diagram) which have been shown to improve outcomes [36] (Fig. 4).

Extracorporeal Life Support (ECLS)

ECLS if available should be performed in high-risk PE and cardiogenic shock with cardiac arrest as a lifesaving procedure. Cardiopulmonary support with venoarterial extracorporeal membrane oxygenation (ECMO) should be considered in patients that have failed catheter or systemic thrombolytics, or who are deteriorating so rapidly that cardiopulmonary arrest is imminent. These patients usually demonstrate severe and worsening shock despite therapy directed at reducing clot burden and use of vasopressor agents. There is no published randomized controlled data comparing ECMO to other treatments of high-risk PE; however, numerous observational reports have indicated favorable outcomes [37]. And, among all ECMO indications, the treatment of PE remains one of ECMO's most successful uses [38]. The general duration of ECMO in these patients is typically 4–6 days and can be used in combination with systemic thrombolysis, catheter-directed therapy, or surgical embolectomy providing cardiopulmonary support while the clot burden resolves. Despite this, mortality remains high in patients treated with ECLS in the range of 40–60%.

Prevention

The need for thromboprophylaxis is based upon the high incidence of venous thromboembolism in high-risk patients. The apparent need for adequate prophylaxis may be further magnified within the critically ill patient because of limited cardiopulmonary reserve. Although intensive, non-invasive surveillance may be an alternative to prophylaxis, tests such as duplex ultrasonography have only moderate sensitivity in asymptomatic high-risk patients [10]. Furthermore, patients with primary pelvic thrombosis leading to PE will not be identified by this approach.

Optimal prophylaxis for high-risk medical and surgical patients has been defined by randomized studies with appropriate guidelines developed. However, appropriate prophylaxis has been underutilized, and thus successful minimization of this disease has not been achieved. Most patients with low and moderate risk of VTE would benefit from either unfractionated heparin, low-molecular-weight heparin, or intermittent pneumatic compression devices. However, patients at high risk for VTE should be treated with low-molecular-weight heparin if possible [39]. The use of

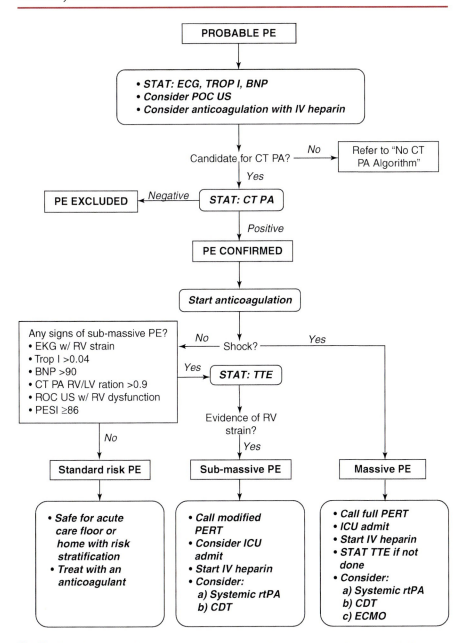

Fig. 4 Algorithm for rapid assessment, diagnosis, and classification of pulmonary embolism

low-molecular-weight heparin in this patient population reduces the risk of VTE by greater than 25% in comparison to unfractionated heparin. However, this reduction in the rate of VTE has only led to modest benefit in high-risk trauma patients with a rate between 4 and 28% [40]. As a result, despite limited data, some experts continue to advocate prophylactic IVC filter placement. Although placement may reduce in the incidence of PE, the rate of DVT is significantly increased in this patient population.

Conclusion

The definition and treatment of pulmonary embolism, especially massive PE, are coming into focus with new studies and clearer guidelines. However, there continues to be a general paucity of high-quality evidence for deciding among treatment modalities especially in the area of submassive PEs. As this knowledge gap fills in, it will be important to continue leaning on the expertise of institutional PERTs to guide clinical decision making in higher-risk PEs.

References

1. Silverstein MD, et al. Trends in the incidence of deep vein thrombosis and pulmonary embolism: a 25-year population-based study. JAMA Intern Med. 1998;158(6):585–93.
2. Tagalakis V, et al. Incidence of and Mortality from Venous Thromboembolism in a Real-world Population: The Q-VTE Study Cohort. Am J Med. 2013;126(9):832.e13–21.
3. Sharifi M, et al. Pulseless electrical activity in pulmonary embolism treated with thrombolysis (from the "PEAPETT" study). Am J Emerg Med. 2016;34(10):1963–7.
4. Jaff MR, et al. Management of massive and submassive pulmonary embolism, iliofemoral deep vein thrombosis, and chronic thromboembolic pulmonary hypertension: a scientific statement from the American Heart Association. Circulation. 2011;123(16):1788–830.
5. Kearon C, et al. Antithrombotic therapy for VTE disease: CHEST guideline and expert panel report. Chest. 2016;149(2):315–52.
6. Singh B, et al. Diagnostic accuracy of pulmonary embolism rule-out criteria: a systematic review and meta-analysis. Ann Emerg Med. 2012;59(6):517–520.e4.
7. Wells PS, et al. Use of a clinical model for safe management of patients with suspected pulmonary embolism. Ann Intern Med. 1998;129(12):997–1005.
8. Klok FA, et al. Simplification of the revised Geneva score for assessing clinical probability of pulmonary embolism. Arch Intern Med. 2008;168(19):2131–6.
9. Nagel SN, et al. Age-dependent diagnostic accuracy of clinical scoring systems and D-dimer levels in the diagnosis of pulmonary embolism with computed tomography pulmonary angiography (CTPA). Eur Radiol. 2019;29:4563–71.
10. Cipolle MD, et al. The role of surveillance duplex scanning in preventing venous thromboembolism in trauma patients. J Trauma Acute Care Surg. 2002;52(3):453–62.
11. PIOPED Investigators. Value of the ventilation/perfusion scan in acute pulmonary embolism. Results of the prospective investigation of pulmonary embolism diagnosis (PIOPED). JAMA. 1990;263(20):2753.
12. Stein PD, et al. Diagnostic pathways in acute pulmonary embolism: recommendations of the PIOPED II Investigators. Radiology. 2007;242(1):15–21.
13. Moores L, et al. Pulmonary Embolism Severity Index and troponin testing for the selection of low-risk patients with acute symptomatic pulmonary embolism. J Thromb Haemost. 2010;8(3):517–22.
14. Klok FA, Mos IC, Huisman MV. Brain-type natriuretic peptide levels in the prediction of adverse outcome in patients with pulmonary embolism: a systematic review and meta-analysis. Am J Respir Crit Care Med. 2008;178(4):425–30.

15. Sanchez O, et al. Prognostic value of right ventricular dysfunction in patients with haemodynamically stable pulmonary embolism: a systematic review. Eur Heart J. 2008;29(12):1569–77.
16. Barbar S, et al. A risk assessment model for the identification of hospitalized medical patients at risk for venous thromboembolism: the Padua Prediction Score. J Thromb Haemost. 2010;8(11):2450–7.
17. Spyropoulos AC, et al. Predictive and associative models to identify hospitalized medical patients at risk for VTE. Chest. 2011;140(3):706–14.
18. Cronin M, et al. Completion of the updated Caprini risk assessment model (2013 version). Clin Appl Thromb Hemost. 2019;25:1076029619838052.
19. Jiménez D, et al. Simplification of the pulmonary embolism severity index for prognostication in patients with Acute Symptomatic Pulmonary Embolism Simplified Pulmonary Embolism Severity Index. JAMA Intern Med. 2010;170(15):1383–9.
20. Robertson L, Jones LE. Fixed dose subcutaneous low molecular weight heparins versus adjusted dose unfractionated heparin for the initial treatment of venous thromboembolism. Cochrane Database Syst Rev. 2017;(2):CD001100.
21. Konstantinides SV, et al. 2014 ESC guidelines on the diagnosis and management of acute pulmonary embolism: The Task Force for the Diagnosis and Management of Acute Pulmonary Embolism of the European Society of Cardiology (ESC) endorsed by the European Respiratory Society (ERS). Eur Heart J. 2014;35(43):3033–73.
22. Groetzinger LM, et al. Apixaban or rivaroxaban versus warfarin for treatment of submassive pulmonary embolism after catheter-directed thrombolysis. Clin Appl Thromb Hemost. 2018;24(6):908–13.
23. Kearon C, et al. Antithrombotic therapy for VTE disease: antithrombotic therapy and prevention of thrombosis: American College of Chest Physicians evidence-based clinical practice guidelines. Chest. 2012;141(2):e419S–96S.
24. Konstantinides S, et al. Comparison of alteplase versus heparin for resolution of major pulmonary embolism. Am J Cardiol. 1998;82(8):966–70.
25. Goldhaber SZ, et al. Alteplase versus heparin in acute pulmonary embolism: randomised trial assessing right-ventricular function and pulmonary perfusion. Lancet. 1993;341(8844):507–11.
26. Meyer G, et al. Fibrinolysis for patients with intermediate-risk pulmonary embolism. N Engl J Med. 2014;370(15):1402–11.
27. Wan S, et al. Thrombolysis compared with heparin for the initial treatment of pulmonary embolism: a meta-analysis of the randomized controlled trials. Circulation. 2004;110(6):744–9.
28. Chodakowski JD, Courtney DM. Pulmonary embolism critical care update: prognosis, treatment, and research gaps. Curr Opin Crit Care. 2018;24(6):540–6.
29. Kline JA, et al. Randomized trial of inhaled nitric oxide to treat acute pulmonary embolism: the iNOPE trial. Am Heart J. 2017;186:100–10.
30. Summerfield DT, et al. Inhaled nitric oxide as salvage therapy in massive pulmonary embolism: a case series. Respir Care. 2012;57(3):444–8.
31. Piazza G, et al. A prospective, single-arm, multicenter trial of ultrasound-facilitated, catheter-directed, low-dose fibrinolysis for acute massive and submassive pulmonary embolism: the SEATTLE II study. J Am Coll Cardiol Intv. 2015;8(10):1382–92.
32. Kuo WT, et al. Pulmonary embolism response to fragmentation, embolectomy, and catheter thrombolysis (PERFECT): initial results from a prospective multicenter registry. Chest. 2015;148(3):667–73.
33. Rivera-Lebron B, et al. Diagnosis, treatment and follow up of acute pulmonary embolism: consensus practice from the PERT Consortium. Clin Appl Thromb Hemost. 2019;25:1076029619853037.
34. Aymard T, et al. Massive pulmonary embolism: surgical embolectomy versus thrombolytic therapy—should surgical indications be revisited? Eur J Cardiothorac Surg. 2012;43(1):90–4.
35. Azari A, et al. Surgical embolectomy versus thrombolytic therapy in the management of acute massive pulmonary embolism: short and long-term prognosis. Heart Lung. 2015;44(4):335–9.
36. Rosovsky R, et al. Changes in treatment and outcomes after creation of a pulmonary embolism response team (PERT), a 10-year analysis. J Thromb Thrombolysis. 2019;47(1):31–40.

37. Pasrija C, et al. Triage and optimization: a new paradigm in the treatment of massive pulmonary embolism. J Thorac Cardiovasc Surg. 2018;156(2):672–81.
38. Carroll BJ, et al. Clinical features and outcomes in adults with cardiogenic shock supported by extracorporeal membrane oxygenation. Am J Cardiol. 2015;116(10):1624–30.
39. Geerts WH, et al. Prevention of venous thromboembolism: American College of Chest Physicians evidence-based clinical practice guidelines. Chest. 2008;133(6):381S–453S.
40. Geerts WH, et al. A comparison of low-dose heparin with low-molecular-weight heparin as prophylaxis against venous thromboembolism after major trauma. N Engl J Med. 1996;335(10):701–7.

Empyema and Effusions

Andreas Hecker, Winfried Padberg, Timothy Browder, and David A. Spain

Pleural Empyema

Introduction

Pleural empyema is defined as pus in the pleural cavity. Initially described more than 2500 years ago, the incidence of pleural empyema in the USA doubled at the end of the last decade. Despite the advantages in the field of microbiology, antimicrobial therapy, and modern surgical treatment, the mortality of pleural empyema remains unacceptably high. Compared to uncomplicated pneumonia, any parapneumonic effusion is associated with an increased mortality. Once detected, any delay in drainage of a pleural empyema leads to a dramatically higher mortality rate. One-year mortality after diagnosis of a pleural empyema is 20% and even 30% in the elderly population, respectively [1, 2]. Most common in the childhood and the growing population of frail and elderly patients, the thoracic surgeon is increasingly confronted with immunocompromised patients suffering from a pleural empyema. This book chapter provides an overview on the most important aspects of modern diagnostics and therapeutic approaches in this important field of acute care in thoracic surgery.

Epidemiology and Pathogenesis

Up to 57% of the patients suffering from pneumonia requiring hospitalization present with a complicated pleural effusion (Light class >3, see below), which is an independent risk factor for a dramatically increased morbidity and mortality [3]. In 4–5%, a chest tube insertion and drainage of the effusion are necessary, which is the sufficient therapeutic approach in 2/3 of the cases. In the other patients, a complicated pleural empyema requires surgical therapy.

While normally the pleural space is a thin (10 µm) fluid film containing serum-equivalent glucose and protein levels, an infection of the lung parenchyma induces an increased permeability of the mesothelial cell monolayer and an exudation of sterile fluid into the pleural cavity (simple parapneumonic effusion) [4]. Secondarily bacteria or fungi can invade the effusion through the damaged vascular endothelium and mesothelium (complicated parapneumonic effusion) and thus lead to a switch to typical biochemical characteristics of a pleural infection or fibropurulent empyema. Alternatively, any primary bacterial infection of the pleural cavity can affect the mesothelial monolayer. By cell debris, bacterial components, and inflammatory mediators, a loss of mesothelial integrity can lead to an accumulation of pleural fluid and the recruitment of pro-inflammatory cells. The homeostasis inside the pleural cavity shifts to a pro-coagulant milieu. Fibrin depositions on both the visceral and parietal pleural surface lead to septation and typical loculated effusions with important impact on the therapeutic approach. Later, fibrin deposits and growth factors from the mesothelium induce a fibroproliferation, which results in the formation of a fibrotic cortex and empyema chambers. At the end stage of pleural infection, the progression can summit in an entrapment of the lung with a restricted mobility due to a solid fibrous cortex.

Pleural empyema is mainly caused by community-acquired pneumonia (CAP) (about 2/3 of empyema), although the rate of empyema development is relatively higher in cases of hospital-acquired pneumonia (HAP). Furthermore, pleural empyema often occurs in cases of thoracic trauma, previous pleural drainage, infradiaphragmatic surgery (e.g. splenectomy, cholecystectomy, biliopancreatic surgery) or infection, esophageal perforation, pneumothorax, and lung abscess with concomitant sepsis. The subgroup of patients with pleural empyema after thoracic surgical intervention is at high risk for complicated pleural empyema. Figure 1 summarizes risk factors for the development of pleural empyema such as pre-existing diabetes mellitus (22%, typically *Klebsiella pneumoniae*), immunodeficiency (typically *Staphylococcus aureus*, MRSA, fungi), malignancy, or poor dental hygiene (typically anaerobes) [3, 5]. Depending on the etiology, the spectrum of the underlying bacteria is diverse with aerobic microorganisms as the most frequent followed by anaerobes and mixed cultures. While streptococci are typical bacteria in case of CAP, HAP is often caused by staphylococci (18%), including bacteria with an increased rate of antibiotic resistance (MRSA; 28%). Prognosis is poor in patients with HAP, mixed infection, and exceptionally worse if *Klebsiella pneumoniae* is detected in pleural empyema, which is predominantly found in patients with diabetes mellitus [5].

Empyema and Effusions

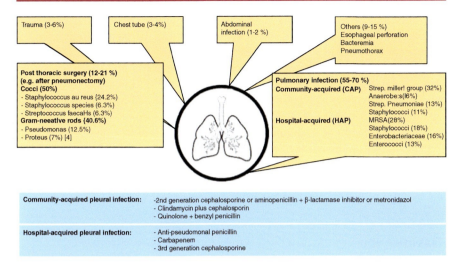

Fig. 1 Etiology of pleural empyema. Underlying diseases and predisposing factors for the development of pleural empyema. Pneumonia is the most frequent reason for (complicated) effusions, which could result in a pleural empyema. Initial antimicrobial treatment options are shown both for community-acquired and hospital-acquired empyema. Figure drawn by author Dr. Andreas Hecker

Diagnosis

Patients with an infected pleural cavity typically present with cough, fever, sputum, and chest pain often combined with anemia and fatigue. Due to the fact that these symptoms are often masked or even missing in the elderly, the rate of underdiagnosis is higher in this population. Once an infection is suspected, it is supported by elevated infection parameters in the laboratory examination. The chest X-ray imaging in the posteroanterior and the lateral positions is usually performed, although the lateral chest radiographs are more likely to detect pleural fluid in the posterior costophrenic angle. In this context, ultrasound is an important and highly sensitive bedside tool to examine the pleural cavity [7], to estimate the amount of pleural fluid, and to determine any echogenicity as a sign of an exudative effusion. Fluid septations and/or loculations could be detected as signs of a progressed stage disease associated with an increased mortality. Contrast-enhanced computed tomography (CT) is the gold standard for the detection and evaluation of a pleural empyema and furthermore enables to analyze its etiology. While thickening of the pleura is found in 56% of cases with exudative parapneumonic pleuritis, this raises to 86–100% in pleural empyemas. The so-called "split pleural sign" (pleural thickness and separation of both pleural layers) is pathognomonic of empyema on CT scan. CT allows the differentiation between pneumonic effusion/pleural empyema and a peripheral pulmonary abscess and detects patients with a malignant pulmonary tumor with concomitant pleural effusion.

Ultrasound-guided sampling is one further important tool to analyze (and to monitor) the macroscopic and microscopic quality of the pleural fluid, which is strongly recommended by the guidelines of the British Thoracic Society (BTS) [4]. Analysis of its biochemical characteristics (pH, glucose level, lactate dehydrogenase [LDH] level) allows a classification of the pleural effusion and could indicate any progress in cases of repetitive sampling. The most powerful clinical indicator for chest tube insertion is a pleural fluid pH < 7.2.

The confirmation of a certain bacterial infection is still low, and using conventional culturing methods, the detection of bacteria is successful in 53–60% only [3]. In cases of a community-acquired empyema, the rate of positivity is 28% [8]. Modern nucleic acid amplification testing can provide a moderate increase in detecting bacteria in another 10–15% [9, 10].

Classification

To provide an adequate, stage-directed therapeutic approach, a classification of pleural empyema is essential. Different classification systems are established and mainly focus on parapneumonic etiology of a pleural empyema. Nevertheless, these classification systems are helpful tools for everyday clinical use to estimate the current clinical status of the patient with an empyema caused by other etiologies.

The classification of the *American Thoracic Society (ATS) (1962)* divides empyema in three phases, which merge into each other and thus reflect the typical disease progress in untreated cases. The *exudative phase (Phase I)* is characterized by a fluid accumulation inside the pleural space. Cell count is typically low and the lung is re-expandable, if the pleural fluid is drained. Invasion of polymorphonuclear leukocytes, pus and fibrin deposits at the pleural layers and in the exudate are characteristic features of the so-called *fibropurulent/intermediate phase (Phase II)*. The infectious source is encapsulated and restricted to the pleural space by these pathophysiological mechanisms which inhibit an expansion of the lung and thus require a more complex therapeutic approach. In the *organized phase (Phase III)*, fibroblast growth leads to an "entrapped lung" with fibrotic connections between lung, diaphragm, and the chest wall. This phase can progress to a spontaneous perforation and drainage of the pleural empyema through the chest wall *(empyema necessitatis)* or into the bronchial tree *(bronchopleural fistula)*.

The *"Light criteria"* are helpful to classify a patient according to clinical parameters such as radiographic signs (thickening of the pleura, loculations, etc.), biochemical markers (pH, LDH, glucose), and microbiological characteristics (Gram stain, positive culture) [11, 12]. This goes in line with the risk-stratifying classification of the *American College of Chest Physicians (ACCP),* which also focusses on these three diagnostic parameters, but emphasizes the importance of pH for the clinical and pathophysiological progress of pleural empyema [13]. Any increased bacterial metabolism inside the pleural cavity leads to a reduced pH and glucose concentration and increases the LDH content.

Table 1 The RAPID score including renal function, age of the patient, quality of the pleural fluid, source of infection and the nutritional/dietary status is an evaluation of the prognosis in the fibro-purulent phase of pleural empyema

Parameter	Measure	Score
Renal	Urea <5 mM	0
	Urea 5–8 mM	1
	Urea >8 mM	2
Age	<50 years	0
	50–70 years	1
	>70 years	2
Pleural fluid	Non-purulent	0
	Purulent	1
Infection source	Community-acquired	0
	Hospital-acquired	1
Dietary	Albumin >27 g/L	0
	Albumin <27 g/L	1
RAPID score	Mortality in % (MIST 1)	Hospital stay (days)
0–2	1	10
2–4	12	15
5–7	51	18

With permission Reichert M, Hecker M, Witte B, et al. (2017) Stage-directed therapy of pleural empyema. Langenbeck's Arch. Surg

Based on the results of the Multicenter Intrapleural Sepsis Trial (MIST 1), Rahman et al. published a scoring system with independent predictors for a poor outcome in the fibropurulent pleural empyema [14]. In this phase (according to ATS phase II), the RAPID (renal, age, purulence of the pleural fluid, infection source and dietary status) score could predict if the patient bears the risk for surgical intervention, increased mortality, and increased length of hospital stay (Table 1).

Treatment

Adequate modern therapy of a pleural empyema is an interdisciplinary challenge for internal medicine, surgery, and intensive care. Any delayed or inadequate therapy could lead to dramatically increased mortality and morbidity. At the onset of empyema, adequate antimicrobial therapy is the gold-standard treatment. According to the Tarragona strategy ("hit hard and early"), the broad-spectrum antibiotic is narrowed and adapted to the results of bacterial culture or alternative modern DNA-based methods [4, 15]. In case of HAP, the typical in-hospital spectrum of bacteria and their resistances should be included into the discussion and must lead to the involvement of an antibiotic steward. While in early phases, pleural effusions (Light class 1) should resolve with antibiotic therapy alone, more complicated effusions, which extend >10 mm up to 50% of the hemithorax (Light class 2, ACCP class 2), could require repetitive thoracocentesis [3, 11]. Additionally to an emptying of the pleural cavity, a permanent microbial and biochemical monitoring of the pleural fluid is recommended. If disease progresses (at least since Light class 4, ACCP 3), a chest tube insertion is standard care. Higher stages of pleural empyema are characterized by the formation of loculations and septae. Typically, if the empyema extends to more than 40% of the hemithorax or if Light class is ≥5, the multiloculated chambers either require the adjunctive application of fibrinolytics (e.g. streptokinase 250,000–500,000 IU/day for 3–7 days, or urokinase 80,000–100,000 IU/day for 3–5 days) to cleave fibrinous septations or should lead to surgical debridement. The potential effects of fibrinolysis inside the pleural cavity are controversially discussed in the literature [16–18]. While in the MIST 1, no differences were observed (intrapleural streptokinase vs. placebo) in complicated intrapleural infections, MIST2 could detect benefits of intrapleural fibrinolysis plus DNA-cleavage (tissue plasminogen activator t-PA plus DNase vs. placebo) [1]. Here, the effective concentrations were 5 mg DNase and 10 mg t-PA repetitive applied on 3 days twice daily (clamping the chest tube for 1 h after application). Local side effects such as hemorrhage, fever, and chest pain should be monitored carefully during application. While the effectiveness of medical or interventional treatment is critically discussed in the literature at that stage of progressive empyema, the video-assisted thoracoscopic surgery (VATS) approach allows a secure and rapid treatment of the fibropurulent pleural infection. As reported by Wait et al., minimally invasive breakdown of fibrinous septae and membranes, evacuation of the pleural cavity, and surgical decortication have been shown to be more effective and beneficial compared to catheter-directed fibrinolytic therapy (VATS vs. streptokinase) [19]. While the rapid VATS approach leads to decreased duration of chest tube drainage, length of hospital stay, and treatment costs, these positive effects disappear, if VATS is performed after intrapleural fibrinolysis failed. The scientific evidence led to the recent guideline recommendation of the European Association for Cardio-Thoracic Surgery (EACTS) that surgery is the method of choice for empyema ATS stages 2 and 3 [20], while the intrapleural fibrinolytic therapy is an optional alternative for fibropurulent empyemas (Fig. 2).

About one third of the patients suffering from pleural empyema require surgical drainage of the pleural cavity. Operation is indicated if the pleural drainage does not lead to an adequate re-expansion of the lung if sepsis persists despite medical therapy. Surgical therapy is based on three elements a) drainage of infected pleural fluid collections, b) debridement of fibrin deposits (ATS phase II), and c) decortication of a fibrotic cortex (ATS phase III). While the minimally invasive approach (VATS) is the gold standard for the fibropurulent pleural empyema, the evidence for its use in organized empyema is still weak. While open decortication of the visceral and parietal pleura is the standard approach, the increasing experience in the field of minimally invasive surgery led to multiple publications on the feasibility of VATS for phase III empyema as well. Potential beneficial effects of VATS are improved pulmonary function, quality of life, and decreased postoperative pain and length of hospital stay. The quality and efficiency of surgical pleural source control itself is comparable between VATS and open surgery in stage II and III empyema. Nevertheless, prospective randomized trials evaluating the two approaches are still missing. Typically, VATS is performed in an anterior (three-port) access as described

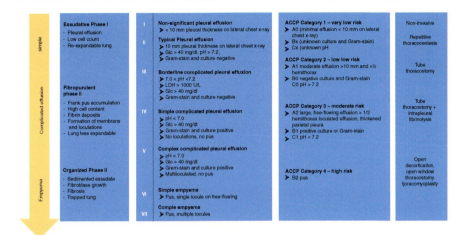

Fig. 2 For the development of a pleural empyema, a clinical progression is typical. This is reflected in the most common classifications, which allow a stratification of the patients into the different stages. In case of progression, these phases merge into each other. With permission Reichert M, Hecker M, Witte B, et al. (2017) Stage-directed therapy of pleural empyema. Langenbeck's Arch. Surg

in the literature. Although the minimally invasive approach is recommended both in stage II and III empyema, conversion to open surgery should be performed, if an inadequate decortication and lack of pulmonary re-expansion are observed during the VATS procedure. Typical, risk factors for conversion include delayed surgical intervention or lack of experience in minimally invasive surgery.

In cases of empyema, chest tube insertion followed by decortication should lead to adequate re-expansion and regeneration of the lung. Due to the chronic character of pleural empyema due to tuberculosis, it must be excluded as the causative agent.

One of the most challenging empyemas of the pleural cavity, the so-called post-pneumonectomy empyema, has a mortality rate of up to 40%, if it occurs within 3 months after surgery ("early post-pneumonectomy empyema"). Typically, the post-pneumonectomy empyema is associated with a broncho-pleural fistula, which has the typical risk factors: postoperative ventilation, right-sided pneumonectomy, wide resection, residual R1-resection, preoperative radiotherapy, and diabetes mellitus. Initial rapid drainage of the pleural cavity is lifesaving and mandatory to prevent the remaining contralateral lung from infection and aspiration of pus.

The so-called open-window thoracostomy followed by continuous drainage and lavage can be an effective surgical approach. Nevertheless, the closure of the bronchopleural fistula, covered by vital tissue such as major omentum (omentopexy) or muscular flaps (thoracomyoplasty, e.g., dorsal latissimus, major pectoralis muscle), provides permanent repair and a reinforcement of the bronchial stump. Clagett established the sequential three-stage procedure for this special type of pleural empyema; after the open-window thoracotomy, repetitive lavage and debridement of the thoracic cavity are followed by closure of the chest after irrigating the pleural cavity with antibiotic solution [21]. This technique was modified by Schneiter et al.; the debridement and lavage of the pleural cavity as well as the plastic reconstruction of the bronchial stump are performed as described above [22], then packing of the pleural cavity combined with chest tube insertion and negative pressure therapy is established. Every 48 h, the patients undergo a redo-thoracotomy with change of the packs. With a success rate of 97.3% and a 90-day mortality of 4%, this modified Clagett procedure has the best outcome for this complicated disease [23]. Modern vacuum-assisted closure (VAC) systems allow an open-window procedure with implantation of VAC sponges and optional instillation of antiseptic/antibiotic solutions for complex pleural empyema. Interestingly, literature reveals that the negative pressure therapy (up to −125 mmHg) does not increase the rate of parenchymal fistula or intrathoracic bleeding and thus is indicated also in cases of bronchopleural fistula. Based on the vacuum sealing, a reduction of the empyema cavity by granulation, angioneogenesis, and pulmonary re-expansion on one hand and an eradication of the pleural infection on the other hand leads to adequate results.

Pleural Effusion

Introduction

Acute care surgeons are frequently asked to evaluate patients with pleural effusions. The potential causes for effusions can be diverse, resulting from localized thoracic disease or as a manifestation of systemic disease. In the United States, the four most common causes of pleural effusion are congestive heart failure, bacterial pneumonia, malignancy, and pulmonary embolus [24]. Infectious causes within the pleural cavity have been previously discussed in this chapter; therefore, this portion of the chapter will focus on the pathophysiology, signs, symptoms, evaluation, and management of non-infected plural effusions.

Plural Space Physiology

There is some overlap between the infected and non-infected pathophysiologic process of pleural effusion; however, there are some significant differences worth noting. As noted previously, a 10-μm glycoprotein-rich fluid layer lies between the visceral and parietal pleural surfaces, and this constitutes the pleural space. The normal volume of plural fluid is approximately 0.1–0.2 mL/kg and mostly acellular. The blood supply to the parietal pleura is primarily from branches of the intercostal arteries. The visceral pleura derives its blood supply from the bronchial and pulmonary arterial systems. Lymphatic flow through the pleural space occurs from the lung parenchyma to the lymphatic channels (1–6 μm stomata) located on the visceral and parietal pleura [25].

In disease states, excess production of pleural fluid or decreased absorption is responsible for the generation of effusions. The pathologic processes causing fluid accumulation most often originate from the thoracic cavity but can be related to systemic fluid overload or extension of subdiaphragmatic disease as well. Examples of infradiaphragmatic pathology include cholecystitis, hepatic hydrothorax, and pancreatitis. The most common resulting symptom of pleural fluid accumulation is dyspnea and may be related to decreased tidal volume from mass effect, reduced diaphragmatic movement, or underlying cardiac and lung pathology.

Evaluation of Plural Effusion

Pleural effusions can be the result of a heterogenous group of processes, and the clinical scenario is helpful in determining the cause of the effusion. Signs or symptoms of infection, history malignancy, or associated medical diseases such as cardiac failure, kidney, or liver disease can be helpful in determining the underlying cause. The workup begins with a complete history and physical exam. A review of systems should elicit local symptoms such as pain, dyspnea, or cough and systemic findings such as fever or weight loss.

As was discussed with pleural empyema, chest radiographs and thoracic ultrasound are important diagnostic tools for the initial evaluation and management of effusions [6]. Significant effusions (200 mL) are generally seen on chest X-rays as blunting of the costophrenic angle. A lateral decubitus film can confirm the effusion to be free flowing and may be able to identify as little as 50 mL of fluid. Loculated effusions are difficult to diagnose from a standard chest radiograph. Ultrasound can be useful in detecting loculated fluid and may also determine an appropriate site for thoracentesis. Most often a computed axial tomography (CT) scan is indicated as useful in the evaluation of pleural effusions. The size and the location of the effusion can be determined, and the CT scan also gives information regarding associated underlying parenchymal and plural abnormalities.

Clinical judgment as a physician is highly protective of identifying clinical causes for transudative and exudative effusions. If the history, physical exam, and imaging studies result in a definitive clinical diagnosis, appropriate medical therapy is frequently effective and invasive diagnostic procedures are typically not necessary. If further workup is indicated, the first invasive modality should be thoracentesis. Due to its safety and efficacy, ultrasound is now recommended for guidance of thoracentesis for pleural effusion. The initial goal of plural fluid analysis is to distinguish between transudative effusions and exudative effusions. The most common etiologies of each type of effusion are listed in Table 2.

The visual appearance of the aspirated fluid can often confirm the clinical diagnosis of the effusion. Fluid with a white milky appearance indicates either a chylothorax or an empyema, food particles are diagnostic of an esophageal perforation, and blood may narrow the differential diagnosis to hemothorax or malignancy. Once aspirated, the plural fluid is sent for pleural chemistry, microbiologic analysis,

Table 2 Common pleural effusion etiologies

	Transudate	Exudate
Frequent	Heart failure	Malignancy
	Liver failure	Infection
		Parapneumonic
Less common	Renal failure	Pancreatitis
	Pulmonary embolus	Rheumatoid
		Autoimmune medications

as well as cytology. Light's criteria are used to determine whether the fluid is transudative or exudative. An exudate is defined by one of the following criteria: pleural fluid lactate dehydrogenase (LDH) level > 200 IU/L, pleural fluid LDH/serum LDH > 0.6, or a ratio of pleural fluid protein to serum protein >0.5 [10]. Other specific analysis can be run on the fluid if clinical suspicion warrants. Malignant cells on cytologic evaluation indicate an underlying malignancy causing the effusion. The specificity of cytologic analysis is high, but the sensitivity of a single evaluation can be as low as 50% [26]. If fluid analysis identifies an exudate and the diagnosis remains unclear, the next diagnostic maneuvers should be bronchoscopy and video-assisted thoracoscopy (VATS). During thoracoscopy, direct plural biopsy is performed and also therapeutic interventions, including evacuation of the effusion either with or without pleurodesis.

A transudative plural effusion indicates that the effusion is the result of a systemic pathologic process, separate from thoracic pathology. This transudative pleural effusion has a low protein content and is most often caused by a medical condition that leads to volume overload, such as renal failure, heart failure, and hypoalbuminemia. In the United States, a transudative effusion occurs most commonly secondary to congestive heart failure [27]. In contrast, exudative pleural effusions have a higher protein content and indicate a local plural process. As noted above, there are multiple causes for exudative effusions, but they are most commonly due to malignancy or infection. The distinction becomes important as the different etiologies necessitate different treatment approaches. Transudative effusions are generally managed by maximal medical therapy for the underlying disease.

Treatment

The management of pleural effusion is focused on relief of symptoms. Small and asymptomatic effusions with a clear etiology may only require observation. An example of this may be immediately following cardiac surgery. The majority of these resolve spontaneously without invasive therapy. The accurate diagnosis of the underlying disease is crucial to initiating the appropriate medical therapy. The majority of transudative effusions will improve, and many will completely resolve when treated with maximal medical therapy. For those patients with persistent small effusions but improved symptoms, observation without drainage may be appropriate. If the diagnosis remains unclear, then the effusion should be aspirated for diagnostic purposes [28].

Symptomatic or complicated pleural effusions should have early drainage of the plural fluid (Fig. 3). The two initial options for drainage are thoracentesis and tube thoracostomy. The choice of drainage is dependent on the viscosity of the plural fluid, location, volume, and general condition of the patient. The use of thoracentesis to aspirate fluid from the thorax can be used as a diagnostic or therapeutic maneuver. The removal of fluid should improve patient symptoms and the fluid sent for analysis as previously described. Potentially, a single therapeutic aspiration may be an appropriate option for long-term management. Slow fluid re-accumulation may require further aspirations, but this strategy of recurrent aspirations should be used with caution. There is a substantial cumulative risk of procedural complications and the introduction of infection. The amount of fluid aspirated at one time should be limited to 1.5 L or less. Aspirating more than this amount increases the risk of re-expansion pulmonary edema [29]. Acute chest pain is also an indication

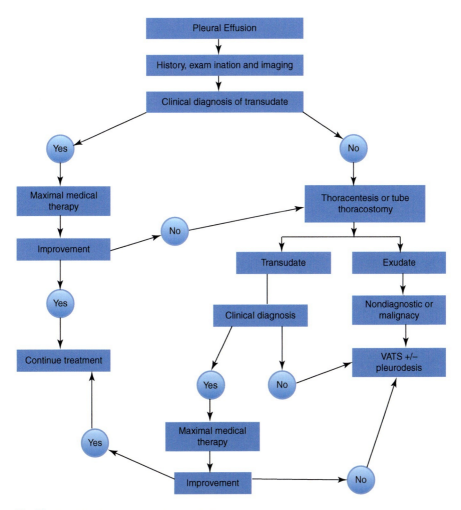

Fig. 3 Algorithm for treatment of pleural effusion

to stop drainage because this is a sign of lung entrapment [30]. An alternative initial drainage procedure for benign pleural effusions is the placement of a tube thoracostomy. Typically, a size 24–28 French chest tube should be placed in the posterior costophrenic recess. Cases refractory to initial therapy or thought to be secondary to malignancy will require further intervention such as pleurodesis with or without the addition of VATS. Thoracoscopy allows direct plural biopsy and also the potential for therapeutic intervention, including evacuation of the effusion either with or without the use of pleurodesis.

Pleurodesis is a treatment that obliterates the pleural space by creating fibrosis of the pleura. The therapeutic goal is to prevent the reaccumulation of effusion after drainage. For the procedure to be successful, the parietal and visceral pleura must be in contact. If the lung cannot fully expand after drainage, then sclerosis should not be attempted. Sclerosing agents must be instilled directly into the plural space to create pleurodesis. Many agents have been used in both malignant effusions and benign effusions. Multiple studies comparing different sclerosants have found that talc is the most effective agent [31–33]. Typically, 5 g of talc are installed into the plural space to induce sclerosis either as a suspension in 50–100 mL of normal saline through a chest tube or a via direct poudrage at thoracoscopy. Following the installation of sclerosant, the chest drain should be removed at 24 h. Early removal has been shown to shorten the duration of hospital stay without decreasing the efficacy of the pleurodesis [34].

The amount of effusion drainage prior to pleurodesis may impact the efficacy of the procedure. Thoracoscopy can typically evacuate more effusion than bedside thoracostomy. The ability to distribute the sclerosant over the pleural surface may also vary depending on the method used. A Cochrane review of thoracoscopic versus chest tube pleurodesis demonstrated an improved outcome using thoracoscopy, with a relative risk of non-recurrence of 1.19 (95% confidence interval, 1.04–1.36) [31]. Another large study of 611 patients reported on the outcomes of thoracoscopic talc pleurodesis. Radiographic improvement was seen in 68.6% and symptomatic improvement in 89.1% immediately after drainage. Sixty-eight percent of the patients in the study had benign a fusions and reported a success rate of 77% [35]. Although thoracoscopic drainage and pleurodesis appear to have superior outcome, the treatment of symptomatic pleural effusions should be individualized by a patient's functional status. Patients with poor functional status may have procedure-related morbidity and mortality related to thoracoscopy. The use of indwelling pleural catheters may be an option in this patient population. There is extensive evidence supporting the use of indwelling pleural catheters for the outpatient management of malignant pleural effusions but minimal evidence showing benefit in non-malignant effusions [36]. Further discussion of indwelling catheters is beyond the scope of this chapter.

References

1. Rahman NM, Maskell NA, West A, et al. Intrapleural use of tissue plasminogen activator and DNase in pleural infection. N Engl J Med. 2011;365(6):518–26. https://doi.org/10.1056/nejmoa1012740.

2. Nielsen J, Meyer CN, Rosenlund S. Outcome and clinical characteristics in pleural empyema: a retrospective study. Scand J Infect Dis. 2011;43(6–7):430–5. https://doi.org/10.3109/00365548.2011.562527.
3. Reichert M, Hecker M, Witte B, et al. Stage-directed therapy of pleural empyema. Langenbecks Arch Surg. 2017;402(1):15–26.
4. Roberts HSA, Davies RJO, Davies CWH, Gleeson FV. BTS guidelines for the management of pleural infection [2] (multiple letters). Thorax. 2004;59(2):178.
5. Chen KY, Hsueh PR, Liaw YS, et al. A 10-year experience with bacteriology of acute thoracic empyema: emphasis on Klebsiella pneumoniae in patients with diabetes mellitus. Chest. 2000;117(6):1685–9. https://doi.org/10.1378/chest.117.6.1685.
6. Ingelfinger JR, Feller-Kopman D, Light R. Pleural disease. N Engl J Med. 2018;378(8):740–51.
7. Sperandeo M, Filabozzi P, Varriale A, et al. Role of thoracic ultrasound in the assessment of pleural and pulmonary diseases. J Ultrasound. 2008; https://doi.org/10.1016/j.jus.2008.02.001.
8. Park CK, Oh HJ, Choi HY, et al. Microbiological characteristics and predictive factors for mortality in pleural infection: a single-center cohort study in Korea. PLoS One. 2016;11(8):e0161280. https://doi.org/10.1371/journal.pone.0161280.
9. Bedawi EO, Hassan M, Rahman NM. Recent developments in the management of pleural infection: a comprehensive review. Clin Respir J. 2018;12(8):2309–20.
10. Maskell NA, Batt S, Hedley EL, et al. The bacteriology of pleural infection by genetic and standard methods and its mortality significance. Am J Respir Crit Care Med. 2006;174(7):817–23. https://doi.org/10.1164/rccm.200601-074OC.
11. Light RW. A new classification of parapneumonic effusions and empyema. Chest. 1995;108(2):299–301. https://doi.org/10.1378/chest.108.2.299.
12. Muers M. Streptokinase for empyema. Lancet. 2005;349(9064):1491–2. https://doi.org/10.1016/s0140-6736(05)62094-6.
13. Colice GL, Curtis A, Deslauriers J, et al. Medical and surgical treatment of parapneumonic effusions: an evidence-based guideline. Chest. 2000;118(4):1158–71. https://doi.org/10.1378/chest.118.4.1158.
14. Rahman NM, Kahan BC, Miller RF, et al. A clinical score (RAPID) to identify those at risk for poor outcome at presentation in patients with pleural infection. Chest. 2014;145(4):848–55. https://doi.org/10.1378/chest.13-1558.
15. Hecker A, Uhle F, Schwandner T, et al. Diagnostics, therapy and outcome prediction in abdominal sepsis: current standards and future perspectives. Langenbeck's Arch Surg. 2014;399:11–22.
16. Cameron R, Davies HR. Intra-pleural fibrinolytic therapy versus conservative management in the treatment of adult parapneumonic effusions and empyema. Cochrane Database Syst Rev. 2008;(2):CD002312.
17. Tokuda Y, Matsushima D, Stein GH, Miyagi S. Intrapleural fibrinolytic agents for empyema and complicated parapneumonic effusions: a meta-analysis. Chest. 2006;129(3):783–90. https://doi.org/10.1378/chest.129.3.783.
18. Nie W, Liu Y, Ye J, et al. Efficacy of intrapleural instillation of fibrinolytics for treating pleural empyema and parapneumonic effusion: a meta-analysis of randomized control trials. Clin Respir J. 2014;8(3):281–91. https://doi.org/10.1111/crj.12068.
19. Wait MA, Sharma S, Hohn J, Dal Nogare A. A randomized trial of empyema therapy. Chest. 1997;111(6):1548–51. https://doi.org/10.1378/chest.111.6.1548.
20. Scarci M, Abah U, Solli P, et al. EACTS expert consensus statement for surgical management of pleural empyema. Eur J Cardiothorac Surg. 2015;48(5):642–53. https://doi.org/10.1093/ejcts/ezv272.
21. Clagett OT, Geraci JE. A procedure for the management of postpneumonectomy empyema. J Thorac Cardiovasc Surg. 1963;45:141–5.
22. Schneiter D, Grodzki T, Lardinois D, et al. Accelerated treatment of postpneumonectomy empyema: a binational long-term study. J Thorac Cardiovasc Surg. 2008;136(1):179–85. https://doi.org/10.1016/j.jtcvs.2008.01.036.

23. Zaheer S, Allen MS, Cassivi SD, et al. Postpneumonectomy empyema: results after the Clagett procedure. Ann Thorac Surg. 2006;82(1):279–86. https://doi.org/10.1016/j.athoracsur.2006.01.052.
24. Rusch VW. Pleural effusions: benign and malignant. In: Patterson GA, Cooper JD, Deslauriers J, et al., editors. Pearson's thoracic and esophagial surgery. 3rd ed. Philadelphia: Churchill Livingston; 2008. p. 1042–54. (Chapter 85).
25. Wang NS. Anatomy of the pleura. Clin Chest Med. 1998;19(2):229–40. https://doi.org/10.1016/S0272-5231(05)70074-5.
26. Heffner J, Klein J. Recent advances in the diagnosis and management of malignant pleural effusions. Mayo Clin Proc. 2008;83(2):235–50. https://doi.org/10.4065/83.2.235.
27. Kataoka H. Pericardial and pleural effusions in decompensated chronic heart failure. Am Heart J. 2000;139(5):918–23. https://doi.org/10.1016/S0002-8703(00)90026-7.
28. Gonlugur TF, Gonlugur U. Transudated in malignancy: still a role for pleural fluid. Ann Acad Med Singap. 2008;37:760–3.
29. Roberts M, Neville E, Berrisford R, et al. Management of a malignant pleural effusion: British Thoracic Society pleural disease guideline 2010. Thorax. 2010;65(Suppl 2):ii32–40. https://doi.org/10.1136/thx.2010.136994.
30. Huggins JT, Sahn SA, Heidecker J, et al. Characteristics of trapped lung: pleural fluid analysis, manometry, and air-contrast chest CT. Chest. 2007;131(1):206–13. https://doi.org/10.1378/chest.06-0430.
31. Shaw P, Agarwal. Pleurodesis for malignant pleural effusions. Cochrane Database Syst Rev. 2009;(1):CD002916. https://doi.org/10.1002/14651858.CD0002916.pub2.
32. Tan C, Sedrakyan A, Browne J, et al. The evidence on the effectiveness of management for malignant pleural effusions: a systematic review. Eur Cardiothorac Surg. 2006;29(5):829–38. https://doi.org/10.1016/j.ejcts.2005.12.025.
33. Glazer M, Berkman N, Lafair JS, et al. Successful talc slurry pleurodesis in patients with nonmalignant pleural effusion. Chest. 2000;117(5):1404–9. https://doi.org/10.1378/chest.117.5.1404.
34. Goodman A, Davies C. Efficacy of short-term versus long-term chest tube drainage following talc slurry pleurodesis in patients with malignant pleural effusions: a randomized trial. Lung Cancer. 2006;54(1):51–5. https://doi.org/10.1016/j.lungcan.2006.06.004.
35. Steger V, Mika U, Toomes H, et al. Who gains most? A 10-year experience with 611 thoracoscopic talc pleurodeses. Ann Thorac Surg. 2007;83:1940–5.
36. Wilshire C, Gilbert C, Asciak R, et al. Multicenter review of tunneled pleural catheter implementation and use in patients with malignant pleural effusions. Chest. 2018;154(4):523A–4A. https://doi.org/10.1016/j.chest.2018.08.473.

Pericarditis and Pericardial Effusions

Ho H. Phan, Amanda Phares, Gustavo P. Fraga,
and Lindemberg M. Silveira-Filho

Acute Pericarditis

Epidemiology

Pericarditis is the most common disease of the pericardium worldwide. It most commonly affects young adults and middle aged people. The actual incidence of pericarditis is unknown as many cases are mild and resolve without a diagnosis. A few population-based studies in Europe and North America estimate the incidence of pericarditis to range from 3.32 to 27.7 cases per 100,000 person-years [1–3]. The incidence of pericarditis among hospitalized patients is 1.5–2 times more common in men than women. While the highest incidence is in young adults, in-hospital mortality is highest in the elderly population.

H. H. Phan (✉)
Trauma and Acute Care Surgery, Department of Surgery, University of California, Davis, Sacramento, CA, USA
e-mail: hhphan@ucdavis.edu

A. Phares
Department of Surgery, University of California Davis, Sacramento, CA, USA
e-mail: anphares@ucdavis.edu

G. P. Fraga
Department of Surgery, Division of Trauma Surgery, School of Medical Sciences (SMS), University of Campinas (Unicamp), Campinas, São Paulo, Brazil

L. M. Silveira-Filho
Cardiovascular Surgery Unit, Department of Surgery, School of Medical Sciences, State University of Campinas, Campinas, São Paulo, Brazil
e-mail: lmsf@fcm.unicamp.br

© Springer Nature Switzerland AG 2021
J. M. Galante, R. Coimbra (eds.), *Thoracic Surgery for the Acute Care Surgeon*,
Hot Topics in Acute Care Surgery and Trauma,
https://doi.org/10.1007/978-3-030-48493-4_6

Etiology

Acute pericarditis is characterized by polymorphonuclear infiltration, increase in vascularity, and formation of fibrous pericardial adhesions. The pathogenesis of acute pericarditis is still unclear, but more data are suggesting an immune-mediated process.

In developed countries, 80% of the cases of acute pericarditis are determined to be idiopathic [4, 5]. Most of these cases are presumed to be due to a viral etiology. Tuberculosis is still a common cause of acute pericarditis worldwide due to its high prevalence in developing countries. Pericarditis can present with either infectious or non-infectious etiologies. Infectious etiologies include viral, bacterial, fungal, and parasitic. Non-infectious etiologies include neoplasms (most commonly lung, breast, lymphoma, mesothelioma), autoimmune diseases, pericardial injury syndromes (trauma, radiation, post-pericardiotomy syndrome, transmural myocardial infarction), metabolic syndromes (uremia, myxedema, anorexia nervosa), and drugs (particularly hydralazine and procainamide).

Clinical Presentation and Diagnosis

According to the European Society of Cardiology (ESC) guidelines, acute pericarditis is diagnosed when two out of the following four clinical features are present: pericardial chest pain, pericardial rub on clinical examination, characteristic EKG changes, and new or worsening pericardial effusion on echocardiography [6, 7]. According to ESC, incessant pericarditis is defined as pericarditis lasting for more than 4–6 weeks but less than 3 months without remission. Recurrent pericarditis is when pericarditis occurs after a documented first episode of acute pericarditis and a symptom-free interval of 4–6 weeks or longer. Chronic pericarditis is defined as pericarditis lasting more than 3 months.

The most common symptom of pericarditis is the substernal chest pain that may radiate to the left shoulder, arm, and/or jaw. This chest pain often worsens with inspiration, coughing, or lying supine, and may improve with sitting up and leaning forward. This characteristic chest pain is present in 90% of the cases and may have other associated symptoms such as fever, chills, dyspnea, and weakness. The pericardial rub, generally heard best over the left sternal border, louder at inspiration and leaning forward, is highly specific for acute pericarditis. However, it is present in only 1/3 of the cases. Electrocardiographic (EKG) changes, typically widespread ST-segment elevation or PR interval depression, are present in about 60% of patients. These characteristic findings are more common in younger patients and are associated with concomitant myocarditis [5]. As EKG changes naturally evolve throughout the course of pericarditis, the presence of characteristic of EKG findings depends on the timing of diagnosis along the course of disease. Early in the disease course, PR depression or ST elevation may be present. Later in the disease course and in chronic pericarditis, T-wave inversion may be present. In patients who respond rapidly to treatment, there may not be any EKG changes. Thus, the absence of EKG changes does not exclude the diagnosis of pericarditis. Pericardial effusions can be seen on echocardiography in approximately 60% of the cases. Most of the effusions are small or moderate. The presence of large effusions (>20 mm) is a poor prognostic indicator. Because of the similarity in clinical presentation, pericarditis should always be a differential diagnosis in patients being evaluated for acute coronary syndromes.

Other markers of inflammation such as C-reactive protein (CRP) and white blood count (WBC) can also be used as supporting evidence and to follow response to therapy. White blood count is only modestly elevated in patients with idiopathic pericarditis. Highly elevated WBC suggests infectious etiology. C-reactive protein is elevated in about 75% of patients with acute pericarditis and normalizes 1–2 weeks later. Thus, its level is useful for treatment response follow-up [8]. Approximately 30% of patients have concomitant myocarditis, thus assessing markers of myocardial injury such as troponin or creatine kinase is recommended [7]. Although chest X-ray is usually normal in patients with pericarditis, it is routinely recommended to evaluate for pleural involvement. In patients with large pericardial effusions, an enlarged cardiac silhouette on chest X-ray can be seen.

In cases where pericarditis is suspected but not confirmed, cardiac computed tomography (CT) and cardiac magnetic resonance imaging (CMR) might be useful in supporting the diagnosis of pericarditis. The presence of pericardial thickening, contrast-enhanced pericardium on CT, or enhanced pericardial gadolinium uptake on CMR supports the diagnosis of pericarditis. Besides their supportive role, CT and CMR are also useful in evaluating neoplastic disease, congenital abnormality, and calcification in constrictive pericarditis.

Biochemical and cell-count analyses of pericardial fluid do not bring useful information in the majority of patients diagnosed with acute pericarditis. If purulent, tuberculosis, or neoplastic etiologies are suspected, pericardiocentesis should be done and pericardial fluid sent for cell count, biochemical analysis, cytology, culture, and molecular analysis (polymerase chain reaction).

The majority of cases are idiopathic or viral in nature. Specific clinical features may be present at the time of diagnosis that would increase the likelihood of having an etiology other than viral or idiopathic. These predictors are fever >38 °C, subacute onset (symptoms over several days without a clear-cut acute onset), large pericardial effusion (>20 mm on echocardiography), cardiac tamponade, and failure to respond to non-steroidal anti-inflammatory medications within 7 days [7, 9]. These features also increase the likelihood of subsequent complications (recurrence, tamponade, constriction).

Management

Post-Cardiac Injury Syndrome

Post-cardiac injury syndromes (PCIS) are syndromes that include post-traumatic pericarditis, post-myocardial infarction pericarditis, and post-pericardiotomy syndrome (after cardiac surgery). The pathogenesis of PCIS is thought to be an immune-mediated reaction against the injured pericardium. PCIS usually manifests 2–4 weeks after the initial injury. In addition to the typical signs and symptoms of pericarditis, systemic inflammatory indicators such as fever and elevated CRP are also present. Concomitant pleural involvement (pleuritis and pleural effusions) is also common. It is sometimes difficult to differentiate PCIS from post-operative pericardial or pleural effusions. The demonstration of inflammation is critical in differentiating PCIS from post-operative effusions. The main treatment for PCIS is anti-inflammatory therapy (NSAIDs +colchicine).

It is important to differentiate the post-pericardiotomy syndrome from post-operative pericardial effusion after cardiac surgery, as this has treatment implications. Post-operative pericardial effusions are very common after cardiac surgery, and they usually disappear after 7–10 days. Many patients are asymptomatic and NSAIDs' treatment is not indicated as they are ineffective and may be associated with an increased risk of side effects. A small number of patients with large post-operative pericardial effusions may progress to cardiac tamponade and may need pericardial drainage.

Idiopathic, Viral and Immune-Mediated Acute Pericarditis

The treatment for acute pericarditis is non-steroidal anti-inflammatory drugs (NSAIDs). The most common agents used are aspirin, ibuprofen, and indomethacin. The 2015 ESC guidelines provide an outline of recommended dose schedules for these commonly used NSAIDs [7]. Although there is no randomized control trial that would guide the duration of therapy, most experts recommend that NSAID treatment should be maintained until resolution of symptoms and normalization of C-reactive protein [7]. This usually takes 7–10 days, after which tapering of the medications should be considered. To date, there is no randomized controlled trial comparing the efficacy of different NSAIDs used. Proton pump inhibitor during NSAID treatment is recommended for gastric protection [4].

There are strong data to support the use of colchicine in combination with NSAIDs for the treatment of acute pericarditis. The combination of colchicine with NSAIDs has been shown to reduce treatment failure and recurrence compared to treatment with NSAIDs alone [10, 11]. Colchicine is given at the weight-adjusted dose for the duration of 3 months. A loading dose for colchicine is not necessary and should be avoided to minimize adverse events. The most common side effect associated with colchicine is gastrointestinal intolerance, which is reported in up to 10% of patients. Tapering of colchicine is not required but can be considered.

Corticosteroids are recommended as a second-line treatment for patients who have contraindications to NSAIDs or have failed combined therapy with NSAIDs and colchicine as long as infectious etiologies have been excluded. Corticosteroids should be considered as the initial treatment for patients with connective tissue or immune-mediated disorders as etiology for pericarditis. If corticosteroids are considered, they should be given in low to moderate doses (Prednisone 0.2–0.5 mg/kg/day or equivalent) rather than high doses (1.0 mg/kg/day or equivalent) as high doses are associated with higher rate of recurrences and adverse events [7]. Corticosteroids should be continued until resolution of symptoms and normalization of C-reactive protein, after which it can be slowly tapered.

Recurrent Pericarditis

Twenty to 30% of patients treated for acute pericarditis will have recurrent or chronic pericarditis. Treatment of these patients should be targeted at the underlying etiology if there is an identifiable cause (see below). The first-line treatment for recurrent disease remains anti-inflammatory therapy. NSAIDs and colchicine at the dosage used for the initial therapy should be reinstituted. If only NSAIDs were used at the initial episode, then colchicine should be added for the recurrent episode as it has been shown to reduce future recurrence and evolution into chronic disease. Most patients with recurrent disease will have a good response with combination of NSAIDs and colchicine treatment. If the patients have multiple recurrences, the treatment should be maintained as long as the therapy is still effective and the symptoms are not too disabling. If patients no longer have a good response to NSAIDs and colchicine or have disabling symptoms, low-dose corticosteroids can be added. For patients who do not respond to combination treatment and/or corticosteroid treatment, alternative therapies such as azathioprine, intravenous immunoglobulins, and biologic agents (IL-1R inhibitor Anakinra) have been proposed [4].

For patients who present with recurrent refractory disease and no response to any medical therapy, pericardiectomy can be considered as a last treatment option. To date, pericardiectomy as a treatment option for persistent relapsing pericarditis is supported only by retrospective series [12–14]. In the series reported by Khandaker et al., patients with relapsing pericarditis who underwent pericardiectomy were found to have markedly lower relapses compared to patients continuing with medical treatment at 5-year follow-up [13].

Uremic Pericarditis

Pericardial manifestations of end-stage renal failure are pericarditis and chronic pericardial effusion. Uremic pericarditis frequently begins before renal replacement therapy. Up to 30% of patients do not have chest pain, and EKG findings are absent in most patients. The pathogenesis of uremic pericarditis may be related to retention of toxic metabolites and fluid overload. The preferred treatment is dialysis, either peritoneal or hemodialysis. Patients with uremic pericarditis respond rapidly to dialysis, and the majority of the patients will have resolution of chest pain and pericardial effusion [15]. As the pericardial effusions are often hemorrhagic, systemic anticoagulation should be avoided to prevent bleeding into the pericardial space. Some patients with renal failure may develop pericarditis after initiation of dialysis, even with normal BUN and creatinine levels. This condition is called dialysis-associated pericarditis. Increasing the intensity of dialysis in these patients will result in resolution of pericarditis within a couple of weeks. The development of tamponade is a concern, and these patients should undergo careful hemodynamic and echocardiographic monitoring during intensive dialysis. Pericardiocentesis and pericardial drainage are indicated in patients with tamponade or impending tamponade. Anti-inflammatory therapy particularly with indomethacin has been tried with limited success. Indomethacin has been shown to reduce fever without changing the course of pericardial inflammation or effusion [16]. High-dose corticosteroids may be beneficial, but their use is limited due to high risk of recurrence and side effects. In patients who have large effusions or who do not respond to dialysis, pericardiotomy for drainage may be considered, even in the absence of tamponade physiology. Intrapericardial treatment with triamcinolone hexacetonide (50 mg every 6 h for 3 days) can be effective in resolving effusions [17]. In patients with recurrent disease or with constrictive pericarditis, pericardiectomy may be required.

Purulent Pericarditis

Purulent pericarditis is caused by bacterial contamination of the pericardial space after cardiac/thoracic surgery through hematogenous spread or by direct extension of intrathoracic and subdiaphragmatic infections (Fig. 1). It is rare nowadays and is more common in immunosuppressed patients. The most common causative organism is *Staphylococcus aureus*. Other common organisms include *Streptococcus pneumonia*, *Haemophilus influenza*, gram-negative bacteria, and *Candida species*. Clinical features typical of pericarditis are usually present in addition to fever (in virtually all patients) and leukocytosis (in most patients). Accumulation of pus in the pericardial sac can lead to tamponade, and pericardiocentesis helps establish the diagnosis along with pericardial fluid culture. A low pericardial-to-serum glucose ratio and elevated pericardial fluid WBC help differentiate purulent from tuberculous or neoplastic pericarditis.

The treatment for purulent pericarditis involves targeted antibiotic therapy and drainage of the pericardial sac. Drainage of the pericardial sac can be achieved by repeated pericardiocentesis, but thick fluid may drain poorly resulting in loculation of the pericardial space. Better drainage can be achieved by subxiphoid pericardiotomy with placement of drainage catheter. The pericardial catheter can also be used for irrigation and/or for instillation of fibrinolytic therapy. Intrapericardial fibrinolysis therapy has been proposed as an alternative to pericardiectomy [18].

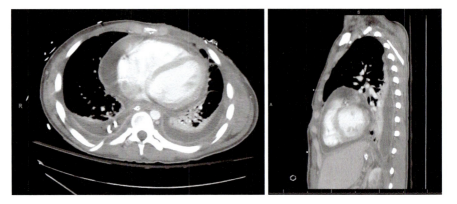

Fig. 1 Purulent pericarditis and bilateraly empyema in a patient who underwent resuscitative thoracotomy, pericardiotomy, repair of left hemidiaphragm, and bowel resection associated with blunt trauma. Microbiological studies revealed *Staphylococcus* and *Candida* species

If drainage is insufficient, infection is persistent or constriction develops, pericardiectomy may be required. Purulent pericarditis is a far more severe disease than other types of pericarditis and frequently demands early, aggressive treatment with pericardiotomy for drainage to avoid complications. Prognosis for purulent pericarditis is poor with reported mortality rate between 20 and 30%.

Tuberculous Pericarditis

Tuberculous pericarditis is rare in the United States due to the low prevalence of tuberculosis but remains the leading cause of pericarditis where tuberculosis is endemic. Pericardial infection may occur via hematogenous spread or via direct extension from lung, bronchial tree, pleura, or adjacent lymph nodes. Tuberculous pericarditis can present in three stages: acute, subacute, and chronic. In the acute phase, serosanguineous effusion and lymphocytic infiltration are present. Protein concentration is high, and tubercle bacilli concentration is low. As the bacilli concentration is low in this phase, the tuberculosis etiology is seldom confirmed. In the subacute phase, granulomatous inflammation with or without caseation and pericardial thickening are present. The chronic stage is characterized by fibrosis, calcification, and constriction.

Clinical presentation varies depending on the phase at diagnosis. The onset of disease may be abrupt, resembling idiopathic pericarditis, or insidious, resembling congestive heart failure. The latter is more common. Pericardiocentesis is recommended for routine evaluation of suspected tuberculous pericarditis. In cases where pericardial fluid analysis is uncertain, pericardial biopsy may be required. In general, the diagnosis of tuberculous pericarditis is established by the detection of tubercle bacilli in smear, culture, or PCR analysis of pericardial fluid and/or detection of tubercle bacilli or caseating granulomas on histological examination of the pericardium. Pericardial fluid high in protein content, increase in leukocyte count with predominance of lymphocyte, elevated adenosine deaminase level, or elevated interferon-gamma level is highly suggestive of tuberculous pericarditis.

The primary treatment for tuberculous pericarditis is multidrug antibiotic treatment, same as the regimen used for pulmonary tuberculosis. The regimen usually consists of rifampin, isoniazid, pyrazinamide, and ethambutol for 2 months followed by isoniazid and rifampin, for a total of 6 months of therapy. Improvement of symptoms is expected within 2–3 weeks of treatment. Adjuvant corticosteroid therapy in patients with tuberculous pericarditis may reduce the incidence of constrictive pericarditis and possibly reduce the need for pericardiectomy [19]. However, the risk of Kaposi sarcoma may increase with use of adjuvant corticosteroid in patients with concomitant HIV infections [20]. In patients with chronic constrictive pericarditis, pericardiectomy may be the only treatment.

Without effective tuberculosis treatment, up to 50% of patients with tuberculous pericarditis will progress to constriction. Timely and effective anti-tuberculosis chemotherapy is the key to reducing the risk of constriction.

Pericardial Neoplasms

Primary pericardial neoplasms are very rare. The most common malignant primary tumor of the pericardium is mesothelioma. It is usually a diffuse disease, encasing the heart and invading the myocardium leading to constriction. Benign tumors of the pericardium include teratoma, lipomas, and fibromas. Benign tumors are not invasive or infiltrative, but they can cause compressive symptoms. Metastatic pericardial neoplasms are more common than primary neoplasms. The most common metastatic malignant tumors of the pericardium are lung cancer, breast cancer, melanoma, lymphomas, and leukemias. Patients with documented malignancy who develop pericardial effusion should raise suspicion for pericardial tumor involvement. However, it is important to note that, in 2/3 of these patients, the pericardial effusions are caused by non-neoplastic etiologies [7]. Imaging studies such as CT, CMR, and PET may be helpful in revealing pericardial tumor involvement. Pericardial fluid analysis and pericardial biopsies are necessary for confirmation of malignant pericardial disease.

The primary treatment for pericardial neoplasms should be directed at the underlying malignancy. Patients with symptomatic effusions or tamponade should undergo pericardial drainage. Reaccumulation of effusions can occur up to 60% of patients. In most of these patients, pericardial and cardiac tumor involvement indicates advanced disease, and management should focus on palliation. Intrapericardial treatment with chemotherapeutic agents (cisplatin for lung cancer, thiotepa for breast cancer) and sclerosing agents (tetracyclines) may reduce recurrences. In patients with radiosensitive tumors such as lymphomas and leukemias, radiation treatment can be effective in controlling malignant pericardial effusions. However, radiation can also cause pericardial and myocardial damage. To reduce reaccumulation of malignant effusions, pericardial windows to allow drainage into the peritoneal or pleural cavity can be created. This option should be considered in advanced neoplastic disease patients with poor prognosis as palliative treatment.

Prognosis

The overall prognosis is very good for patients with idiopathic pericarditis. Approximately 70–80% of patients will be successfully treated with complete resolution during the initial episode. In about 20–30% of patients, incessant or recurrent pericarditis may develop [5]. Cardiac tamponade is rare in idiopathic pericarditis, and it generally occurs at the beginning of the disease process. Constrictive pericarditis as a sequela of viral/idiopathic pericarditis is exceedingly rare (<1%), even in patients with repeated recurrences [7]. In patients diagnosed with specific etiologies, the risk for development of constrictive pericarditis is much higher. The risk of constrictive pericarditis is 3–4% in patients with autoimmune disease and neoplasms, while the risk is as high as 20–35% in patients with tuberculous or purulent pericarditis [8].

Constrictive Pericarditis

Constrictive pericarditis is a condition caused by a reduction in elasticity of the pericardium due to scarring from an inflammatory or infectious process. This loss of elasticity leads to limitations in cardiac filling and cardiac function. Physiologic changes associated with constrictive pericarditis include enhanced ventricular interdependence, early rapid diastolic filling, and reductions in ventricular volumes and stroke volume. Patients usually present with symptoms of right heart failure. Diagnosis is based on signs and symptoms along with characteristic findings on echocardiography, computed tomography, cardiac magnetic resonance, and/or cardiac angiography. Transient forms may be effectively treated using anti-inflammatory medications. The only effective treatment for chronic constrictive pericarditis is pericardiectomy.

Etiology

Constrictive pericarditis can result from a variety of pericardial disorders including viral and bacterial pericarditis and can occur following cardiac surgery or radiation treatment [7]. In a prospective trial in Israel and Italy, 500 patients with acute pericarditis were followed and, overall, less than 2% developed constrictive pericarditis. Only 0.5% of patients with idiopathic or viral pericarditis progressed to constrictive pericarditis, while 3% of patients with connective tissue diseases, 4% of patients with neoplastic processes, 20% of patients with tuberculosis, and 33% of patients with purulent pericarditis progressed to constrictive pericarditis [21]. The time between the predisposing condition and developing constrictive pericarditis is variable. The primary causes differ between developed and developing countries. In developed countries, the most common causes are idiopathic or viral, post-cardiac surgery, and post-radiation therapy. In developing countries, infectious causes are more common with the major cause being tuberculosis [7, 22].

Clinical Presentation and Diagnosis

The most common symptoms of constrictive pericarditis are those of right heart failure such as peripheral edema and hepatomegaly, fluid overload, and dyspnea on exertion. Physical examination findings associated with constrictive pericarditis are elevated jugular venous distension (JVD), pulsus paradoxus, Kussmaul's sign, and a pericardial knock. JVD is the most common physical finding (90% of patients) followed by pericardial knock (50%). Pulsus paradoxus and Kussmaul's sign are uncommon. A pericardial knock is an additional heart sound heard during early diastole. It is usually heard best in the left sternal border and is a result of sudden cessation of ventricular filling. Pulses paradoxus is defined as a decrease in systolic blood pressure more than 10 mmHg with inspiration. It is related to a compensatory decrease in left ventricular volume in response to an increase in right ventricular volume during inspiration. This is a result of enhanced ventricular interdependence from having a fixed overall cardiac volume. Kussmaul's sign is referred to the loss of inspiratory decline in JVD caused by increased atrial pressures. Frequently, patients present with other associated systemic physical findings, especially peripheral edema, ascites, hepatomegaly, and cachexia [22, 23]. Occasionally, patients with idiopathic constrictive pericarditis are referred for diagnosis from gastroenterologists, as the hepatic decompensation may be the first notable sign that prompts investigation.

Constrictive pericarditis is diagnosed by the presenting symptoms of right heart failure and evidence of impaired diastolic filling due to pericardial constriction. Patients presenting with signs and symptoms of constrictive pericarditis should undergo electrocardiography, chest X-ray, and echocardiography [7]. EKG findings seen in constrictive pericarditis include non-specific ST and T wave changes, tachycardia, low voltage, and atrial fibrillation (late sign due to atrial distension) (see Fig. 2) [7, 23]. These EKG findings are seen in 20–40% of patients, and none of them are specific to constrictive pericarditis. Chest X-ray may reveal a ring of calcification around the heart in about 1/3 of patients [7]. This finding is fairly specific for constrictive pericarditis. Echocardiography can identify increased pericardial thickness, bilateral atrial enlargement, and dilated inferior vena cava and hepatic veins. Echocardiographic findings that favor constriction physiology include the characteristic ventricular septal motion abnormality, respiratory variation in mitral inflow velocity, respiratory variation in pulmonary venous flow velocity, preserved or increased mitral annulus velocity, and hepatic vein flow reversal that is more prominent during expiration [7]. The characteristic septal motion abnormality seen in constriction is generally referred to as "septal bounce".

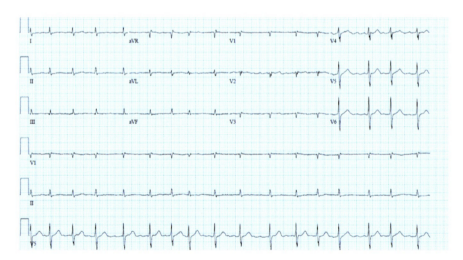

Fig. 2 Electrocardiographic findings of low electrical voltage and atrial fibrillation in a patient with constrictive pericarditis

It is the paradoxical motion of the interventricular septum that deviates toward and then away from the left ventricle during diastole. This is a sign of enhanced ventricular interdependence.

If initial workup is suggestive but not diagnostic for constrictive pericarditis, additional imaging using CT or CMR is recommended. CT findings associated with constrictive pericarditis include increased pericardial thickness, pericardial calcification, bilateral atrial dilation, abnormal shape of the interventricular septum, and dilation of the inferior vena cava (IVC) (see Fig. 3). Sometimes, reversal of contrast flow can be seen in hepatic veins or vena cava. CMR findings include increased pericardial thickness, increased ventricular interdependence, and dilation of the IVC. In addition to their role in supporting the diagnosis, CT and CMR are also very useful for operative planning.

If CT and CMR do not confirm the diagnosis of constrictive pericarditis, cardiac angiography may be needed. Cardiac angiography provides hemodynamic information that can aid in the diagnosis. The key findings seen in cardiac angiography are elevation and equalization of end-diastolic pressures in all chambers, increased right atrial pressure with associated prominent X and Y descents, early diastolic dip followed by a high diastolic plateau (square root sign) on right and left ventricular pressure curves, and enhanced ventricular interdependence seen as mirror-image discordance in systolic pressures between the right and left ventricles during inspiration [7].

The signs and symptoms of constrictive pericarditis overlap with other cardiac disorders, mainly restrictive cardiomyopathy and cardiac tamponade. Medical history is key to differentiating between constrictive pericarditis and restrictive cardiomyopathy as the predisposing conditions are very different between the two. Poor

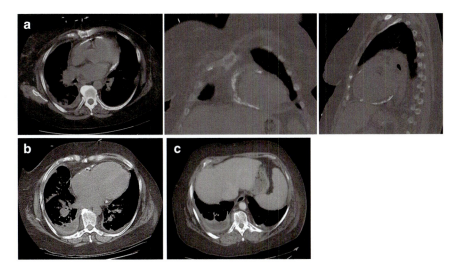

Fig. 3 Computed Tomography showing pericardial calcification (**a**), bilateral atrial enlargement (**b**), and dilation of the inferior vena cava (**c**) in a patient with constrictive pericarditis

Table 1 Diagnosis of constrictive pericarditis and cardiac tamponade

	Constrictive pericarditis	Cardiac tamponade
Presentation	Peripheral edema, hepatomegaly, dyspnea on exertion	Fatigue, dyspnea, syncope, shock
Physical exam	Jugular venous distension, pulses paradoxus, Kussmaul's sign, precordial knock	Tachycardia, hypotension, jugular venous distension, distant heart sounds, pulses paradoxus
EKG	Tachycardia, low voltage, non-specific ST changes, atrial fibrillation	Tachycardia, low voltage, electrical alternans
Chest X-ray	Pericardial calcifications	Normal or enlarged cardiac silhouette
Echocardiogram	Pericardial thickening, bilateral atrial enlargement, dilated IVC and hepatic veins, septal motion abnormality, respiratory variation in mitral inflow velocity and pulmonary venous flow velocity	Pericardial effusion, early diastolic collapse of right ventricle, late diastolic collapse of right and left atria, respiratory variation with mitral and tricuspid flow velocities
CT/MR	Pericardial thickening, pericardial calcifications, bilateral atrial dilation, dilated IVC	Pericardial effusion
Cardiac angiography	Elevation and equalization of end-diastolic pressures in all chambers, increased right atrial pressure, enhanced ventricular interdependence	Elevation and equalization of diastolic pressures in all chambers

filling in restrictive cardiomyopathy is caused by myocardial stiffness leading to poor relaxation and compliance, whereas myocardial relaxation is normal in constrictive pericarditis. On imaging, pericardial thickening supports a diagnosis of constrictive pericarditis, while myocardial thickening supports a diagnosis of restrictive cardiomyopathy. In constrictive pericarditis, the right and left ventricular end-diastolic pressures are equal, while the left ventricular end-diastolic pressure is greater than the right in restrictive cardiomyopathy [7]. The diagnosis of constrictive pericarditis as compared to cardiac tamponade is summarized in Table 1.

Management

Constrictive pericarditis can be divided into three forms, each with a different recommended treatment. Transient constrictive pericarditis is a temporary form of constrictive pericarditis resulting after acute pericarditis and can be treated with anti-inflammatory medications. The constriction ceases after the inflammation resolves, usually after several weeks of anti-inflammatory treatment. Patients diagnosed with early constrictive pericarditis should initially have the underlying disease process treated to reverse the constriction and prevent progression to chronic constrictive pericarditis.

Another form of constrictive pericarditis is effusive–constrictive pericarditis. In this form, cardiac function is limited by both pericardial fluid and the scarred pericardium. Patients are typically misdiagnosed as having cardiac tamponade, and, once the effusion is drained, continue to have signs and symptoms of constrictive pericarditis. A diagnosis of effusive–constrictive pericarditis can be made when the right atrial pressure fails to fall by 50% or to a level below 10 mmHg after pericardiocentesis. Following pericardiocentesis, medical therapy can be targeted to treat the inflammation. Patients with persistent disease should be considered for pericardiectomy.

Chronic constrictive pericarditis, the third form, is treated by pericardiectomy. Pericardiectomy is indicated in patients who have persistent and significant symptoms. The procedure is performed by removing as much pericardium as technically possible, most commonly through a median sternotomy. Operative mortality ranges from 2.5 to 10% depending on the series. Pericardiectomy is technically challenging and should be performed by specialists. In patients with very mild disease, the operative risk outweighs the potential benefit. In patients with advanced disease and long-term history of the constrictive pericarditis, little benefit is seen, and the operative risks are likely higher. These patients might not be offered pericardiectomy due to the high operative risk and are managed instead with medical therapy targeted at symptom reduction. The exact criteria used for selection of patients for pericardiectomy have not been well described.

Cardiac Tamponade

Pericardial tamponade is a condition where the accumulation of pericardial fluid (effusion, pus, or blood) causes compression of cardiac chambers leading to an increase in intracardial pressure, reduced ventricular filling, and decreased cardiac output. The severity of the clinical symptoms and hemodynamic abnormalities depends on the speed of fluid accumulation, the volume of the pericardial fluid, and the compliance of the pericardium. A small amount of fluid can cause tamponade if it accumulates rapidly and the pericardium does not have enough time to distend. A classic example of this is myocardial injury from penetrating trauma resulting in rapid accumulation of blood in the pericardium and compression of the cardiac chambers. In contrast, slowly accumulating effusions, such as those associated with pericarditis, autoimmune conditions, and renal failure, can get very large before hemodynamic instability becomes evident. Regardless of etiology or effusion size, cardiac tamponade is a life-threatening condition that demands prompt and effective treatment.

Etiology

Almost any cause of pericardial effusion can result in tamponade. Etiologies related to a more acute development of tamponade are post-injury (trauma or iatrogenic), post-pericardiotomy syndromes, cardiac rupture (post-myocardial infarction), aortic dissection, idiopathic pericarditis, neoplasms, and granulomatous diseases.

Large volume effusions that develop insidiously over time can evolve into cardiac tamponade, especially when the underlying etiology of pericarditis has not been diagnosed. In these cases, the development of tamponade is less dramatic and less acute. These patients may have pericardial effusions over the period of days to weeks without cardiovascular symptoms. As their effusions continue to develop and the pericardial pressures reach a critical threshold, the patients begin to manifest signs and symptoms of decreased cardiac output. Autoimmune diseases, neoplasms, renal failure, idiopathic pericarditis, granulomatous diseases, and myxedema are some conditions that can present with subacute onset of tamponade.

Clinical Presentation and Diagnosis

Patients with pericardial tamponade may present with symptoms of fatigue and dyspnea. In more severe cases, syncope and shock are the presenting symptoms. A number of findings may be present on physical examination, but none of them alone are highly sensitive or specific. Tachycardia is the result of adrenergic response due to the declining stroke volume and is present in almost all patients. In contrast, the presence of hypotension is more variable. Jugular venous distension is common but may be absent in patients who are severely hypovolemic. Thus, the lack of this finding does not rule out tamponade. Muffled or distant heart sounds due to the damping effect of the pericardial effusion may be present. *Pulsus paradoxus* (a decrease in systolic blood pressure more than 10 mm of Hg during inspiration) is a common finding. It is a sign of exaggerated ventricular interdependence related to a fixed pericardial volume. Inspiratory increase in venous return and right ventricular volume results in compensatory decrease in left ventricular volume, leading to reduced stroke volume and systemic blood pressure. The classic Beck's triad (jugular venous distension, hypotension, and muffling of heart sounds) is only present in 10% of patients [24].

Electrocardiogram may show sinus tachycardia, abnormalities related to pericarditis, and/or low voltage. Electrical alternans refers to beat-to-beat variation in the QRS complexes due to the swinging of the heart within the pericardial fluid. It is a relatively specific indicator of tamponade, but it is rarely seen. Chest X-ray is usually normal, especially in those with acute onset of tamponade. In cases of slowly developing tamponade, the cardiac silhouette can be enlarged with a "water bottle" configuration.

Echocardiography can reliably identify and characterize pericardial effusions and can help differentiate cardiac tamponade from other potential causes of similar clinical presentations. Echocardiographic findings most suggestive of cardiac tamponade are early diastolic collapse of the right ventricle and late diastolic collapse of the right and left atria. Other echocardiographic findings are respiratory variation with reciprocal changes in right and left ventricular volumes and respiratory variation in mitral and tricuspid flow velocities. Cardiac catheterization is usually not used to diagnose cardiac tamponade. If it is performed, it usually demonstrates elevation and equalization of diastolic pressures in all chambers. Inspiratory increase in right-sided pressures with associated reduction in left-sided pressures (*pulsus paradoxus*) may also be observed. The diagnosis of cardiac tamponade as compared to constrictive pericarditis is summarized in Table 1.

Management

Cardiac tamponade is a life-threatening condition that demands prompt and effective treatment. Drainage of the pericardial fluid can be done either by pericardiocentesis or by surgical pericardiotomy. Pericardiocentesis should be performed under echocardiographic guidance to minimize complications and to target the appropriate collection. A drainage catheter should be inserted for ongoing drainage. Pericardiocentesis is generally preferred in hemodynamically unstable patients as it can be performed at bedside and can be achieved quickly. Open surgical drainage has the advantage of allowing direct visualization of the epicardium and manual break-up of loculations for better evacuation of pericardial contents. Open surgical drainage also permits access for pericardial biopsy. Open drainage is generally preferred for hemopericardium due to trauma and purulent pericarditis.

Once tamponade is relieved with drainage, the underlying cause for tamponade must be identified and treated. For trauma victims and patients with aortic dissection or myocardial rupture, emergent surgical intervention is required. It is important to note that general anesthesia and positive pressure ventilation can worsen venous return and hemodynamic collapse. For this reason, these patients should be prepped and ready for incision prior to induction under general anesthesia.

Pericardial Procedures

Pericardiocentesis

Pericardiocentesis is usually performed to investigate the etiology of pericarditis/effusion or to relieve symptoms of cardiac tamponade. The procedure should be accomplished under fluoroscopic or echocardiographic guidance. The latter is preferred and is more commonly employed. Blind pericardiocentesis is very risky and should not be done, except in very rare, immediately life-threatening situations. If blind pericardiocentesis must be done, the subxiphoid approach is recommended. If clinically feasible, the patient should be positioned semi-upright and rotated slightly toward the left. This allows the fluid to concentrate more in the inferior and anterior portion of pericardial space. A long needle is advanced below the xiphoid process and angled 30–45° below the skin surface, aiming slightly toward the left, while the operator aspirates the syringe until pericardial fluid is observed. To help with blind aspiration, a precordial EKG electrode can be attached to the needle to transduce the signal during aspiration. If the needle contacts the cardiac surface, ST changes or negative deflection will appear on the EKG tracing, and this should signal the operator to withdraw the needle slightly (see Fig. 4).

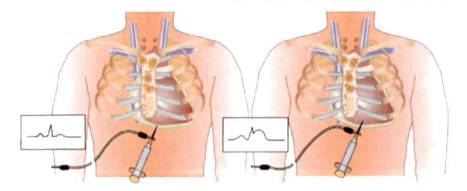

Fig. 4 EKG monitoring showing the change in tracing if the myocardium is contacted with the needle. (From Sadiq, A and Wall, M: Chapter 9 Pericardiocentesis. *In* Falter, F [Ed.], *Bedside Procedures in the ICU*, DOI https://doi.org/10.1007/978-1-4471-2259-3_9, Springer-Verlag London Limited 2012)

For ultrasound-guided pericardiocentesis, echocardiographic evaluation is used to determine the optimal needle entry site, which should be the point on the body that is closest to the transducer probe and where the fluid collection is the largest. With the patient semi-upright and left tilted, the ideal spot is identified using echocardiography, and it is marked as the intended site of entry. This spot is typically found along the left parasternal axis away from the left internal thoracic artery. Insertion of the needle into the fluid collection can either be guided by continuous echocardiographic visualization or guided based on the trajectory of the transducer probe and depth as memorized by the operator. Once the needle is inserted, the extracardiac position can be confirmed by injecting a few milliliters of agitated saline infusion and visualization of bubbles in the pericardial space on echocardiography. Once intrapericardial position is confirmed, the needle is then exchanged over a guidewire with a pigtail catheter, which is left in place for continued drainage. For fluoroscopic guided pericardiocentesis, the needle is usually inserted via the subxiphoid approach toward the heart shadow, while the operator alternates between suction and injection of small amount of diluted contrast, until pericardial fluid is aspirated. The location of the needle is confirmed by injecting contrast medium into the pericardial space prior to exchanging with a guidewire. Multiple fluoroscopic projections should be used to confirm the position of the guidewire prior to placement of the pigtail catheter.

In cases of recurrent effusion, percutaneous balloon pericardial window creation is an option for temporary drainage into the pleural space. In this technique, a balloon dilator threaded over the guidewire is straddled across the pericardium and dilated to create a window in the pericardium. This allows the pericardial fluid to drain into the pleural space where it is absorbed.

Complication rates of pericardiocentesis range from 4 to 10% depending on the method used, operator skills, and clinical settings [7]. Complications can be serious and potentially fatal, including ventricular arrhythmias and laceration of the heart, coronary arteries, internal thoracic arteries, lung, and liver.

Pericardiotomy and Pericardial Biopsy

When the pericardial effusion is large, pericardiocentesis under image guidance is relatively safe. When the effusions are small or loculated or when the character of the fluid is not suitable for pericardiocentesis (such as purulent effusion, fibrin, or clot), open surgical drainage is a safer and more effective approach. With the open approach, pericardial tissue biopsy can also be obtained.

Subxiphoid pericardiotomy can be performed under general anesthesia or local anesthesia with monitored sedation. A vertical incision is made over the xiphoid process toward the upper abdomen, and the rectus abdominis muscle is divided at the linea alba. Once the xiphoid process is exposed, it can be excised or retracted. Dissection is carried cephalad in the substernal space until the inferior surface of the pericardium is encountered. The pericardium is grasped, pulled down, and incised, and drainage of pericardial fluid should be observed. The pericardial fluid should be collected and sent for culture, cytology, cell count, and biochemical analysis. A small portion of the pericardium should also be excised and sent for histological analysis. The pericardial space should now be inspected with direct visualization and digital examination. Adhesions and loculations can be broken up by the operator's finger. Two drainage catheters are placed into the pericardial space (one anterior and one posterior to the heart) through two separate counter incisions. The incision is then closed in layers.

If the pericardial effusion is persistent or recurrent, a transpleural pericardiotomy can be done to allow drainage into the pleural space. This so-called pericardial window can be achieved through a left anterior thoracotomy at the fourth intercostal space. With this exposure, an incision into the pericardium is made and the pericardial fluid is sampled for diagnostic studies. To allow reliable drainage of the effusion into the pleural space, a large portion of the pericardium should be removed when creating the window. Pericardial tissue should also be sent for histological analysis. This procedure can also be accomplished by the video-assisted thoracoscopic approach, using single lung ventilation. Once the pericardial window has been created, temporary drainage catheters are left in both pericardial and pleural spaces. For drainage of purulent pericarditis, the subxiphoid approach is usually preferred to avoid contamination of the pleural space.

In patients' recurrent pericardial effusions associated with metastatic malignancy, pericardial-peritoneal drainage can be achieved by creating a transdiaphragmatic pericardial window or by inserting a large drainage catheter connecting the pericardial sac with the abdomen. The latter is performed with a 15 cm drain inserted half in the pericardial sac and half in the peritoneal cavity, and the drain is secured with a suture at the diaphragm level. This will enable continued drainage of the pericardium into the peritoneum, avoiding repeated interventions.

Pericardioscopy

Pericardioscopy has been suggested by some authors as a diagnostic tool when evaluating pericardial effusions. It can be done at the time of subxiphoid pericardiotomy as an adjunctive technique to allow exploration of the pericardial space. This is accomplished by inserting a rigid or flexible pericardioscope through the pericardiotomy for visual inspection of the pericardium and epicardium and for targeted tissue sampling. The use of pericardioscopy with targeted biopsy in addition to pericardial fluid analysis and open pericardial biopsy may increase diagnostic yield [25]. Percutaneous pericardioscopy under image guidance has also been described by some. This procedure is technically demanding and is only available in a limited number of experienced referral centers [26].

Pericardiectomy

Pericardiectomy is typically indicated for the treatment of recurrent pericarditis refractory to medical treatment or for constrictive pericarditis. Several surgical approaches have been described, including left anterolateral thoracotomy, bilateral thoracotomies, and median sternotomy. The advantage of the left anterolateral thoracotomy is avoidance of a redo median sternotomy. The disadvantage is limited exposure of the right phrenic nerve which could potentially compromise the completeness of pericardial resection. Bilateral thoracotomy approach is associated with higher morbidity and is usually employed for redo surgery or when extension of left anterolateral thoracotomy is needed. Median sternotomy provides the best exposure and is the most common approach used for this operation.

The extent of pericardiectomy is still a matter of controversy. Complete pericardiectomy involves removal of the entire pericardium overlying the heart and great vessels except for the pericardium posterior to the left atrium. Radical pericardiectomy is defined by removal of the anterior portion of the pericardium anterior to the left to right phrenic nerves, the diaphragm portion of the pericardium, and the pericardium posterior to the left phrenic nerve. Anterior pericardiectomy refers to removal of the anterior portion of the pericardium only (phrenic nerve to phrenic nerve). In all cases, care is taken to preserve the phrenic nerves. For patients who undergo pericardiectomy for recurrent pericarditis, the pericardium is inflamed and generally non-calcified and non-adherent to the underlying pericardium. Extensive resection may be more feasible in this group of patients. Since the goal for this indication is to remove as much of inflamed pericardium as possible to prevent recurrent symptoms, effort should be made to be more complete. In patients who undergo pericardiectomy for constrictive pericarditis, heavily calcified and thicken pericardium, sometimes with extension into myocardium, may be encountered. The pericardial space is obliterated, and separation is tedious and technically challenging. More complete resection may be wrought with potential complications. For this reason, some surgeons recommend only anterior pericardiectomy based on the rationale that anterior resection alone can improve constrictive hemodynamics in most patients [27]. On the other hand, others have shown that for constrictive pericarditis, complete resection is associated with superior survival and functional outcome when compared to partial resection [28]. In most large series of pericardiectomy for constrictive pericarditis, the standard technique described is radical pericardiectomy [14, 28, 29].

The depth of resection is also important. In some cases, after removal of the outer layer, a constricting peel overlying the epicardium may still limit ventricular function. Effort should be made to remove this peel to relieve the constriction. If removal is not possible, the epicardial peel may be scored in a checkerboard manner, leaving behind non-contiguous islands of the epicardium. This may be sufficient to allow expansion of the ventricles.

Pericardiectomy can be performed with or without cardiopulmonary bypass. In a large series of 513 pericardiectomies performed over 20 years at the Mayo Clinic, cardiopulmonary bypass was used in 40% of the cases [14]. Hemodynamic support with cardiopulmonary bypass is used in many instances to allow greater manipulation of the heart and to decompress the chambers to facilitate epicardial dissection. Furthermore, in cases when the myocardium is injured during the dissection, repair is easier with cardiopulmonary bypass.

In-hospital mortality for pericardiectomy ranges from 2.5 to 10% [14, 29]. The reported mortality rate is generally lower for pericardiectomy done for recurrent/effusive pericarditis compared to constrictive pericarditis [14]. The most common reason for in-hospital mortality is low cardiac output and post-operative renal failure. Patients who present at time of surgery with advanced hepatic congestion tend to have worse outcomes. The overall 5-, 10-, and 15-year survival of patients undergoing pericardiectomy is reported to be 80%, 60%, and 40%, respectively [14, 30]. The most important variable for long-term outcomes of pericardiectomy is the etiology of constriction. Patients with idiopathic constrictive pericarditis have the best 5- and 10-year survival. Patients with post-radiation pericarditis have the worst long-term outcomes because these patients also have concomitant myocardiopathy and coronary arterial disease [31]. Other conditions associated with worse long-term outcomes include advanced heart failure, poor renal function, abnormal left ventricular function, advanced liver disease, and older age [23].

References

1. Imazio M, Cecchi E, Demichelis B, et al. Myopericarditis versus viral or idiopathic acute pericarditis. Heart. 2008;94:498–501.
2. Kyto V, Sipila J, Rautava P. Clinical profile and influences on outcomes in patients hospitalized for acute pericarditis. Circulation. 2014;130(18):1601–6.
3. Kumar N, Pandey A, Jain P, et al. Acute pericarditis-associated hospitalization in the USA: a nation-wide analysis, 2003–2012. Cardiology. 2016;135(1):27–35.
4. LeWinter MM. Clinical practice. Acute pericarditis. N Engl J Med. 2014;371(25):2410–6.
5. Imazio M, Gaita F. Acute and recurrent pericarditis. Cardiol Clin. 2017;35(4):505–3.
6. Maisch B, Seferovic PM, Ristic AD, et al. Guidelines on the diagnosis and management of pericardial diseases executive summary; Task Force on the diagnosis and management of pericardial diseases of the European Society of Cardiology. Eur Heart J. 2004;25(7):587–610.
7. Adler Y, Charron P, Imazio M, et al. 2015 ESC guidelines for the diagnosis and management of pericardial diseases: The task force for the diagnosis and management of pericardial diseases of the European Society of Cardiology (ESC) Endorsed by: The European Association for Cardio-Thoracic Surgery (EACTS). Eur Heart J. 2015;36(42):2921–64.

8. Imazio M, Brucato A, Maestroni S, et al. Prevalence of C-reactive protein elevation and time course of normalization in acute pericarditis: implication for the diagnosis, therapy, and prognosis of pericarditis. Circulation. 2011;123(10):1092–7.
9. Imazio M, Gaita F, LeWinter M. Evaluation and treatment of pericarditis: a systemic review. JAMA. 2015;314(14):1498–506.
10. Imazio M, Brucato A, Cemin R, et al. A randomized trial of colchicine for acute pericarditis. N Engl J Med. 2013;369(16):1522–8.
11. Lotrionte M, Biondi-Zoccai G, Imazio M, et al. International collaborative systematic review of controlled clinical trials on pharmacologic treatments for acute pericarditis and its recurrences. Am Heart J. 2010;160(4):662–70.
12. Hatcher CR, Logue RB, Logan WD, et al. Pericardiectomy for recurrent pericarditis. J Thorac Cardiovasc Surg. 1971;62(3):371–8.
13. Khandaker MH, Schaff HV, Greason KL, et al. Pericardiectomy vs medical management in patients with relapsing pericarditis. Mayo Clin Proc. 2012;87(11):1062–70.
14. Gillaspie EA, Stulak JM, Daly RC, et al. A 20-year experience with isolated pericardiectomy: analysis of indications and outcomes. J Thorac Cardiovasc Surg. 2016;152(2):448–58.
15. Bentata Y, Hamdi F, Chemlal A, et al. Uremica pericarditis in patients with end stage renal disease: prevalence, symptoms and outcome in 2017. Am J Emerg Med. 2018;36(3):464–6.
16. Spector D, Alfred H, Siedlecki M, et al. A controlled study of the effect of indomethacin in uremic pericarditis. Kidney Int. 1983;24(5):663–9.
17. Busselmeier TJ, Davin TD, Simmons RL, et al. Treatment of intractable uremic pericardial effusion. Avoidance of pericardiectomy with local steroid instillation. JAMA. 1978;240(13):1358–9.
18. Augustin P, Desmard M, Mordant P, et al. Clinical review: intrapericardial fibrinolysis in management of purulent pericarditis. Crit Care. 2011;15(2):220.
19. Strang JI, Kakaza HH, Gibson DG, et al. Controlled trial of prednisolone as adjuvant in treatment of tuberculous constrictive pericarditis in Transkei. Lancet. 1987;2(8573):1418–22.
20. Mayosi BM, Ntsekhe M, Bosch J, et al. Prednisolone and Mycobacterium indicus pranii in tuberculous pericarditis. N Engl J Med. 2014;371(12):1121–30.
21. Imazio M, Brucato A, Maestroni S, et al. Risk of constrictive pericarditis after acute pericarditis. Circulation. 2011;124(11):1270–5.
22. Troughton RW, Asher CR, Klein AL. Pericarditis. Lancet. 2004;363(9410):717–27.
23. Welch TD. Constrictive pericarditis: diagnosis, management and clinical outcomes. Heart. 2018;104(9):725–31.
24. Guberman BA, Fowler NO, Engel PJ, et al. Cardiac tamponade in medical patients. Circulation. 1981;64(3):633–40.
25. Nugue O, Millaire A, Porte H, et al. Pericardioscopy in the etiologic diagnosis of pericardial effusion in 141 consecutive patients. Circulation. 1996;94(7):1635–41.
26. Seferović PM, Ristić AD, Maksimović R, et al. Diagnostic value of pericardial biopsy: improvement with extensive sampling enabled by pericardioscopy. Circulation. 2003;107(7):978–83.
27. Nataf P, Cacoub P, Dorent R, et al. Result of subtotal pericardiectomy for constrictive pericarditis. Eur J Cardiothorac Surg. 1993;7(5):252–5.
28. Chowdhury UK, Subramaniam GK, Kumar AS, et al. Pericardiectomy for constrictive pericarditis: a clinical, echocardiographic, and hemodynamic evaluation of two surgical techniques. Ann Thorac Surg. 2006;81(2):522–9.
29. Cho YH, Schaff HV. Surgery for pericardial disease. Heart Fail Res. 2013;18(3):375–87.
30. George TJ, Arnaoutakis GJ, Beaty CA, et al. Contemporary etiologies, risk factors, and outcomes after pericardiectomy. Ann Thorac Surg. 2012;94(2):445–51.
31. Vistarini N, Chen C, Mazine A, et al. Pericardiectomy for constrictive pericarditis: 20 years of experience at the Montreal Heart Institute. Ann Thorac Surg. 2015;100(1):107–13.

Necrotizing Lung Infections

Jill Streams, Jaclyn Clark, Marc de Moya, and Sharon Henry

Introduction

A 38-year-old male who was a victim of a motor vehicle collision sustained multiple orthopedic and abdominal visceral injuries. These included fractures of the left clavicle, left scapula, left ribs three through five, right distal radius, as well as a grade IV splenic injury. He underwent splenic embolization with re-bleeding requiring a splenectomy and distal pancreatectomy for pancreas necrosis. He had an indolent course with multiple abdominal reoperations and was unable to be extubated. After 21 days in the intensive care unit (ICU), he developed worsening respiratory failure, sepsis, and acute renal failure. Chest X-ray (CXR) (Fig. 1) showed a right lower lobe infiltrate, and computed tomography (CT) revealed a nearly complete necrotic right lower lobe with cavitation (Fig. 2).

Bronchoalveolar lavage (BAL) specimens repeatedly grew methicillin-resistant *Staphylococcus aureus* (MRSA). His pulmonary condition deteriorated, and he was placed on veno-venous extracorporeal membrane oxygenation (ECMO) on hospital on day 25. He spent 15 days on ECMO and a total of 68 days in the ICU. He was treated for 2 months with linezolid therapy. Currently, he is 8 months from his trauma and has chronic dyspnea and productive cough. His baseline saturation at home is 89% and does not use home oxygen. He can walk four blocks without stopping due to shortness of breath. He follows closely with a pulmonologist.

Fig. 1 Right lower lobe infiltrate

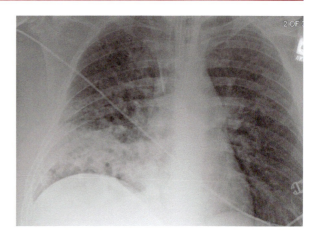

Fig. 2 Right lower lobe necrosis and consolidation

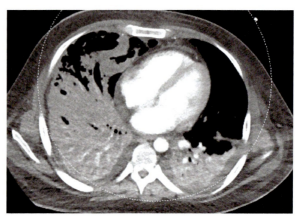

While pneumonia, both community acquired and nosocomial, is a common diagnosis with an annual incidence of approximately 5.6 million cases, over 1 million hospital admissions, and almost 50,000 deaths, necrotizing pneumonia and other necrotizing lung infections (NLI) are rare [1]. The true incidence of necrotizing lung infections is unknown; however, NLI has been estimated to be less than 1% of cases of pneumonia in adult patients. Necrotizing pneumonia is somewhat more common in children with reported rates of 1–7% of all cases of pneumonia [2, 3]. Necrotizing lung infections (NLI) can afflict healthy adults and children, though are more likely in patients with chronic diseases such as diabetes, asthma, and alcohol abuse. Immunosuppression with corticosteroids and other agents confers increased risk of NLI [2].

Reports of necrotizing features of severe pneumonia date back to the late 1800s. Khan identified Rene Laennec, the inventor of the stethoscope, as the first to mention "pulmonary gangrene" in 1821. There was no further mention of the disease in the literature until Sir. William Osler in 1897 recognized that pulmonary necrosis could be a complication of pneumonia, aspiration pneumonia, or pulmonary malignancy [4]. Knight et al. reported the first case series and literature review of necrotizing pneumonia in 1975, compiling 12 cases between 1921 and 1968. Of those patients, the 4 who were managed medically died, whereas the 8 who had surgical treatment lived. The predominant organisms identified were *Klebsiella pneumoniae*, *Streptococcus pneumoniae*, and *Staphylococcus* spp. [5] The first case of necrotizing pneumonia in children was reported in 1994 [3]. A review of necrotizing pneumonia in children reports increasing occurrence of necrotizing pneumonia in recent years [4]. Both adult and pediatric cases of necrotizing lung infections appear to be occurring more frequently in the last 25 years, although some of this increased incidence may be due to improvement in imaging capabilities as computed tomography is much more sensitive for necrosis than traditional radiography [6–8].

Bacteriology and Other Causative Organisms

Certain bacterial etiologies of pneumonia, such as those due to pneumococcus, have higher incidence of necrotizing lung infections. Pande et al. retrospectively reviewed all cases of pneumococcal pneumonia at a VA hospital over 10 years and reported an incidence of 6.6% of necrotizing pneumonia on radiographic imaging [8].

Necrotizing lung infections are a spectrum of disease from lung abscess to pulmonary gangrene. Lung abscesses are usually due to anaerobic oropharyngeal bacteria such as *Bacteroides fragilis*, *Fusobacterium capsulatum*, and *Peptostreptococcus* [9]. Necrotizing pneumonia and pulmonary gangrene are prototypically caused by virulent bacterial infections. The most frequent causative bacteria of NLI are *Staphylococcus aureus* and *Streptococcus pneumoniae* (pneumococcus) [1, 10, 11]. It is postulated that necrotizing pneumonia and pulmonary gangrene develop due to perivascular inflammation causing microvascular and macrovascular thrombosis, respectively. Vascular thrombosis results in ischemic pulmonary parenchyma. Systemically delivered antibiotics fail to reach the malperfused infected lung tissues; however, this is the initial approach to treatment. Ischemic parenchyma then progresses to frank necrosis.

Staphylococcus aureus, both methicillin-sensitive and -resistant strains, is implicated in approximately 2% of all community-acquired pneumonias. However, in several retrospective case series, *S. aureus* was the identified organism in 20–30% of necrotizing pneumonia cases [10, 12]. The Panton–Valentine leukocidin (PVL) was described in 1932 as a Staphylococcal toxin capable of hemolytic, leukocytic, and necrotic action [13]. PVL-producing strains of *S. aureus* have been associated with higher rates of necrotizing lung infections as well as necrotizing soft-tissue infections [14–16].

The other dominant microbe in reported cases of necrotizing lung infection is *Streptococcus pneumonia* [2, 12, 17]. Children and the elderly are particularly vulnerable to pneumococcal infections and subsequent progression to necrotizing infection. The pneumococcal vaccine immunizes against the most common serotypes and has reduced the incidence of pneumococcal pneumonia overall; however, there are multiple non-vaccine serotypes that are associated with a necrotizing course including serotypes 3 and 19A. Despite now being included in the PCV13 vaccine, these serotypes are being reported as the causative organism in some NLI [18] and empyema [19].

Klebsiella pneumoniae is the principal gram-negative microbe isolated with necrotizing lung infections and is seen more often in the adult population. Classical serotype *Klebsiella* remains the prototypical causative organism in aspiration pneumonia, particularly that of patients with concomitant alcohol abuse. *Klebsiella* has been associated with cases of pulmonary gangrene [20]. The aggressive pathogenesis of Klebsiella infections has been postulated to be due to K1/K2 serotype and has been termed "hypervirulent" Klebsiella [21].

Pseudomonas aeruginosa is another aggressive and potentially lethal organism in necrotizing pneumonia. This is believed to be due to infection of vasculature resulting in thrombotic endarteritis [22]. Pseudomonal infections are more often seen in immunocompromised patients or in nosocomial infections. Reimel et al. report 6 out 35 patients undergoing surgical resection for necrotizing lung infections had cultures positive for *Pseudomonas* [12]. More rare causative organisms in NLI include: *Haemophilus influenza, Legionella, Burkholderia pseudomallei* causing melioidosis, *Acinetobacter*, and *Escherichia coli*. *Fusobacterium* is an uncommon etiology but may cause NLI from septic emboli in Lemierre's syndrome. The immunosuppressed patient population is at risk for NLI due to *Mycobacterium* species, *Microascus*, and invasive fungal infections such as *Aspergillus* and *Mucormycosis* [23]. The fungal infections generally follow a more chronic, cavitary course but can present as acute necrotic lung infections [24].

Diagnosis

The clinical findings are non-specific and include fever, cough, chest pain, and shortness of breath. Diagnosing necrotizing pneumonia focuses both on identifying the pathogen responsible as well as defining the presence and extent of necrosis. Septic shock and respiratory failure requiring ventilator support are not uncommon. Sputum cultures can often be contaminated with oropharyngeal flora, so if unrevealing, distal and targeted airway samples can be obtained with bronchoalveolar lavage (BAL). Blood cultures can also be useful—in a French series of 21 pediatric patients, 10 had positive blood cultures [25]. If pleural fluid from an effusion or empyema is drained, it should also be sent for culture. It is important to also send viral studies, including influenza and HIV. White blood cell (WBC) count elevation seen in both necrotizing and non-necrotizing pneumonias is higher in the former as are inflammatory markers including erythrocyte sedimentation rate (ESR) and C reactive protein (CRP) [26].

CXR is the usual initial diagnostic test. Distinguishing necrotizing from non-necrotizing pneumonia is difficult. Consolidation may be evident, but the extent of parenchymal tissue loss is impossible to determine [27] and frequently underestimated on CXR. The right middle and lower and the left lower lobes are most commonly involved. CXR may identify other complications of pneumonia such as pleural effusion, empyema, and pneumothorax from bronchopleural fistula (BPF). Contrast-enhanced computed tomography (CT) is the preferred and most sensitive diagnostic test [11]. Typical findings include consolidation with areas of decreased enhancement and small cavities [27]. As liquefaction progresses, these small cavities can coalesce to form larger ones, which can become gangrenous [11]. Processes that lead to bronchial obstruction can mimic the findings of necrotizing pneumonia. Examples include foreign bodies or underlying carcinoma. Bronchoscopy is helpful in excluding these conditions.

Treatment and Surgical Indications

The mainstay of treatment for necrotizing lung infections is appropriate and early antibiotic therapy directed at the causative organisms and supportive care including ICU admission and mechanical ventilation as needed [2, 10]. Delays in initiation of antibiotics can result in substantial morbidity and mortality. Antibiotic therapy should be guided by local resistance patterns for initial broad-spectrum coverage. Sputum cultures, tracheal aspirates, or bronchoalveolar lavage samples can then be used to tailor antibiotic therapy. Percutaneous drainage of necrotic tissue is not recommended. Tubes can be difficult to place because of the inflammatory response or become obstructed with necrotic material and can result in bronchopleural fistulae. However, failure to respond to maximal medical management should prompt discussion of surgical intervention [12, 28–31].

Treatment of pleural-based infectious processes, such as parapneumonic effusion and empyema, can initially be accomplished with tube thoracostomy. Image-guided drainage may be necessary as the development of loculations within the pleural space and parenchymal to chest wall adhesions is common and can sequester fluid collections despite adequate chest tube placement. Fibrinolytic agents can be administered via chest tube to facilitate drainage of loculated pleural fluid with varying degrees of success but with increased concern for bleeding complications. Lack of source control in the pleural space can result in ongoing sepsis. Patients may require operative intervention, either thoracoscopically or via thoracotomy, for complete evacuation of the pleural space.

The inflammatory process of necrotizing lung infections can result in the development of a fibrinous rind on the visceral and parietal pleural surfaces. This thickened pleural "peel" prevents the adequate expansion of lung parenchyma and frequently requires decortication. Acute care surgeons should be well versed in decortication by both thoracoscopic and open thoracotomy approaches. Thoracoscopic surgical intervention requires the patient is physiologically capable of tolerating single lung ventilation, which many NLI patients are often not. The principle of decortication is meticulous and complete removal of the pleural rind encasing the affected lung while minimizing underlying parenchymal injury.

As pulmonary infection progresses and lung parenchyma becomes necrotic, the terminal bronchiole cells lyse and expose the bronchial system to the pleural space, leading to pneumothorax. Pneumothorax can be managed with tube thoracostomy in most cases. As parenchymal healing and remodeling occurs, the exposed bronchial tree can seal; however, large segmental necrosis can erode into larger caliber bronchi and result in the development of bronchopleural fistulas (BPF). Formation of BPF can result in sudden tension pneumothorax if the pressurization of the pleural space is not alleviated emergently. Large BPF can result in acute respiratory failure due to preferential ventilation through the BPF into the pleural space. BPF can also lead to inability to ventilate despite being on positive pressure ventilation. Bronchopleural fistulas can be managed non-operatively with tube thoracostomy and/or endobronchial valves with varying degrees of success [32–34], but may require operative intervention if persistent. Endobronchial valves are one-way valves that allow expiratory passage of air but no inspiratory ventilation, effectively sealing off the leaking bronchial tree in BPF. There are numerous surgical techniques for the treatment of BPF including parenchymal resection, lobectomy, and Eloesser flaps that are beyond the scope of this chapter.

Refractory hypoxia, despite advanced ventilator modes such as airway pressure relase ventilation (APRV) with lung protective low tidal volumes, should prompt evaluation for extracorporeal membrane oxygenation (ECMO). Evaluation and cannulation for ECMO should be performed by specialized teams with experience in ECMO including a critically care trained intensivist. Options for ECMO include peripheral and central cannulation, as well as catheter-based cannulas such as Avalon or Crescent. ECMO has been reported for both pediatric and adult cases of necrotizing pneumonia with good results [35–39]. ECMO may also be used as a bridge through surgical intervention for patients unable to tolerated single lung ventilation.

When necrotic lung parenchyma is driving an ongoing clinical picture of sepsis, then consideration for resection is indicated. Of note, there are no guidelines for which patients should undergo resection or recommendations on when in the clinical course this should occur. Axial imaging can help delineate diffuse versus localized necrosis and thus the extent of resection necessary. Peripheral necrosis and small abscesses can be debrided or excised with wedge resections. Larger areas or more centralized necrosis may require formal lobectomy. Pneumonectomy is reserved for extensive necrosis but has been reported in both children and adult patients with acceptable outcomes [12, 25, 29, 31, 40].

Retrospective reviews of necrotizing lung infections show relatively good outcomes with surgical resection. The largest case series was reported by Reimel et al. with the results of 35 patients at a single institution undergoing surgical resection for NLI ranging from wedge resection to pneumonectomy. They report an 8.5% mortality rate, with all mortalities occurring in patients requiring preoperative mechanical ventilation [12]. A German case series of 20 patients with NLI undergoing surgical intervention reported 13 patients required lobectomy and 4 patient required pneumonectomy; the overall mortality in this series was 15% [29]. A similar review of 26 cases in Taiwan also reported a post-operatively mortality of 15% [30].

In a small series of necrotizing lung infections, 10 of 14 patients with pulmonary necrosis underwent surgical resection with 100% survival, while 4 patients treated with medical management alone all died [35].

Conclusion

Necrotizing lung infections (NLI) are rare occurrences; however, they can be devastating if not managed appropriately. NLI represent a spectrum of disease from lung abscess to pulmonary gangrene. The most common causes of NLI are *Staphylococcus aureus* and *Streptococcus pneumoniae* (pneumococcus). The mainstay of treatment is the early and aggressive use of appropriate antibiotics. If the infection extends to the pleural space causing an effusion or an empyema, drainage of the pleural space is necessary. If drainage of the pleural space fails or if sepsis is not controlled with antibiotics, then surgical debridement or drainage is needed. These patients require a multi-disciplinary team to provide optimal critical care and often times have long-term pulmonary dysfunction.

References

1. Centers for Disease Control and Prevention. https://www.cdc.gov/nchs/fastats/pneumonia.htm.
2. Krutikov M, Rahman A, Tiberi S. Necrotizing pneumonia (aetiology, clinical features and management). Curr Opin Pulm Med. 2019;25(3):225–32.
3. Kerem E, et al. Bacteremic necrotizing pneumococcal pneumonia in children. Am J Respir Crit Care Med. 1994;149(1):242–4.
4. Khan FA. Pulmonary gangrene occurring as a complication of pulmonary tuberculosis. Chest. 1980;77(1):76–80.
5. Knight L, et al. Massive pulmonary gangrene: a severe complication of Klebsiella pneumonia. Can Med Assoc J. 1975;112(2):196–8.
6. Masters IB, Isles AF, Grimwood K. Necrotizing pneumonia: an emerging problem in children? Pneumonia (Nathan). 2017;9:11.
7. Sawicki GS, et al. Necrotising pneumonia is an increasingly detected complication of pneumonia in children. Eur Respir J. 2008;31(6):1285–91.
8. Pande A, et al. The incidence of necrotizing changes in adults with pneumococcal pneumonia. Clin Infect Dis. 2012;54(1):10–6.
9. Kuhajda I, et al. Lung abscess-etiology, diagnostic and treatment options. Ann Transl Med. 2015;3(13):183.
10. Chatha N, Fortin D, Bosma KJ. Management of necrotizing pneumonia and pulmonary gangrene: a case series and review of the literature. Can Respir J. 2014;21(4):239–45.
11. Tsai YF, Ku YH. Necrotizing pneumonia: a rare complication of pneumonia requiring special consideration. Curr Opin Pulm Med. 2012;18(3):246–52.
12. Reimel BA, et al. Surgical management of acute necrotizing lung infections. Can Respir J. 2006;13(7):369–73.
13. Panton PN, Valentine FCO. Staphylococcal toxin. Lancet. 1932;219(5662):506–8.
14. Gillet Y, et al. Factors predicting mortality in necrotizing community-acquired pneumonia caused by Staphylococcus aureus containing Panton-Valentine leukocidin. Clin Infect Dis. 2007;45(3):315–21.

15. Hoppe PA, et al. Severe infections of Panton-Valentine leukocidin positive Staphylococcus aureus in children. Medicine (Baltimore). 2019;98(38):e17185.
16. Takigawa Y, et al. Rapidly progressive multiple cavity formation in necrotizing pneumonia caused by community-acquired methicillin-resistant Staphylococcus aureus positive for the Panton-Valentine Leucocidin gene. Intern Med. 2019;58(5):685–91.
17. Hammond JM, et al. Severe pneumococcal pneumonia complicated by massive pulmonary gangrene. Chest. 1993;104(5):1610–2.
18. Alkan G, et al. Necrotizing pneumonia caused by Streptococcus pneumoniae serotype 3 despite PCV13. Arch Argent Pediatr. 2019;117(2):e155–7.
19. Grijalva CG, et al. Increasing incidence of empyema complicating childhood community-acquired pneumonia in the United States. Clin Infect Dis. 2010;50(6):805–13.
20. Knight L, Fraser RG, Robson HG. Massive pulmonary gangrene: a severe complication of Klebsiella pneumonia. Can Med Assoc J. 1975;112(2):196–8.
21. Shon AS, Bajwa RP, Russo TA. Hypervirulent (hypermucoviscous) Klebsiella pneumoniae: a new and dangerous breed. Virulence. 2013;4(2):107–18.
22. Karmy-Jones R, Vallières E, Harrington R. Surgical management of necrotizing pneumonia. Clin Pulm Med. 2003;10(1):17–25.
23. Taton O, et al. Necrotizing Microascus tracheobronchitis in a bilateral lung transplant recipient. Transpl Infect Dis, 2018;20(1).
24. Bassetti M, Bouza E. Invasive mould infections in the ICU setting: complexities and solutions. J Antimicrob Chemother. 2017;72(Suppl_1):i39–47.
25. Krishnadasan B, et al. Surgical management of lung gangrene. Can Respir J. 2000;7(5):401–4.
26. Lemaitre C, et al. Necrotizing pneumonia in children: report of 41 cases between 2206 and 2011 in a French tertiary care center. Pediatr Infect Dis J. 2013;10:1146–9.
27. Seo H, et al. Clinical relevance of necrotizing change in patients with community-acquired pneumonia. Respirology. 2017;3:551–8.
28. Chatha N, et al. Management of necrotizing pneumonia and pulmonary gangrene: a case series and review of literature. Can Respir J. 2014;21(4):239–45.
29. Schweigert M, et al. Surgical therapy for necrotizing pneumonia and lung gangrene. Thorac Cardiovasc Surg. 2013;61(7):636–41.
30. Tsai YF, Tsai YT, Ku YH. Surgical treatment of 26 patients with necrotizing pneumonia. Eur Surg Res. 2011;47(1):13–8.
31. Ayed AK, Al-Rowayeh A. Lung resection in children for infectious pulmonary diseases. Pediatr Surg Int. 2005;21(8):604–8.
32. Toth JW, et al. Endobronchial occlusion with one-way endobronchial valves: a novel technique for persistent air leaks in children. J Pediatr Surg. 2015;50(1):82–5.
33. Hance JM, Martin JT, Mullett TW. Endobronchial valves in the treatment of persistent air leaks. Ann Thorac Surg. 2015;100(5):1780–5; discussion 1785–6.
34. Gudbjartsson T, Helgadottir S, Ek L. One-way endobronchial valve for bronchopleural fistula after necrotizing pneumonia. Asian Cardiovasc Thorac Ann. 2013;21(4):498–9.
35. Lavoue S, et al. Extracorporeal circuit for Panton-Valentine leukocidin-producing Staphylococcus aureus necrotizing pneumonia. Med Mal Infect. 2016;46(6):314–7.
36. Merlo A, et al. Venovenous extracorporeal membrane oxygenation and pulmonary resection for necrotizing pneumonia. Ann Thorac Surg. 2019;107(2):e115–7.
37. Noah MA, et al. Panton-Valentine leukocidin expressing Staphylococcus aureus pneumonia managed with extracorporeal membrane oxygenation: experience and outcome. Crit Care Med. 2010;38(11):2250–3.
38. Stroud MH, et al. Successful use of extracorporeal membrane oxygenation in severe necrotizing pneumonia caused by Staphylococcus aureus. Pediatr Crit Care Med. 2007;8(3):282–7.
39. Martens T, et al. Deep hypothermic extracorporeal membrane oxygenation cannula exchange in a child with necrotic pneumonia. Perfusion. 2020;5(2):169–71.
40. Gerdung CA, et al. Pneumonectomy in a child with multilobar pneumatocele secondary to necrotizing pneumonia: case report and review of the literature. Case Rep Pediatr. 2019;2019:2464390.

Incidental Pulmonary Nodule

Fabio Ramponi, Cino Bendinelli, Joseph M. Galante, Luis Godoy, and Anna Xue

Part 1: Incidental Finding on Imaging

Fabio Ramponi and Cino Bendinelli

Identification and Prediction Models

Incidental pulmonary nodules are detected on chest imaging performed for unrelated reasons including trauma admissions. When diagnosed in asymptomatic individuals older than 35 years and without past history of other malignancies, the management pathway is aimed to prompt diagnosis (or exclusion) of lung cancer. Both patients' clinical features and nodules characteristics should guide the clinician toward invasive testing or imaging follow-up. When the lung incidentaloma is first detected by plain chest X-ray, a 1-mm thin-section computed tomography (CT) of the chest using low-radiation technique is mandatory to properly characterize the morphology of the lesion and seek the presence of other nodules, mediastinal lymphadenopathy, and pleural effusions. Comparison with previous imaging, if available, is crucial to observe any lesion progression.

F. Ramponi · C. Bendinelli
Department of Traumatology, John Hunter Hospital, University of Newcastle, Newcastle, NSW, Australia
e-mail: Cino.Bendinelli@hnehealth.nsw.gov.au

J. M. Galante (✉)
Davis Medical Centre, University of California, Davis, Sacramento, CA, USA
e-mail: jmgalante@ucdavis.edu

L. Godoy · A. Xue
Section of General Thoracic Surgery, Department of Surgery, University of California, Davis Health, Sacramento, CA, USA
e-mail: lagodoy@ucdavis.edu; ahxue@ucdavis.edu

© Springer Nature Switzerland AG 2021
J. M. Galante, R. Coimbra (eds.), *Thoracic Surgery for the Acute Care Surgeon*, Hot Topics in Acute Care Surgery and Trauma, https://doi.org/10.1007/978-3-030-48493-4_8

A solitary pulmonary nodule is defined as a well-defined lesion surrounded by normal lung parenchyma of less than small 30 mm in maximum diameter [6, 7] (Fig. 1a). Lesions larger than 30 mm are defined lung masses and carry a higher risk of being malignant. According to their morphology, lung nodules are classified as solid or subsolid; the latter are divided in pure ground-glass and part solid nodules, depending on the presence of some solid component (Fig. 1b). Finally, when multiple nodules are detected, attention is directed to the evolution of the most suspicious one; when countless 1–4 mm nodules are encountered, we refer to "miliary nodules" as seen in tuberculosis.

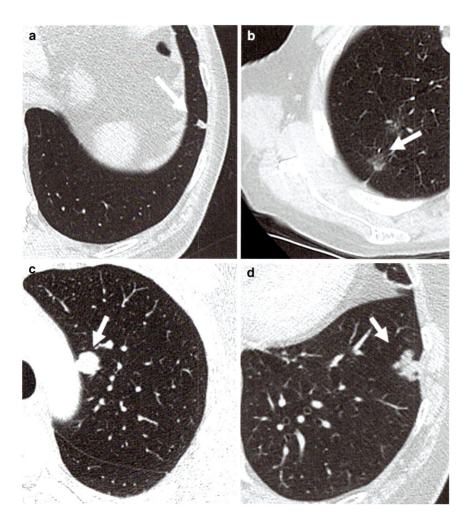

Fig. 1 (**a**) Seven millimeter nodule of the posterior segment of the left lower lobe incidentally found in a 67-year-old male lifelong smoker; (**b**) 12 mm ground-glass nodule of the right upper lobe; (**c**) 15 mm calcified nodule of the left upper lobe incidentally diagnosed in a 52 year-old former smoker; frozen section of a wedge biopsy revealed hamartoma; (**d**) 20 mm spiculated nodule of the left lower lobe; pathology showed adenocarcinoma of the lung

Table 1 Differential diagnosis for solitary pulmonary nodules

Malignant	Benign
Bronchogenic carcinoma	*Infectious granuloma*
Adenocarcinoma	Histoplasmosis
Squamous Cell Carcinoma	Coccidioidomycosis
Large Cell Carcinoma	Tuberculosis
Small Cell Carcinoma	Atypical mycobacteria
Metastatic lesions	Cryptococcosis
Breast	Blastomycosis
Head and neck	*Benign neoplasm*
Melanoma	Hamartoma
Colon	Lipoma/fibroma/neurofibroma
Kidney	Leiomyoma/angioma
Sarcoma	*Vascular*
Germ cell tumor	A-V malformation
Pulmonary carcinoid	Pulmonary varix and infarct
Lymphoma	*Inflammatory*
Miscellaneous	Wegener's granulomatosis
Plasmacytoma	Rheumatoid nodules
Schwannoma	Sarcoidosis

If the main differential diagnosis for incidental pulmonary nodules is between benign or malignant etiology (Table 1), only tissue biopsy can definitely confirm the diagnosis. Data from lung cancer screening studies in North America show that the majority of lesions detected on CT in high-risk population are benign in nature [8], so the incidence of malignant nodules in the average- or low-risk population should be well below 1% (relative risk of 0.15 in never smoker compared to heavy smoker for solid nodules) [26]. On the other hand, the risk of pulmonary metastasis in patients with extra-thoracic malignancies diagnosed with lung nodules is as high as 25% [9].

Among nodules of malignant etiology, primary lung cancer is mostly represented by adenocarcinoma (50%) followed by squamous cell carcinoma (20–25%) and large cell carcinoma (10%) [7]. Pulmonary metastases are typically from melanoma, sarcoma, and carcinomas of colon, breast, kidney, and testicles [10]. Finally, carcinoid tumors, typical and atypical, despite being usually cherry-like endobronchial lesions, can appear in 20% of cases as peripheral nodules. Infectious granulomas represent the majority (80%) of benign nodules, with fungal (histoplasmosis, coccidioidomycosis) and mycobacterial pathogens (tuberculous and non) most frequently responsible for well-demarcated, fully, or centrally calcified nodules (Fig. 2). Slow growing pulmonary hamartomas represents 10% of benign nodules; they can contain cartilage, fat, muscle, and myxomatous tissue. While the classic "pop-corn" calcifications are present in a minority of chest X-ray, the presence of calcium alternating with fat is a pathognomonic feature on high-resolution CT (Fig. 1c). Less common benign neoplasms are fibromas, leiomyomas, and hemangiomas, and they lack radiological diagnostic attributes [11].

Benign nodules of vascular origin should not be biopsied! Arteriovenous malformations are common in hemorrhagic syndrome like Osler–Weber–Rendu and present with lobulated margins and classic feeding/draining vessels. Pulmonary

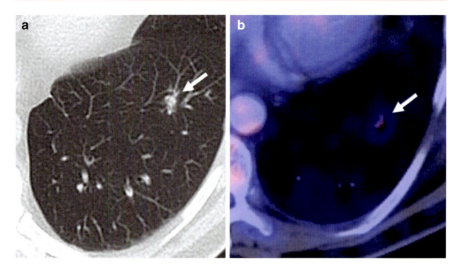

Fig. 2 (**a**) Eleven millimeter solid nodule of the superior segment of the left lower lobe, showing only mild FDG avidity on PET (**b**). Pathology showed necrotizing granuloma

infarcts, varices, and contusions can also present as lung nodules. Furthermore, pulmonary nodules can be the presenting feature of a systemic inflammatory disease like Wegener's granulomatosis, rheumatoid arthritis, sarcoidosis, and amyloidosis.

Assessment of clinical and radiographic features along with quantitative predictive models is used complementarily to determine the odds of malignancy: low probability (<5%), intermediate probability (5–65%), and high probability (>65%) [7, 12]. Important clinical traits associated with the malignant nature of solitary nodules are advanced age [13] and the presence of risk factors for lung cancer (cigarette smoking, family history, female sex, emphysema, prior malignancy, and asbestos exposure) [14].

According to the 2017 Fleischner Society guidelines, CT chest is the gold-standard imaging modality in the initial evaluation of malignancy risk [6]; low-radiation technique (1.5 mSv) with helically acquired 1 mm thin-section volumetric scanning is the most reliable method for assessing major nodule features: size, location, growth, density, borders, and presence of calcium and fat (Table 2).

Iodinated intravenous contrast is sometimes used if a vascular origin is suspected. Nodule *size* measured as the average of the long and short axis rounded to the nearest millimeter [6] is an independent predictor for malignancy, with the risk increasing form less than 1% in nodules smaller than 5 mm to above 50% in lesions larger than 20 mm [8].

According to their *density*, pulmonary nodules can be classified in solid (more common) or subsolid, the latter having higher chance of being early stage preinvasive adenocarcinoma [8, 15, 16]. Subsolid nodules have less then soft tissue density; they are divided in pure ground-glass or part-solid depending on the absence or presence of solid component (Fig. 1b). This latter feature is an important predictor

Table 2 Distinguishing radiological features for solitary pulmonary nodules

Nodule etiology	Distinguishing features
Granuloma	Smooth margins
	Solid of lamellated calcifications
Carcinoid	Lobulated margins
	Dystrophic, eccentric calcifications
Hamartoma	Lobulated margins
	Calcifications in rings and arcs
	Fat
AVM	Lobulated margins
	Infrequent calcifications
	Feeding/draining vessels
Lung Cancer Metastasis	Spiculated, lobulated or smooth margins
	Dystrophic calcifications
	Large lesions with necrosis
	Cavitation in SCC and Adenocarcinoma
AIS/MIA	≤5 mm of atypical adenomatous hyperplasia
	Ground-glass opacity
	Well-demarcated margins
	Part-solid nodule
	Cystic space
	Focal extension to pleura

AVM arteriovenous malformation, *AIS* adenocarcinoma in situ, *MIA* minimally invasive adenocarcinoma

of malignancy especially if newly developed during surveillance [8]. Solid lesions smaller than 8 mm (Fig. 1a) are more difficult to biopsy, not reliable on PET, and less likely to be malignant, hence usually followed up with serial CT [11]. For solid nodules, growth is defined as an increase in size >2 mm [17]; the volume doubling time (VDT) of most malignant nodules is between 20 and 400 days [11, 18], with slower growth for pulmonary carcinoid and adenocarcinoma in situ (Fig. 3). For subsolid nodules, growth can be identified also as an increase in density or increase in size of the solid component; their median VDT is generally slower being around 813 days for pure ground-glass, 457 days for part-solid compared to 149 days for solid lesions [19].

Both calcifications and fat can help identify benign nodules particularly pulmonary hamartoma when chondroid calcium shows "popcorn" distribution; prior infections, in particular histoplasmosis and TB, mostly show central, diffuse, or lamellated pattern of calcification. Spiculated or lobular margins (due to growth of malignant cells along the pulmonary interstitium at different rates) and upper lobe location are mostly seen in malignant nodules [8] (Fig. 1d), while typically benign nodules have a well-defined smooth border. Intravenous iodinated contrast can help identify benign from malignant nodules; the latter in fact enhance more than 20 Hounsfield units while benign lesion shows less contrast uptake [20].

CT images can be integrated with Positron Emission Tomography using 18-Fludeoxyglucose (18-FDG PET); this will provide valuable functional information based on the increased glucose uptake and glycolysis of cancer cells. The value

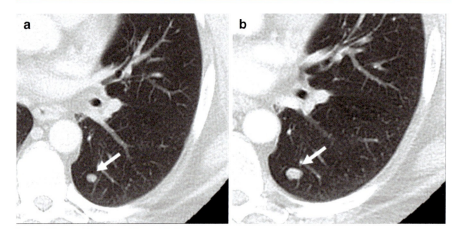

Fig. 3 (**a**) Six millimeter nodule of the posterior segment of the left lower lobe; CT follow-up in 9 months showed increase in size to 9 mm (**b**). Pathology revealed metastatic squamous cell carcinoma

of PET/CT, although limited in solid nodules smaller than 8 mm and in subsolid lesions, is universally accepted in helping to differentiate malignant versus benign nodules and in staging malignant process. The latter in fact are usually not FDG-avid, and in general, a standardized uptake value (SUV) > 2.5 is associated with high likelihood of malignancy [7]. Recent data on PET suggest a sensitivity of 89% and specificity of 75% for detecting cancer [21]; the main limitation on PET/CT is in populations with endemic infectious lung disease because both infection and inflammation can give false-positive results. On the contrary, early stage adenocarcinoma and carcinoid tumors are less metabolically active and can result in false-negative study.

Quantitative predictive models combine clinical information with radiological features of the lung lesion to assess the risk of malignancy; they represent a useful tool for nodules between 8 and 30 mm in size. Older models like the one introduced by the Mayo Clinic in the late 1990s [22] derived data mostly from chest X-ray findings to estimate the probability of malignancy (http://www.chestx-ray.com/index.php/calculators/spn-calculator). The addition of nodule volume to the original six independent predictors (age, history of smoking and cancer, nodule diameter, speculation, and upper lobe location) increased the model accuracy [23]. More recently, the Brock model (http://www.brocku.ca/cancerpredictionresearch) has been validated using the data from the British Columbia Cancer Agency study [8]. This model showed excellent discrimination between benign and malignant lesions even for nodules ≤10 mm when used within a higher-risk population. Incorporating nodule attenuation as a variable, the Brock model has an advantage with early stage adenocarcinoma which often presents as subsolid or part-solid nodule. Similarly, the Veteran Administration Cooperative model, derived from CT or PET data on 375 veterans, performs well within high-risk populations and incorporates time since quitting smoking among the predictors [24].

The diagnostic management of incidental solitary pulmonary nodules needs to be tailored to the individual patient according to the pre-test clinical probability of lung cancer, the individual risk of invasive biopsy or surgery, and most importantly patient preferences [7]. A more aggressive approach aimed to resection of solitary nodules, although exposing patients to the unnecessary surgical risk of removing benign lesions, results in early diagnosis and cure of pre-invasive stage lung cancer associated with 5-year survival up to 80% [11, 25]. Prolonged CT surveillance instead can cause crucial delays in the diagnosis and malignant lesions which might progress to a non-curable stage.

In 2017, the Fleischner Society management updated the guidelines on management of solitary pulmonary nodules [6].

Solid nodules are managed according to their size and the individual risk of lung cancer; for solitary or multiple pulmonary nodules <6 mm (<100 mm^3), no follow-up is required for low-risk patients, while in high-risk individuals, a follow-up CT might be repeated at 12 months in nodules with suspicious morphology and upper lobe location. For single nodules 6–8 mm (100–250 mm^3) in size, an initial follow-up CT is recommended at 6–12 months; in low-risk patients, surveillance can be safely discontinued at 12–18 months if the nodule shows stability. In high-risk patients, repeated imaging at 18–24 months is recommended given an estimated average risk of malignancy of 2% [8]. For same size, multiple nodules, the largest or most suspicious nodule (dominant), should be used as a guide; metastasis should be highly suspected especially with peripheral and lower zones distribution. For this reason, an earlier first follow-up is suggested at 3–6 months. For single nodules >8 mm (>250 mm^3), the risk of malignancy is around 3%; a CT follow-up at 3 months, work-up with PET/CT, and tissue biopsy are all recommended according to size, morphology, and comorbidities.

Single *subsolid nodules* <6 mm (<100 mm^3) in size generally don't require any follow-up, except for extremely suspicious lesions in high-risk patient where surveillance for up to 4 years may be warranted. For pure ground-glass nodules larger than 6 mm, initial follow-up is recommended at 6–12 months (especially for nodules >10 mm and with bubbly lucencies) and thereafter every 2 years until 5 years. Part-solid nodules larger than 6 mm require close follow-up at 3–6 months and then annually for a minimum of 5 years to assess stability of the solid component; when the solid component of a part-solid nodule is larger than 6 mm and growing with suspicious morphology (lobulated margins or cystic component), the likelihood of malignancy and metastasis increases: PET/CT, biopsy, and resection are recommended (Fig. 4). Multiple subsolid nodules, especially if smaller than 6 mm, should be followed up in 3–6 months and most likely are of infectious origin. If at least one nodule is larger than 6 mm and persistent after 3–6 months, the possibility of multiple adenocarcinoma should be considered; decisions should be made according to the progress of the dominant lesion.

Once an incidental pulmonary nodule is diagnosed, the choice is between imaging surveillance and tissue biopsy. FDG PET/CT is useful in refining the probability of malignancy in solid nodules >8 mm (or subsolid with solid component >8 mm)

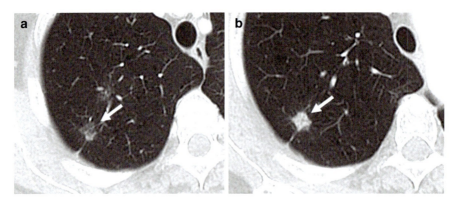

Fig. 4 (**a**) Twelve millimeter ground-glass nodule of the right upper lobe; (**b**) follow-up at 12 months showed increase in both absolute size and size of the solid component

and in staging the mediastinum; it is not helpful in pure ground-glass lesions. FDG-avid nodules should be biopsied; non-avid lesions can be triaged to CT surveillance.

Non-surgical tissue diagnosis is preferred in patients with a nodule at intermediate or high risk of malignancy but who are not surgical candidates for lung resection; non-invasive methods like washing, lavage, or brushing can occasionally be diagnostic of malignancy, but bronchoscopic or transthoracic technique is more often selected according to the nodule location. For large (>20 mm) centrally located lesion, radial endobronchial ultrasound-guided transbronchial biopsy (R-EBUS-TBB) shows a diagnostic sensitivity of 73–85% [27]. Conventional bronchoscopic-guided transbronchial biopsy (TBB) is used where EBUS is not available.

CT-guided transthoracic needle biopsy (TTNB) has sensitivity and specificity >90% and 99% for malignancy even for lesion <10 mm [28]; both core biopsy and needle aspiration are performed at the same time. Almost a third of TTNB will be non-diagnostic for nodules smaller than 6 mm; in this instance, malignancy cannot be excluded and additional biopsies or ongoing CT surveillance is necessary as almost half of those will show cancer [28]. Needle biopsy carries the risk of pneumothorax in up to 17% of cases. This is usually treated conservatively, and a chest tube is needed in only a minority of cases; older patients with emphysema and centrally located lesions are at higher risk [29]. Other possible but rare complications are hemoptysis and other hemorrhage requiring intervention, especially in patients on dual antiplatelet therapy.

When the result of a needle biopsy is inconclusive in patients at intermediate or high risk of lung cancer, surgical wedge biopsy is the gold standard for diagnosis of a solitary pulmonary nodule [30]. Video-assisted thoracoscopy (VATS) is usually the initial approach, especially for peripheral lesions that can be localized by visual inspection; deeper lesions can be challenging to be identified and might require localization technique such as hook wires, micro-coils, or percutaneous injection of methylene blue. When digital palpation is necessary, a mini-thoracotomy and wedge resection is the safer approach. Diagnosis is made by intraoperative frozen section analysis; if positive for non-small cell lung cancer, the gold-standard therapy for stage I and II disease is a radical lobectomy (open or VATS) with mediastinal lymph nodes sampling (at least three stations for N1 and N2 nodes) to complete pathological staging. If the patient's pre-operative respiratory function is limited, an anatomical segmentectomy with lymph node sampling is an alternative therapy. Frozen section is less accurate with lesion <1.1 cm, with early stage pre-invasive adenocarcinoma and with carcinoid tumors. Finally, if the initial frozen section is negative but further formal pathology analysis shows malignancy, a completion lobectomy with curative intent is indicated for stage I and II disease.

Part 2: Intraoperative Pulmonary Lesion

Joseph M. GalanteLuis Godoy, and Anna Xue

Bullous Disease

A lung bulla is defined as an air-space more than 1 cm in diameter regardless of its pathogenesis [31]. Causes of bullous lung disease include cigarette smoking, inhaled drug abuse, alpha-1 antitrypsin deficiency, Marfan syndrome, and Ehlers–Danlos syndrome [32]. Bullous lung disease can be classified into several major categories based on the condition of the surrounding lung parenchyma. Bullous emphysema refers to the formation of bullae that coalesce due to progressive loss of alveolar attachments and form within emphysematous lung parenchyma. Bullae within otherwise normal lungs are often singular and surrounded by morphologically normal lung tissue. These are classified as simple bullae. This category is far less common than bullous emphysema.

Giant bullous emphysema (GBE) or vanishing lung syndrome (VLS), a primary bullous disease of the lung, or Type I bullous disease is defined as a large bulla occupying at least one-third of a hemithorax. This is a rare syndrome with no identifiable underlying etiology [33]. The upper lobes are most often involved, and the presence of subpleural bullae is a dominant feature. It tends to affect younger male smokers usually in their fourth decade. Giant lung bullae have a large impact on respiratory mechanics [34] and make ventilator management difficult in patients undergoing mechanical ventilation.

Even in non-traumatic cases, it is a diagnosis that frequently leads to misperception. Thus, during initial trauma evaluation, where time is of the essence and the team has limited knowledge of the patient's past medical history, GBE can easily be misdiagnosed as pneumothorax. We recommend that in patients who have suspected pneumothorax, if they are clinically stable, imaging studies should be performed prior to any chest tube insertion. Performing CT scans on these patients can avoid catastrophic complications.

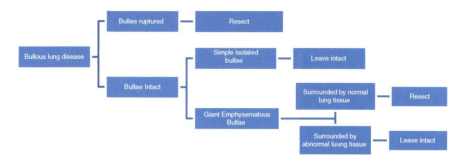

Fig. 5 Proposed algorithm for management of bullous lung disease

When encountered intraoperatively, the operating surgeon should assess the surrounding lung quality as well as whether the bullae are intact or ruptured. Ruptured bullae will inevitably lead to large air leaks, especially in patients requiring ventilator support. If the surrounding lung tissue is of poor quality, we suggest the utilization of reinforced staple loads. If the Bullae are intact and considered simple, we recommend leaving the bullae intact. Giant emphysematous bullae can create a challenge in the post-operative patient. The significant impact on respiratory mechanics can lead to difficulties in ventilator management even when the bullae are intact. If GBE is encountered intraoperatively, we recommend careful evaluation of the surrounding lung parenchyma. If the surrounding lung tissue is normal, then the GBE-affected area can be resected. The elimination of the bullous disease will allow the remaining "normal" lung to expand and may potentially provide a benefit to the patient similar to that seen in lung volume reduction surgery. Often times, however, the surrounding lung parenchyma is also affected. If the bullae are intact and the surrounding lung tissue is diseased, the bullae should be left intact. Resection bullous disease in this setting may lead to prolonged air leaks and a potential for alveolar-pleural fistulization which can be difficult to manage (Fig. 5).

Lung Masses

A lung mass is defined as a growth in the lung parenchyma that is greater than 3 cm in diameter. This should be distinguished from a lung nodule which is 3 cm or less in diameter. Morphologically lung masses can be classified as solid or subsolid. Etiology of lung mass can be either benign or malignant (Table 3) [35].

Given the multitude of possible etiologies of an incidentally identified lung nodule or mass as well as the potential complexity of additional work up including dedicated imaging and follow-up, we recommend consulting chest specialists such as pulmonologists and/or thoracic surgeons. In the emergency setting, lesions that are incidentally found should be resected only if absolutely necessary in order to accomplish the goals of the immediate lifesaving procedure.

Table 3 Malignant and benign lung masses

Malignant	Benign	
Primary lung malignancy	*Infectious granuloma*	*Vascular*
Adenocarcinoma	Coccidioidomycosis	Arteriovenous malformation
Squamous cell carcinoma	Tuberculosis	Hematoma
Small cell carcinoma	Histoplasmosis	Pulmonary infarct
Large cell carcinoma	Cryptococcosis	
Pulmonary carcinoid	Blastomycosis	*Congenital*
		Bronchogenic cyst
Metastatic lesions	*Other infections*	
	Pulmonary abscess/septic emboli	*Inflammatory*
Extranodal lymphoma	Aspergillus	Rheumatoid
	Pneumocystis jirovecii	Sarcoidosis
	Echinococcus cyst	Granulomatosis with polyangiitis
	Ascariasis	
	Benign neoplasm	
	Lipoma	
	Hamartoma	
	Fibroma	
	Neurofibroma	
	Leiomyoma	
	Angioma	
	Schwannoma	

Chronic Effusion/Trapped Lung

Pleural effusions may be found incidentally on imaging as some may be asymptomatic, although patients may also present with dyspnea on exertion, dry cough, and/or pleuritic chest pain. A pleural effusion is an excess accumulation of fluid in the pleural space and may be transudative or exudative. Examples of transudative pleural effusions include heart failure, nephrotic syndrome, hypothyroidism, and hypoalbuminemia. Exudative pleural fluid may be due to malignancy, pneumonia (parapneumonic), tuberculosis, rheumatoid arthritis, and systemic lupus erythematous, among other inflammatory conditions [36]. The Light's criterion (Table 4) is used to determine whether the pleural fluid is exudative versus transudative [37].

CT chest with IV contrast (for patients without renal impairment) is usually the imaging of choice to evaluate pleural effusion and/or trapped lung. Thoracentesis for free-flowing pleural effusions may be attempted with or without image guidance and the fluid sent for cytology, gram stain, and culture. For complex or loculated pleural effusions, pleural effusions with evidence of thick rind, or for patients without symptomatic improvement after thoracentesis, consulting Pulmonology and/or Thoracic Surgery early is recommended as additional interventions including chest tube placement, intrapleural fibrinolytic therapy, and/or surgical decortication, may be indicated [38]. However, in chronic pleural effusion/trapped lung, even if surgical decortication is performed, the lung may not fully re-expand and the patient may not have symptomatic improvement (Fig. 6). In the trauma setting, an incidentally encountered chronic pleural effusion/trapped lung should only be decorticated if decortication will provide the necessary exposure to properly address the traumatic injuries.

Table 4 (*Made by authors*) Differentiating transudative and exudative effusions are critical to diagnosis and treatment of pleural effusions

	Transudate	Exudate
Appearance	Serous	Cloudy
WBC	Low	High
Protein (g/dL)	<3	>3
Protein:serum ratio	<0.5	>0.5
Lactate dehydrogenase (LDH) (IU/L)	Low	High
LDH:serum ratio	High	Low

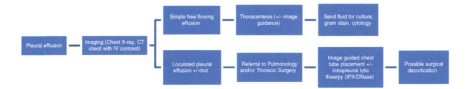

Fig. 6 Management of pleural effusions

Pleural Plaques

Pleural plaques are areas of accumulated hyalinized collagen fibers mostly found on the parietal pleural and are most commonly associated with asbestos exposure [39]. Bilateral pleural plaques, especially, are more likely to be associated with asbestos exposure than unilateral plaques. On chest radiograph, they are characteristically seen along the chest wall and along the diaphragm (Fig. 7) [40]. Prior chest wall trauma, old empyemas/loculated pleural effusions, tuberculosis, and chronic or recurrent hemothoraces may cause a similar appearance on radiograph; however, these can be distinguished from asbestos plaques by histology [41]. The majority of patients with pleural plaques are asymptomatic and are diagnosed incidentally on imaging or during chest surgery. Pleural plaques, however, may be a risk factor for developing cancer in asbestos-exposed patients. In most cases, incidentally encountered pleural plaques in the operating room should not be resected. However, these pleural plaques should be biopsied to rule out possible mesothelioma or other malignancy. Referral to a pulmonologist may also be warranted, and consideration should also be given to undergo formal pulmonary function testing.

Traumatic Pulmonary Pseudocyst

Traumatic pulmonary pseudocysts can develop in the lung parenchyma after chest trauma and appear as cystic or cavitary lesions on chest radiographs or CT scans. They are formed by interlobar interstitial connective tissue without epithelial lining or bronchial wall elements [42]. On CT imaging, they appear as thin-walled cystic lesion(s) with air-space consolidation of the surrounding lung parenchyma [43].

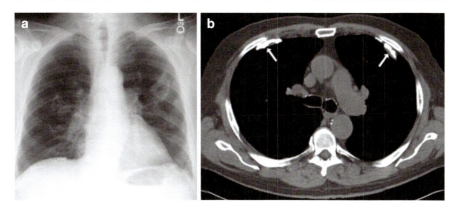

Fig. 7 (**a**) Calcified asbestos-related pleural plaques on frontal chest radiograph. (**b**) Calcified asbestos-related pleural plaques on CT

These pseudocysts are rare and more often seen in children likely due to the physiology of their chest wall compliance allowing a larger transmission of force to the lung parenchyma in blunt injury [44]. Clinically, patients may be asymptomatic, have associated chest pain and hemoptysis, or develop fulminant respiratory failure [45]. When found incidentally, similar appearing lung lesions such as lung abscess, tuberculosis, bronchogenic cyst, pulmonary sequestration, and/or primary lung malignancy should be ruled out. Uncomplicated pseudocysts that are decreasing in size can usually be managed conservatively. However, pseudocysts may rupture or become infected necessitating additional intervention including bronchoscopy, chest tube placement, or antibiotics. Surgery resection usually requiring a lobectomy of the affected lobe is usually reserved for patients with extensive necrotic lung parenchyma, large abscesses, airway hemorrhage, or failure to respond to conservative treatment.

Cavitary Lung Lesions

A lung cavitary lesion is defined radiographically as a lucency contained within an area of pulmonary consolidation, mass, or nodule with thick walls >4 mm (Fig. 8) [46]. Etiology includes both infectious causes such as tuberculosis, lung abscess/necrotizing pneumonia, pulmonary coccidioidomycosis, septic emboli (i.e. from endocarditis), and non-infectious causes such as granulomatosis with polyangiitis, sarcoidosis, rheumatoid arthritis, pulmonary embolism leading to infarction, and malignancy (i.e. bronchogenic carcinoma). If a cavitary lesion is detected on a plain chest radiograph, a subsequent CT chest should be obtained for further evaluation of the lesion. The appearance of the cavitary lesion on imaging studies can assist in determining the etiology of the lesion including wall thickness, location in upper lobes/multiple lobes, and associated mediastinal lymphadenopathy [47]. Additional work up may include respiratory cultures, blood cultures, and antigen/antibody

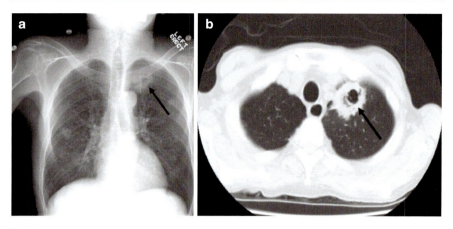

Fig. 8 (**a**) Typical X-ray appearance of a left upper lobe cavitary lesion. (**b**) CT scan showing left upper lobe cavitary lesion

testing. Due to the wide spectrum of both infectious and non-infectious causes of cavitary lung lesions, resection is usually not recommended without an established diagnosis. If encountered incidentally in the operating room, consideration may be given for obtaining microbiological and/or pathological samples of the lesion(s). Subsequent follow-up with chest specialists is recommended.

Empyema

An empyema is an infection of the pleural space with an exudative effusion containing thick pus and fibrin products forming loculations and most often occurs secondary to parapneumonic effusions [48]. Any pleural effusion with presence of bacteria on fluid gram stain or culture is considered to be an empyema. The evolution of a parapneumonic effusion/empyema is in three phases with the first being the exudative stage in which sterile pleural fluid develops due to inflammation. The second phase is the fibrinopurulent stage in which a fibrinous peel develops on the visceral and parietal pleura and affects lung expansion. The third phase is the organizing stage in which there is an ingrowth of fibroblasts and capillaries into the peel [37]. Imaging is crucial in diagnosing empyemas. Plain chest radiographs are often the initial imaging performed with subsequent CT chest with contrast for further evaluation. A "split pleura sign" (Fig. 9) is seen on CT with thickening and enhancement of the visceral and parietal pleura and separation of the pleura by an effusion (Fig. 9) [49]. In the appropriate clinical setting, this sign is highly suggestive of empyema. When an empyema is suspected, broad-spectrum antibiotics should be initiated immediately. Chest tube thoracostomy should also be performed and the pleural fluid sent for gram stain and culture. Administration of intrapleural fibrinolytics (tPA and DNase) via the chest tube is commonly trialed for chemical debridement [50]. Daily plain chest radiographs

Fig. 9 Split pleura sign indicative of loculated empyema

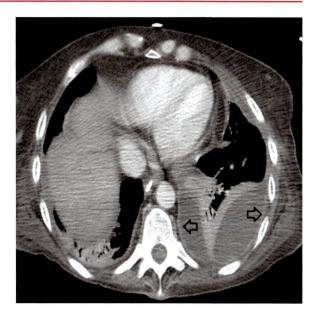

should be obtained to evaluate for radiographic improvement. If there is no radiographic improvement, thoracic surgery should be consulted for consideration of surgical decortication.

Empyema Necessitans

Empyema necessitans is the extension of a pleural infection (i.e. empyema) out of the thoracic cavity and into the adjacent chest wall and surrounding soft tissues [51]. Most commonly, the extension is to the chest wall but can also involve other tissues including pericardium and peritoneum. This is a rare complication and occurs due to inadequate treatment of an empyema or in the setting of prior thoracic surgery or trauma and is most commonly due to *Mycobacterium tuberculosis* [52]. CT chest is the recommended imaging modality to assess the extent of the infection. Due to its appearance, empyema necessitans may be mistaken for an isolated chest wall abscess; however, imaging will classically also demonstrate the presence of an empyema that is communicating with the extra thoracic infection (Fig. 10). Needle aspiration of both the intrapleural and extrapleural lesion may be considered and the aspirate sent for gram stain, culture, and cytology [53]. Chest specialists should be involved early in the management of empyema necessitans. Treatment strategies include antibiotics as well as open or closed drainage and/or surgical decortication to obliterate the infected chest cavity and restore pulmonary function [54]. Clinicians should also rule out primary chest wall lesions and primary lung malignancies which may have similar radiographic appearances.

Massive Hemoptysis

Massive hemoptysis is described as a large amount of expectorated blood or bleeding at a rapid rate and may be a potentially lethal condition that requires immediate attention [55]. There are differences in the criteria used to define massive hemoptysis, but life-threatening hemoptysis is generally considered to be hemoptysis requiring blood transfusion, intubation, airway obstruction, hypoxemia with $PaO_2 < 60$ mmHg, and/or hemodynamic instability [55]. Overall, the risk of mortality from massive hemoptysis is correlated with the rate of bleeding. Prior to undergoing any invasive procedures to control bleeding, the patient's airway should be secured, and the patient should be stabilized. The non-bleeding lung should be protected if possible, however recognizing that this may not be possible in certain trauma patients [56]. Flexible bronchoscopy is the initial diagnostic procedure of choice in massive hemoptysis patients as it is often readily available, can be performed at the bedside, and may localize the site of bleeding [57]. Once the patient is stabilized, consideration should be given to obtain imaging including plain chest radiography and CT as CT can provide information regarding vascular anatomy that may be useful for patients who eventually undergo bronchial artery embolization. Temporizing strategies such as bronchial blocking, balloon tamponade, deploying and inflating PA catheter into smaller bronchi, and endobronchial instillation of hemostatic agents have all been described with varying levels of success [56, 58, 59]. Interventional radiology bronchial artery embolization is now often used in the management of massive hemoptysis with a reported success rate of 60–90% [60, 61]. Surgery is usually reserved for instances when the aforementioned approaches fail and in cases of chest trauma (Fig. 10).

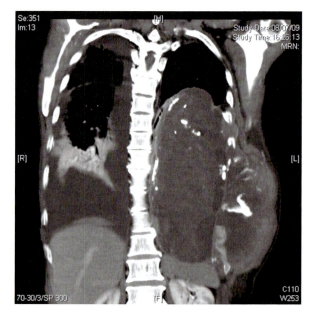

Fig. 10 Empyema necessitans showing communication between intrathoracic empyema and extrathoracic soft tissue. (Courtesy of Dr. J Yeung, Radiopaedia.org, rID: 13415)

Table 5 Intralobar versus extralobar pulmonary sequestration

Features	Intralobar	Extralobar
Frequency	Common, 80% of pulmonary sequestration	Uncommon
Onset	Presents later in childhood or adulthood with recurrent infections	Diagnosed in neonatal period, often incidental but may present with respiratory distress, infection, cyanosis
Gender (male:female)	1:1	4:1
Location	60% left lung, lower lobes (posterior basal segment)	90% left lung, predominantly lower lobes
Pleura	Share common pleura with normal lung parenchyma	Has separate lining of pleura
Arterial supply	70% thoracic aorta	45% thoracic aorta
Venous drainage	Pulmonary veins, but also via azygos, portal vein, superior/inferior vena cava	Most commonly via systemic veins
Associated anomalies	Uncommon	Common

Congenital Pulmonary Sequestration

Congenital pulmonary sequestration is a lung anomaly in which a mass of dysplastic lung tissue develops which does not have a connection with the tracheobronchial tree, has a variant arterial blood supply from the thoracic aorta, the abdominal aorta, intercostal arteries, internal thoracic artery, or subclavian artery, and venous drainage to the pulmonary vessels, the superior/inferior vena cava, or azygos vein [62]. There are two types of pulmonary sequestration, intralobar and extralobar (Table 5) [62–64].

Chest CT is the imaging modality of choice to diagnose and evaluate sequestrations. Angiography is also crucial to evaluate aberrant arterial supply and venous drainage of pulmonary sequestrations. Treatment with surgical resection is recommended for symptomatic patients with recurrent infections, hemoptysis, and/or congestive heart failure. Extralobar sequestrations have separate pleura and can usually be resected while sparing normal lung parenchyma while intralobar sequestration will often require segmentectomy or lobectomy. Pre-operative planning with careful review of angiography is crucial as pre-resection endovascular embolization of aberrant arterial supply may be indicated to avoid catastrophic hemorrhage intraoperatively [34]. This variation in blood supply is important especially in the acute care setting as congenital pulmonary sequestration may be encountered intraoperatively and potentially mistaken for contused or injured lung.

References

1. DeGrauw X, Annest JL, Stevens JA, Xu L, Coronado V. Unintentional injuries treated in hospital emergency departments among persons aged 65 years and older, United States, 2006–2011. J Saf Res. 2016;56:105–9.

2. Andrawes P, Picon AI, Shariff MA, et al. CT scan incidental findings in trauma patients: does it impact hospital length of stay? Trauma Surg Acute Care Open. 2017;2(1):e000101. https://doi.org/10.1136/tsaco-2017-000101.
3. Salim A, Sangthong B, Martin M, Brown C, Plurad D, Demetriades D. Whole body imaging in blunt multisystem trauma patients without obvious signs of injury: results of a prospective study. Arch Surg. 2006;141:468–73.
4. Sampson MA, Colquhoun KB, Hennessy NL. Computed tomography whole body imaging in multi-trauma: 7 years experience. Clin Radiol. 2006;61:365–9.
5. Seah MK, Murphy CG, McDonald S, Carrothers A. Incidental findings on wholebody trauma computed tomography: experience at a major trauma centre. Injury. 2016;47:691–4.
6. MacMahon H, Naidich DP, Goo JM, et al. Guidelines for management of incidental pulmonary nodules detected on CT images: from the Fleischner Society 2017. Radiology. 2017;284(1):228–43. Epub 2017 Feb 23.
7. Gould MK, Donington J, Lynch WR, et al. Evaluation of individuals with pulmonary nodules: when is it lung cancer? Diagnosis and management of lung cancer, 3rd ed: American College of Chest Physicians evidence-based clinical practice guidelines. Chest. 2013;143(5 Suppl):e93S–120S.
8. McWilliams A, Tammemagi MC, Mayo JR, et al. Probability of cancer in pulmonary nodules detected on first screening CT. N Engl J Med. 2013;369(10):910.
9. Cahan WG, Shah JP, Castro EB. Benign solitary lung lesions in patients with cancer. Ann Surg. 1978;187(3):241.
10. Seo JB, Im JG, Goo JM, et al. Atypical pulmonary metastases: spectrum of radiologic findings. Radiographics. 2001;21(2):403.
11. Ost D, Fein AM, Feinsilver SH. Clinical practice. The solitary pulmonary nodule. N Engl J Med. 2003;348(25):2535.
12. Balekian AA, Silvestri GA, Simkovich SM, et al. Accuracy of clinicians and models for estimating the probability that a pulmonary nodule is malignant. Ann Am Thorac Soc. 2013;10(6):629.
13. Trunk G, Gracey DR, Byrd RB. The management and evaluation of the solitary pulmonary nodule. Chest. 1974;66(3):236.
14. Gohagan J, Marcus P, Fagerstrom R, et al. Baseline findings of a randomized feasibility trial of lung cancer screening with spiral CT scan vs chest radiograph: the Lung Screening Study of the National Cancer Institute. Chest. 2004;126(1):114.
15. Henschke CI, Yankelevitz DF, Mirtcheva R, et al. CT screening for lung cancer: frequency and significance of part-solid and nonsolid nodules. AJR Am J Roentgenol. 2002;178(5):1053.
16. Ohtsuka T, Watanabe K, Kaji M, et al. A clinicopathological study of resected pulmonary nodules with focal pure ground-glass opacity. Eur J Cardiothorac Surg. 2006;30(1):160–3. Epub 2006 May 24.
17. Bankier AA, MacMahon H, Goo JM, et al. Recommendations for measuring pulmonary nodules at CT: a statement from the Fleischner Society. Radiology. 2017;285(2):584.
18. Song YS, Park CM, Park SJ, et al. Volume and mass doubling times of persistent pulmonary subsolid nodules detected in patients without known malignancy. Radiology. 2014;273(1):276.
19. Hasegawa M, Sone S, Takashima S, et al. Growth rate of small lung cancers detected on mass CT screening. Br J Radiol. 2000;73(876):1252.
20. Swensen SJ, Viggiano RW, Midthun DE, et al. Lung nodule enhancement at CT: multicenter study. Radiology. 2000;214(1):73.
21. Deppen SA, Blume JD, Kensinger CD, et al. Accuracy of FDG-PET to diagnose lung cancer in areas with infectious lung disease: a meta-analysis. JAMA. 2014;312(12):1227.
22. Swensen SJ, Silverstein MD, Ilstrup DM, et al. The probability of malignancy in solitary pulmonary nodules. Application to small radiologically indeterminate nodules. Arch Intern Med. 1997;157(8):849.
23. Mehta HJ, Ravenel JG, Shaftman SR, et al. The utility of nodule volume in the context of malignancy prediction for small pulmonary nodules. Chest. 2014;145(3):464.

24. Gsould MK, Ananth L, Barnett PG, et al. A clinical model to estimate the pretest probability of lung cancer in patients with solitary pulmonary nodules. Chest. 2007;131(2):383–8.
25. Allen MS, Darling GE, Pechet TT, et al. Morbidity and mortality of major pulmonary resections in patients with early-stage lung cancer: initial results of the randomized, prospective ACOSOG Z0030 trial. Ann Thorac Surg. 2006;81(3):1013.
26. Samet JM, Avila-Tang E, Boffetta P, et al. Lung cancer in never smokers: clinical epidemiology and environmental risk factors. Clin Cancer Res. 2009;15(18):5626–45.
27. Steinfort DP, Khor YH, Manser RL, et al. Radial probe endobronchial ultrasound for the diagnosis of peripheral lung cancer: systematic review and meta-analysis. Eur Respir J. 2011;37(4):902.
28. Fontaine-Delaruelle C, Souquet PJ, Gamondes D, et al. Negative predictive value of transthoracic core-needle biopsy: a multicenter study. Chest. 2015;148(2):472–80.
29. Lee SM, Park CM, Lee KH, et al. C-arm cone-beam CT-guided percutaneous transthoracic needle biopsy of lung nodules: clinical experience in 1108 patients. Radiology. 2014;271(1):291.
30. Allen MS, Deschamps C, Lee RE, et al. Video-assisted thoracoscopic stapled wedge excision for indeterminate pulmonary nodules. J Thorac Cardiovasc Surg. 1993;106(6):1048.
31. Adam A, Dixon AK, Grainger RG, Allison DJ. Grainger & Allison's diagnostic radiology: a textbook of medical imaging. Philadelphia: Churchill Livingstone/Elsevier; 2008.
32. Stern EJ, Webb WR, Weinacker WA, Muller NL. Idiopathic giant bullousemphysema (vanishing lung syndrome): imaging findings in nine patients. AJR. 1994;162:279–82.
33. Fraser RG, Peter Paré JA. Diagnosis of diseases of the chest (Third Edition). Crit Care Med. 1990;18(9):1052.
34. O'Donnell DE, Webb KA, Bertley JC, Chau LK, Conlan AA. Mechanisms of relief of exertional breathlessness following unilateral bullectomy and lung volume reduction surgery in emphysema. Chest. 1996;110(1):18–27.
35. Weinberger S, McDermott S. Diagnostic evaluation of the incidental pulmonary nodule. In: Post TW (Ed). Waltham, MA: UpToDate; 2010.
36. Light RW, Macgregor MI, Luchsinger PC, Ball WC Jr. Pleural effusions: the diagnostic separation of transudates and exudates. Ann Intern Med. 1972;77(4):507–13.
37. Yu H. Management of pleural effusion, empyema, and lung abscess. Semin Intervent Radiol. 2011;28(1):75–86.
38. Karkhanis VS, Jyotsna MJ. Pleural effusion: diagnosis, treatment, and management. Open Access Emerg Med. 2012;4:31–52. https://doi.org/10.2147/OAEM.S2994.
39. Torigian DA, Miller WT. Radiology secrets plus. 3rd ed. St. Louis: Mosby; 2011.
40. Antonietta MM, et al. Incidental and underreported pleural plaques at chest CT: do not miss them-asbestos exposure still exists. BioMed Res Int. 2017;2017:6797826.
41. Wick MR, Allen TC, Ritter JH, Matsubara O. Pseudoneoplastic lesions of the lungs and pleural surfaces, practical pulmonary pathology: a diagnostic approach. 3rd ed. Amsterdam: Elsevier; 2018. p. 643–664.e3.
42. Gupta N, et al. Traumatic pulmonary pseudocyst. Int J Crit Illness Inj Sci. 2013;3(2):155–8.
43. Suchocki PV, Stull MA, Twigg HL, et al. Am J Roentgenol. 1990;154:1323–4.
44. Sorsdahl OA, Powell JW. Cavitary pulmonary lesions following non penetrating chest trauma in children. Am J Roentgenol Radium Therapy Nucl Med. 1965;95:118–24.
45. Chon SH, Lee CB, Kim H, Chung WS, Kim YH. Diagnosis and prognosis of traumatic pulmonary pseudocysts: a review of 12 cases. Eur J Cardiothorac Surg. 2006;29:819–23.
46. Hansell DM, Bankier AA, MacMahon H, McLoud TC, Müller NL, Remy J. Fleischner Society: glossary of terms for thoracic imaging. Radiology. 2008;246(3):697–722.
47. Gadkowski LB, Stout JE. Cavitary pulmonary disease. Clin Microbiol Rev. 2008;21(2):305–33.
48. Ahmed O, Zangan S. Emergent management of empyema. Semin Intervent Radiol. 2012;29(3):226–30.
49. Kraus GJ. The split pleura sign. Radiology. 2007;243(1):297–8.

50. Temes RT, Follis F, Kessler RM, Pett SB Jr, Wernly JA. Intrapleural fibrinolytics in management of empyema thoracis. Chest. 1996;110(1):102–6.
51. Ahmed SI, Gripaldo RE, Alao OA. Empyema necessitans in the setting of pneumonia and parapneumonic effusion. Am J Med Sci. 2007;333(2):106–8.
52. Ho ML, Gutierrez FR. Chest radiography in thoracic polytrauma. AJR Am J Roentgenol. 2009;192(3):599–612.
53. Gomes MM, et al. Empyema necessitans: very late complication of pulmonary tuberculosis. BMJ Case Rep. 2013;2013:bcr2013202072.
54. Akgül AG, Örki A, Örki T, Yüksel M, Arman B. Approach to empymea necessitatis. World J Surg. 2011;35:981.
55. Radchenko C, et al. A systematic approach to the management of massive hemoptysis. J Thorac Dis. 2017;9(Suppl 10):S1069–86.
56. Solomonov A, Fruchter O, Zuckerman T, et al. Pulmonary hemorrhage: a novel mode of therapy. Respir Med. 2009;103:1196–200.
57. Sakr L, Dutau H. Massive hemoptysis: an update on the role of bronchoscopy in diagnosis and management. Respiration. 2010;80:38–58.
58. Jolliet P, Soccal P, Chevrolet JC. Control of massive hemoptysis by endobronchial tamponade with a pulmonary artery balloon catheter. Crit Care Med. 1992;20:1730–2.
59. Tsukamoto T, Sasaki H, Nakamura H. Treatment of hemoptysis patients by thrombin and fibrinogen-thrombin infusion therapy using a fiberoptic bronchoscope. Chest. 1989;96:473–6.
60. Fernando HC, Stein M, Benfield JR, et al. Role of bronchial artery embolization in the management of hemoptysis. Arch Surg. 1998;133:862–6.
61. Fruchter O, Schneer S, Rusanov V, et al. Bronchial artery embolization for massive hemoptysis: long-term follow-up. Asian Cardiovasc Thorac Ann. 2015;23:55–60.
62. Yucel O, Gurkok S, Gozubuyuk A, et al. Diagnosis and surgical treatment of pulmonary sequestration. Thorac Cardiovasc Surg. 2008;56(3):154–7.
63. Micallef SP, Grech V, Sammut P, DeGiovanni JV. 3 year old with chronic wet cough: intralobar bronchopulmonary sequestration. Images Paediatr Cardiol. 2016;18(2):5–10.
64. Gerle R, Jaretzki A, Ashley C, Berne A. Congenital bronchopulmonary-foregut malformation-pulmonary sequestration communicating with the gastrointestinal tract. N Engl J Med. 1968;278:1413–9.

Chylothorax

Laura Godat, Todd W. Costantini, and Kimberly A. Davis

Introduction

Chylothorax is a result of injury to the thoracic duct leading to leakage of chyle or lymph into the chest. Bartolet first described chylothorax in 1633, followed by Quincke's description of the first traumatic chylothorax in 1875 [1]. Eighty years later, in 1953, Bressler et al. [2] described the first chylothorax following esophageal resection. Chyle from the intestines and lymph from the liver, abdominal wall, and bilateral lower extremities drain into the thoracic duct to be carried into circulation at a rate of 1.5–2.5 L a day and as high as 4 L a day depending on diet and medications [1, 3, 4]. Transport of alimentary fats into systemic circulation is a key function of the thoracic duct. Chyle is composed of chylomicrons, triglycerides, cholesterol, fat-soluble vitamins, and albumin. Other components include lymphocytes, immunoglobulins, and digestive enzymes [3]. Thoracic duct injuries leading to chylothorax, though rare, are important to understand as they are associated with significant morbidity and mortality.

The vast majority of "traumatic" thoracic duct injuries are associated with thoracic surgery, mainly esophagectomies. The incidence of chylothorax after esophagectomy ranges from 1 to 9% and carries an associated mortality in more recent studies of up to 29% [5–16]. These iatrogenic cases account for 80% of traumatic thoracic duct injuries, the other 20% are due to non-iatrogenic trauma including

L. Godat · T. W. Costantini (✉)
Division of Trauma, Surgical Critical Care, Burns and Acute Care Surgery, Department of Surgery, University of California-San Diego School of Medicine, San Diego, CA, USA
e-mail: lgodat@ucsd.edu; tcostantini@ucsd.edu

K. A. Davis
Division of General Surgery, Trauma, and Surgical Critical Care, Department of Surgery, Yale School of Medicine, New Haven, CT, USA
e-mail: Kimberly.davis@yale.edu

© Springer Nature Switzerland AG 2021
J. M. Galante, R. Coimbra (eds.), *Thoracic Surgery for the Acute Care Surgeon*, Hot Topics in Acute Care Surgery and Trauma,
https://doi.org/10.1007/978-3-030-48493-4_9

blunt and penetrating injuries [17]. The most common non-traumatic cause of chylothorax is lymphoma [18]. Early recognition and treatment are critical to optimizing outcomes for these patients.

Acute chylothorax results in local respiratory effects due to the resultant pleural effusion and associated atelectasis with presenting symptoms of cough, dyspnea, or chest pain. Rapid loss of chyle can also result in hypovolemia and respiratory distress [3, 19]. Prolonged chylothorax can lead to chronic depletion of chyle which is associated with immunosuppression, due to loss of immunoglobulins, T lymphocytes, and proteins into the pleural space. The chyle itself is bacteriostatic, and though these patients are at increased risk of infections, they rarely have infected effusions [19, 20]. Electrolyte disturbances can include hyponatremia, hypocalcemia, and metabolic acidosis [3, 4, 19].

Anatomy

Thoracic duct anatomy can be variable; therefore, it is important to understand the potential anatomic variations in the treatment of duct injuries that lead to chylothorax. Jean Pecquet discovered the thoracic duct in 1651, describing the true transport system of intestinal chyle [21]. The lymphatic system is made up of lymphatic vessels, lymph nodes, and the cisterna chyli which deliver chyle to the thoracic duct. The thoracic duct is a 2–3 mm structure. From the abdomen it enters the right chest posterior to the median arcuate ligament between the aorta and azygos vein. It then courses cephalad in the aortoesophageal groove of the posterior mediastinum, when at the level of the fourth to sixth thoracic vertebra, it crosses midline to the left [3, 17, 22]. The duct continues cephalad, posterior to the arch of the aorta, then anterior to the left subclavian artery. Next, it makes a turn inferolateral over the anterior scalene inserting into the junction of the left internal jugular and left subclavian vein. This classic description is found in 40–60% [23, 24] of the population. Duct anatomy is variable, and in an anatomic cadaver study, it was found that in seven of eight cadavers, the thoracic duct did not enter the chest as a single duct but formed above the level of the diaphragm from multiple abdominal tributaries [24]. Other anatomic variations include duplication of the duct. Figure 1 demonstrates the basic anatomical variations of the thoracic duct as it ascends the chest.

Etiology

The causes of chylothorax are many and can be divided into traumatic and non-traumatic. The traumatic causes include iatrogenic, mainly thoracic surgical procedures, and non-iatrogenic. Non-iatrogenic causes include penetrating or blunt trauma, or significant coughing or straining. Non-traumatic causes include neoplasms, infectious disease, or other congenital diseases like sarcoidosis [17, 25, 26]. The traditional thought was that lymphomas made up two-thirds of all chylothorax [26–28]. However, in a review of 203 patients by Doerr et al., trauma was found to

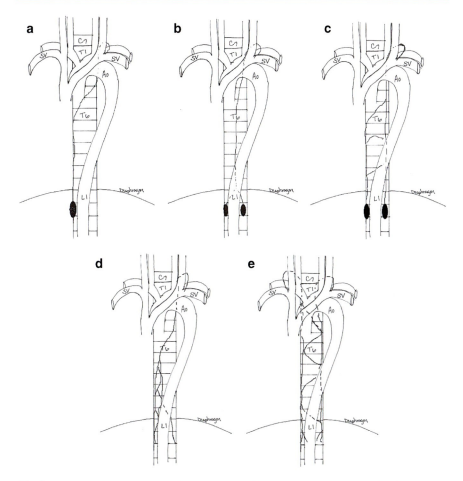

Fig. 1 Anatomic depiction of the thoracic duct and anatomic variations. (**a**) Classic anatomic distribution, (**b–e**) anatomic variations. *SV* subclavian vein, *Ao* aorta, *CC* cisternachyli. (Artwork by LN Godat. Adapted from Chalret du Rieu et al. [3] and Defize et al. [23])

cause nearly 50% of chylothorax, and only 17% were due to malignancies, a majority of which were due to lymphoma. The overwhelming majority of traumatic chylothorax were due to surgical procedures, including central line insertion [26]. Table 1 lists multiple potential causes for chylothorax.

Diagnosis

Presenting symptoms for patients with chylothorax are non-specific and include dyspnea, chest pain, cough, and the presence of a pleural effusion on chest imaging. Diagnosis of chylothorax requires sampling of the pleural fluid, either via thoracentesis or chest tube drainage (Table 2). Chylothorax should be considered for any

Table 1 Causes of chylothorax [17, 19, 26]

Traumatic		Non-traumatic	
Non-iatrogenic	Iatrogenic	Malignancy	Diseases
• Stab wounds • Gun shot wounds • Childbirth • Forceful emesis or cough • Blunt chest trauma • Blunt spine trauma • Weight-lifting • Yawning	• Thoracic surgery • Mediastinal excisions • Sympathectomy • Esophagectomy • Head and neck surgery • Radical neck dissection • Cervical lymph node biopsy • Radiation • Central venous catheterization • Pacemaker insertion • Congenital heart surgery	• Lymphomas • Chronic lymphocytic leukemia • Metastatic disease	• Sarcoidosis • Hemangiomatosis • Lymphangioleiomyomatosis • Filariasis • Amyloidosis • Tuberculosis • Retrosternal goiter • Superior vena cava obstruction • Congenital lymphatic disorders • Benign tumors • Congestive heart failure • Chylous ascites • Idiopathic

Table 2 Characteristics of pleural fluid in chylothorax

Color	Milky/serosanguinous
Cell differential	Lymphocytes predominate
Chylomicrons	Present
LDH	Low
Protein	High
Pleural triglycerides	>110 mg/dL
Pleural fluid: Serum triglycerides	>1.0
Pleural cholesterol	<200 mg/dL

pleural effusion that is milky in appearance; however, not all chylothorax will have the same appearance as the character of chyle can be altered by dietary fat consumption. The presence of hemothorax can also obscure the diagnosis of chylothorax as the pleural fluid may have a bloody character. Chylous effusions contain chylomicrons in the pleural fluid by definition. Diagnostic criteria for chylothorax using pleural fluid analysis include pleural fluid triglyceride levels >110 mg/dL. Pleural fluid cholesterol level of <200 mg/dL is consistent with chylothorax and favors against pseudochylothorax [29]. A ratio of pleural fluid to serum triglycerides >1.0 is also diagnostic of a chylothorax [22].

Imaging

Multiple different imaging techniques may be utilized to diagnose and/or attempt to localize the source of thoracic duct leak causing chylothorax [30]. Chest X-ray can identify the presence of pleural effusion and follow its drainage and potential recurrence. It can also be used to follow the position of drainage catheters or tubes during routine drainage of the effusion. Chest X-ray cannot differentiate between simple pleural effusion, hemothorax, and chylothorax. Ultrasound also cannot differentiate chylothorax from a simple pleural effusion nor detect the source of chyle leakage but can be useful for image-guided drainage of the pleural effusion.

Several imaging modalities can be considered to localize and map the lymphatics. Lymphangiography can be performed to access the lymphatic tree for subsequent imaging. This invasive imaging technique requires expertise to either cannulate the pedal lymphatics or an inguinal lymph node. Most commonly, ultrasound guidance is utilized to access the inguinal lymph node for injection of oil-based contrast material that is subsequently visualized using fluoroscopy or magnetic resonance lymphangiography [31, 32]. These imaging techniques are often able to identify the site of chyle leak or identify variations in lymphatic anatomy that can guide interventions aimed at treating the chyle leak [33]. Magnetic resonance imaging (MRI) can be used to map the lymphatic system when conventional lymphangiography fails. Standard MRI can identify the thoracic duct and cisterna chyli in most patients and potentially provides valuable anatomic information for planning operative intervention in patients with chylothorax.

Treatment

Non-surgical Management

Initial treatment of the chylothorax is directed at drainage of the pleural effusion to help relieve the symptoms of dyspnea and to allow lung re-expansion. As chyle is not a viscous fluid, appropriate chest drainage can be accomplished using small bore chest tubes or pigtail catheters (<20 French) [34]. Non-operative treatment of chylothorax focuses on limiting chyle production through dietary modifications while the pleural effusion is drained from the chest. Daily chest tube outputs should be measured to assess for improvement in chyle drainage and the potential need to escalate therapy for non-resolving chylothorax. In many patients, spontaneous closure of the lymphatics can occur with subsequent resolution of the chylous effusion. Prior studies have demonstrated variable success rates after treatment with non-surgical management with chylothorax resolution ranging from 28 to 100% [9, 14, 35–38].

Dietary modifications can be initiated for patients with chylothorax to attempt to decrease chyle production. Initial conservative treatment should focus on dietary modifications to limit fat intake as decreased intake of long-chain triglycerides can decrease the production of chyle [39]. If dietary modifications are unsuccessful, patients may be kept *nil per os* (NPO) while placing them on total parenteral nutrition (TPN) to address their nutritional needs. Adjuncts such as octreotide or somatostatin have been used as adjuncts to attempt to speed the closure of the chyle leak [40]. Octreotide has been shown to reduce lymphatic fluid excretion and has been shown in small series to promote resolution of chyle drainage in refractory chylothorax in the pediatric population [41, 42].

Chemical pleurodesis can also be considered for patients with persistent chylothorax or for those patients that are not good operative candidates. Use of chemical agents such as talc has been demonstrated to have good efficacy in resolving chylothorax by eliminating the potential space for the chyle to collect in the pleural space [43].

Surgical Management

Traditionally, the main indication for surgical intervention is failure of medical management, which may be difficult to define [44]. The timing of surgical intervention is also of some debate, with increasing interest in earlier intervention. A recent study from the Mayo Clinic supports the idea of early reoperation [45], based on the observation that 89% of patients with chylothorax after esophagectomy eventually required operative intervention. Recognizing that it is very difficult to predict whether a chylous leak would spontaneously heal, early surgical repair may be the treatment of choice to prevent the complications associated with chyle leaks including fat depletion, dehydration, hypoproteinemia, loss of fat-soluble vitamins, and immunologic compromise within 8 days despite optimal supportive care [46]. Techniques to control chyle leaks focus on disruption of the thoracic duct proximal to the area of leak or injury. They range in invasiveness from percutaneous embolization of the thoracic duct, to minimally invasive techniques including thoracoscopic and laparoscopic approaches, all the way to thoracotomy or laparotomy.

Reoperation is recommended in case of persistent leak rates greater than 1000 mL/day over 5 days of strict starvation, failure of the chyle output to decrease over a 2-week period, evidence of loculated chylothorax with fibrin clots and incarcerated lungs, or the presence of nutritional or metabolic complications [47]. However, immediate reoperation may be indicated to expedite recovery and minimize hospital stay if chest tube drainage is more than 500 mL during the first 24 h after complete oral intake cessation and TPN [48–52]. Prompt surgical intervention should also be considered as sufficient T-cell depletion to cause immunosuppression occurs within 8 days of chyle drainage [53]. Results of surgery are much poorer when nutritional and metabolic complications have set in [11].

Thoracic Duct Embolization

Thoracic duct embolization (TDE) to treat chylothorax is increasingly utilized. Access to the lymphatic system is either via pedal lymphangiography or ultrasound-guided intranodal lymphangiography followed by trans-abdominal catheterization of the cisterna chyli. Using this access, a catheter is advanced into the thoracic duct. Contrast is then injected through the catheter to confirm the site of injury or leak [54]. The thoracic duct is embolized below the leak [55]. The embolization is performed using a combination of platinum embolization coils and N-BCA glue

(Trufill, Cordis, Hialeah, Florida, USA) [55]. The success rate varied from 77 to 84% [56]. This approach may be associated with chronic diarrhea or abdominal swelling as a delayed complication in up to 15% cases [57].

In cases in which thoracic duct catheterization is technically unsuccessful, thoracic duct needle disruption can be performed as previously described [38, 58]. Using this technique, the retroperitoneal lymphatics are disrupted using "twiddling motion with the needle" [58]. Traumatic disruption of the lymphatic vessels results in controlled venous bleeding into the lymphatic vessels with subsequent formation of blood clots and local inflammation, which close the leak.

Video-Assisted Thoracoscopic Ligation

Video assisted thoracoscopic surgical (VATS) techniques may represent a good alternative to thoracotomy in the treatment of chylothorax. This technique offers easier access to the entire pleural cavity without the potential morbidity of thoracotomy. Clips are applied to the thoracic duct at the level of the aortic hiatus or to the specific site of thoracic duct injury. Mass ligature of the tissue in the region of the thoracic duct may also be performed with large clips. VATS can also be used for chemical pleurodesis, fibrin glue application, or high-frequency ultrasonic coagulation of the thoracic duct without clipping [59]. However, VATS is not always an applicable method as the patients may not always tolerate one lung anesthesia due to their comorbidities. In some cases, postoperative adhesions may limit exposure in the operating field, especially when the surgery is delayed [60].

Thoracotomy

The classic surgical approach is thoracotomy, usually on the right side, with ligation of the thoracic duct at the aortic hiatus as described by Lampson [61]. Ligation of the thoracic duct at this level has the advantage of stopping flow from any damaged accessory ducts that might not have been recognized. In a unilateral chylothorax, the chest is best approached from the side of the effusion. Pleurectomy and mechanical pleurodesis have been described as complementary procedures to surgical ligation. These procedures may disrupt the collateral subpleural or intercostal lymphatic network leading to an intractable chyle leak [50, 62, 63].

Transabdominal Approaches

Transabdominal ligation of the thoracic duct can be associated with lower morbidity [64]. The method of ligation by the abdominal route has been well described by Schumacher et al. [65]. Because the thoracic duct is fragile, the fibro-fatty tissue between the aorta and the azygos vein should be included in the ligation. Two or three sutures are often required, as there may be two to three channels just above the cisterna chyli [7]. There has also been a recent case report using laparoscopic thoracic duct clipping for persistent chylothorax after extrapleural pneumonectomy which supports use of the abdominal route as potential access to ligate the duct with less morbidity [66].

Complications

Drainage of chyle into the pleural space can lead to several adverse sequelae. First, high output chylothorax can be associated with hypovolemia due to the potentially significant (>1 L/day) volume loss associated with larger effusions. As chyle fluid is rich in fat, protein, and electrolytes, persistent chylothorax can lead to malnutrition. Adequate nutritional support during treatment of chylothorax is required to replace electrolyte imbalance, vitamin deficiency, and to provide adequate caloric support [67]. Chylothorax can be associated with decreased immune function due to persistent loss of T-lymphocytes and immunoglobulins into the pleural space. This relative immunosuppression can predispose patients with chylothorax to infectious complications [68]. Finally, Yellow Nail syndrome is a rare complication of chyle leak and chylothorax. This syndrome, classified by the presence of yellow nails, extremity lymphedema, and pleural effusions, occurs as a result of poor lymphatic drainage.

Conclusion

Initial efforts at diagnosing and treating chylothorax are directed at chest tube drainage to relieve respiratory symptoms caused by the pleural effusion. Non-surgical treatments for chylothorax can include dietary modifications directed at limiting lymph flow. Pleurodesis is a frequently utilized adjunct to limit the potential space for chylothorax to collect. Many patients will require surgical management that includes thoracic duct embolization or ligation using either minimally invasive or open surgical techniques. Chylothorax should be treated aggressively to limit dehydration, electrolyte abnormalities, malnutrition, and immune consequences that occur in patients with ongoing chyle leak.

References

1. Wemyss-Holden SA, Launois B, Maddern GJ. Management of thoracic duct injuries after oesophagectomy. Br J Surg. 2001;88(11):1442–8.
2. Bressler S, Wiener D, Thompson SA. Traumatic chylothorax following esophageal resection. J Thorac Surg. 1953;26(3):321–4.
3. Chalret du Rieu M, Baulieux J, Rode A, Mabrut JY. Management of postoperative chylothorax. J Visc Surg. 2011;148(5):e346–52.
4. Sriram K, Meguid RA, Meguid MM. Nutritional support in adults with chyle leaks. Nutrition. 2016;32(2):281–6.
5. Brinkmann S, Schroeder W, Junggeburth K, Gutschow CA, Bludau M, Hoelscher AH, et al. Incidence and management of chylothorax after Ivor Lewis esophagectomy for cancer of the esophagus. J Thorac Cardiovasc Surg. 2016;151(5):1398–404.
6. Lai FC, Chen L, Tu YR, Lin M, Li X. Prevention of chylothorax complicating extensive esophageal resection by mass ligation of thoracic duct: a random control study. Ann Thorac Surg. 2011;91(6):1770–4.
7. Mishra PK, Saluja SS, Ramaswamy D, Bains SS, Haque PD. Thoracic duct injury following esophagectomy in carcinoma of the esophagus: ligation by the abdominal approach. World J Surg. 2013;37(1):141–6.

8. Shah RD, Luketich JD, Schuchert MJ, Christie NA, Pennathur A, Landreneau RJ, et al. Postesophagectomy chylothorax: incidence, risk factors, and outcomes. Ann Thorac Surg. 2012;93(3):897–903; discussion 904.
9. Dugue L, Sauvanet A, Farges O, Goharin A, Le Mee J, Belghiti J. Output of chyle as an indicator of treatment for chylothorax complicating oesophagectomy. Br J Surg. 1998;85(8):1147–9.
10. Rao DV, Chava SP, Sahni P, Chattopadhyay TK. Thoracic duct injury during esophagectomy: 20 years experience at a tertiary care center in a developing country. Dis Esophagus. 2004;17(2):141–5.
11. Merigliano S, Molena D, Ruol A, Zaninotto G, Cagol M, Scappin S, et al. Chylothorax complicating esophagectomy for cancer: a plea for early thoracic duct ligation. J Thorac Cardiovasc Surg. 2000;119(3):453–7.
12. Alexiou C, Watson M, Beggs D, Salama FD, Morgan WE. Chylothorax following oesophagogastrectomy for malignant disease. Eur J Cardiothorac Surg. 1998;14(5):460–6.
13. Bolger C, Walsh TN, Tanner WA, Keeling P, Hennessy TP. Chylothorax after oesophagectomy. Br J Surg. 1991;78(5):587–8.
14. Cerfolio RJ, Allen MS, Deschamps C, Trastek VF, Pairolero PC. Postoperative chylothorax. J Thorac Cardiovasc Surg. 1996;112(5):1361–5; discussion 5–6.
15. Hulscher JB, van Sandick JW, de Boer AG, Wijnhoven BP, Tijssen JG, Fockens P, et al. Extended transthoracic resection compared with limited transhiatal resection for adenocarcinoma of the esophagus. N Engl J Med. 2002;347(21):1662–9.
16. Kranzfelder M, Gertler R, Hapfelmeier A, Friess H, Feith M. Chylothorax after esophagectomy for cancer: impact of the surgical approach and neoadjuvant treatment: systematic review and institutional analysis. Surg Endosc. 2013;27(10):3530–8.
17. Pillay TG, Singh B. A review of traumatic chylothorax. Injury. 2016;47(3):545–50.
18. Hillerdal G. Chylothorax and pseudochylothorax. Eur Respir J. 1997;10(5):1157–62.
19. McGrath EE, Blades Z, Anderson PB. Chylothorax: aetiology, diagnosis and therapeutic options. Respir Med. 2010;104(1):1–8.
20. Dumont AE, Mayer DJ, Mulholland JH. The suppression of immunologic activity by diversion of thoracic duct lymph. Ann Surg. 1964;160:373–83.
21. Pecquet J. New anatomical experiments. London: Octavian; 1653.
22. Nair SK, Petko M, Hayward MP. Aetiology and management of chylothorax in adults. Eur J Cardiothorac Surg. 2007;32(2):362–9.
23. Johnson OW, Chick JF, Chauhan NR, Fairchild AH, Fan CM, Stecker MS, et al. The thoracic duct: clinical importance, anatomic variation, imaging, and embolization. Eur Radiol. 2016;26(8):2482–93.
24. Defize IL, Schurink B, Weijs TJ, Roeling TAP, Ruurda JP, van Hillegersberg R, et al. The anatomy of the thoracic duct at the level of the diaphragm: a cadaver study. Ann Anat - Anatomischer Anzeiger. 2018;217:47–53.
25. Talwar A, Lee HJ. A contemporary review of chylothorax. Indian J Chest Dis Allied Sci. 2008;50(4):343–51.
26. Doerr CH, Allen MS, Nichols FC III, Ryu JH. Etiology of chylothorax in 203 patients. Mayo Clin Proc. 2005;80(7):867–70.
27. Sassoon CS, Light RW. Chylothorax and pseudochylothorax. Clin Chest Med. 1985;6(1):163–71.
28. Valentine VG, Raffin TA. The management of chylothorax. Chest. 1992;102(2):586–91.
29. Staats BA, Ellefson RD, Budahn LL, Dines DE, Prakash UB, Offord K. The lipoprotein profile of chylous and nonchylous pleural effusions. Mayo Clin Proc. 1980;55(11):700–4.
30. Expert Panel on Vascular Imaging and Interventional Radiology, Majdalany BS, Murrey DA Jr, Kapoor BS, Cain TR, et al. ACR Appropriateness Criteria((R)) chylothorax treatment planning. J Am Coll Radiol. 2017;14(5S):S118–S26.
31. Kiang SC, Ahmed KA, Barnes S, Abou-Zamzam AM Jr, Tomihama RT. Direct contrast-enhanced magnetic resonance lymphangiography in the diagnosis of persistent occult chylous effusion leak after thoracic duct embolization. J Vasc Surg Venous Lymphat Disord. 2019;7(2):251–7.

32. Nadolski G. Nontraumatic chylothorax: diagnostic algorithm and treatment options. Tech Vasc Interv Radiol. 2016;19(4):286–90.
33. Jayasinghe SA, Srinivasa RN, Hage AN, Gemmete JJ, Majdalany BS, Chick JFB. Thoracic duct embolization: analysis of practice patterns. Ann Vasc Surg. 2018;52:168–75.
34. Light RW. Pleural controversy: optimal chest tube size for drainage. Respirology. 2011;16(2):244–8.
35. Graham DD, McGahren ED, Tribble CG, Daniel TM, Rodgers BM. Use of video-assisted thoracic surgery in the treatment of chylothorax. Ann Thorac Surg. 1994;57(6):1507–11; discussion 11–2.
36. Marts BC, Naunheim KS, Fiore AC, Pennington DG. Conservative versus surgical management of chylothorax. Am J Surg. 1992;164(5):532–4; discussion 4–5.
37. Cope C. Management of chylothorax via percutaneous embolization. Curr Opin Pulm Med. 2004;10(4):311–4.
38. Itkin M, Kucharczuk JC, Kwak A, Trerotola SO, Kaiser LR. Nonoperative thoracic duct embolization for traumatic thoracic duct leak: experience in 109 patients. J Thorac Cardiovasc Surg. 2010;139(3):584–9; discussion 9–90.
39. Takuwa T, Yoshida J, Ono S, Hishida T, Nishimura M, Aokage K, et al. Low-fat diet management strategy for chylothorax after pulmonary resection and lymph node dissection for primary lung cancer. J Thorac Cardiovasc Surg. 2013;146(3):571–4.
40. Bryant AS, Minnich DJ, Wei B, Cerfolio RJ. The incidence and management of postoperative chylothorax after pulmonary resection and thoracic mediastinal lymph node dissection. Ann Thorac Surg. 2014;98(1):232–5; discussion 5–7.
41. Bellini C, Cabano R, De Angelis LC, Bellini T, Calevo MG, Gandullia P, et al. Octreotide for congenital and acquired chylothorax in newborns: a systematic review. J Paediatr Child Health. 2018;54(8):840–7.
42. Roehr CC, Jung A, Proquitte H, Blankenstein O, Hammer H, Lakhoo K, et al. Somatostatin or octreotide as treatment options for chylothorax in young children: a systematic review. Intensive Care Med. 2006;32(5):650–7.
43. Cho HJ, Kim DK, Lee GD, Sim HJ, Choi SH, Kim HR, et al. Chylothorax complicating pulmonary resection for lung cancer: effective management and pleurodesis. Ann Thorac Surg. 2014;97(2):408–13.
44. Misthos P, Kanakis MA, Lioulias AG. Chylothorax complicating thoracic surgery: conservative or early surgical management? Updat Surg. 2012;64(1):5–11.
45. Sieczka EM, Harvey JC. Early thoracic duct ligation for postoperative chylothorax. J Surg Oncol. 1996;61(1):56–60.
46. Machleder HI, Paulus H. Clinical and immunological alterations observed in patients undergoing long-term thoracic duct drainage. Surgery. 1978;84(1):157–65.
47. Merrigan BA, Winter DC, O'Sullivan GC. Chylothorax. Br J Surg. 1997;84(1):15–20.
48. Haniuda M, Nishimura H, Kobayashi O, Yamanda T, Miyazawa M, Aoki T, et al. Management of chylothorax after pulmonary resection. J Am Coll Surg. 1995;180(5):537–40.
49. Le Pimpec-Barthes F, D'Attellis N, Dujon A, Legman P, Riquet M. Chylothorax complicating pulmonary resection. Ann Thorac Surg. 2002;73(6):1714–9.
50. Fahimi H, Casselman FP, Mariani MA, van Boven WJ, Knaepen PJ, van Swieten HA. Current management of postoperative chylothorax. Ann Thorac Surg. 2001;71(2):448–50; discussion 50–1.
51. Orringer MB, Bluett M, Deeb GM. Aggressive treatment of chylothorax complicating transhiatal esophagectomy without thoracotomy. Surgery. 1988;104(4):720–6.
52. Paul S, Altorki NK, Port JL, Stiles BM, Lee PC. Surgical management of chylothorax. Thorac Cardiovasc Surg. 2009;57(4):226–8.
53. Breaux JR, Marks C. Chylothorax causing reversible T-cell depletion. J Trauma. 1988;28(5):705–7.
54. Nadolski G, Itkin M. Thoracic duct embolization for the management of chylothoraces. Curr Opin Pulm Med. 2013;19(4):380–6.

55. Nadolski GJ, Itkin M. Feasibility of ultrasound-guided intranodal lymphangiogram for thoracic duct embolization. J Vasc Interv Radiol. 2012;23(5):613–6.
56. Chen E, Itkin M. Thoracic duct embolization for chylous leaks. Semin Intervent Radiol. 2011;28(1):63–74.
57. Laslett D, Trerotola SO, Itkin M. Delayed complications following technically successful thoracic duct embolization. J Vasc Interv Radiol. 2012;23(1):76–9.
58. Cope C, Kaiser LR. Management of unremitting chylothorax by percutaneous embolization and blockage of retroperitoneal lymphatic vessels in 42 patients. J Vasc Interv Radiol. 2002;13(11):1139–48.
59. Takeo S, Yamazaki K, Takagi M, Nakashima A. Thoracoscopic ultrasonic coagulation of thoracic duct in management of postoperative chylothorax. Ann Thorac Surg. 2002;74(1):263–5.
60. Kanakis MA, Misthos P, Kokotsakis JN, Lioulias AG. Chylothorax complicating thoracic aortic surgery. J Card Surg. 2011;26(4):410–4.
61. Lampson RS. Traumatic chylothorax; a review of the literature and report of a case treated by mediastinal ligation of the thoracic duct. J Thorac Surg. 1948;17(6):778–91.
62. Akaogi E, Mitsui K, Sohara Y, Endo S, Ishikawa S, Hori M. Treatment of postoperative chylothorax with intrapleural fibrin glue. Ann Thorac Surg. 1989;48(1):116–8.
63. Mares DC, Mathur PN. Medical thoracoscopic talc pleurodesis for chylothorax due to lymphoma: a case series. Chest. 1998;114(3):731–5.
64. Mason PF, Ragoowansi RH, Thorpe JA. Post-thoracotomy chylothorax—a cure in the abdomen? Eur J Cardiothorac Surg. 1997;11(3):567–70.
65. Schumacher G, Weidemann H, Langrehr JM, Jonas S, Mittler J, Jacob D, et al. Transabdominal ligation of the thoracic duct as treatment of choice for postoperative chylothorax after esophagectomy. Dis Esophagus. 2007;20(1):19–23.
66. Tsubokawa N, Hamai Y, Hihara J, Emi M, Miyata Y, Okada M. Laparoscopic thoracic duct clipping for persistent chylothorax after extrapleural pneumonectomy. Ann Thorac Surg. 2012;93(5):e131–2.
67. Servelle M, Nogues C, Soulie J, Andrieux JB, Terhedebrugge R. Spontaneous, post-operative and traumatic chylothorax. J Cardiovasc Surg. 1980;21(4):475–86.
68. Wasmuth-Pietzuch A, Hansmann M, Bartmann P, Heep A. Congenital chylothorax: lymphopenia and high risk of neonatal infections. Acta Paediatr. 2004;93(2):220–4.

Part II

Trauma

Rib Fractures and Chest Wall Injury

Federico Coccolini, Michelle Hamel, Francesco Favi, and John Mayberry

Demographics, Epidemiology and Clinical Significance

Rib fractures are one of the most common injuries found in blunt chest trauma occurring in 10% of all trauma patients and 30% of patients with significant thoracic trauma [1]. The majority of rib fractures are associated with blunt traumatic mechanisms like motor vehicle crashes and falls, but less commonly with repetitive muscle contraction that occurs during athletic activity and heavy lifting or with prolonged coughing [2–4]. Multiple complications are associated with rib fractures including pneumonia, hemothorax, pneumothorax, acute respiratory distress syndrome (ARDS), solid organ injury, acute and chronic pain, decreased quality of life and prolonged disability [5–8]. More than a third of patients with rib fractures suffer complications, and patients are more likely to experience complications with increased age (>65 years), ≥3 rib fractures, chronic lung disease, use of anticoagulation, oxygen saturation <90% on admission, higher injury severity score (ISS) or lower rib fractures [9–12]. Overall mortality from rib fractures is 12% and is higher in elderly patients (22%) [1, 6]. Patients are more likely to die from rib fractures with older age (≥45 years), multiple rib fractures, and pre-existing heart or lung disease and if the patient develops pneumonia [13, 14].

F. Coccolini (✉)
General, Emergency and Trauma Surgery, Pisa University Hospital, Pisa, Italy

M. Hamel
Acute Care Surgery, Sharp Memorial Hospital, San Diego, CA, USA
e-mail: Michelle.Hamel@sharp.com

F. Favi
General, Emergency and Trauma Surgery, Bufalini Hospital, Cesena, Italy

J. Mayberry
Acute Care Surgery, Sharp Memorial Hospital, San Diego, CA, USA

St Lukes Wood River Medical Center, Ketchum, ID, USA
e-mail: john.mayberry@idahosurgeons.net

Chest Wall Injury Biomechanics

Upon inspiration, 12 pairs of ribs pivot upwards and outwards, the sternum rises anteriorly and superiorly, and the diaphragms contract inferiorly to expand the chest cavity. This biomechanical coordination of the thoracic skeleton, the layered intercostal muscles, the diaphragm and the external muscles of respiration is remarkably complex and discriminatory. Intrathoracic pressure produced by the chest wall and diaphragms fluctuates a mere 2–3 cm water during quiet breathing and 50–300 cm water during exertion and reaches heights of 400 cm water during a Valsalva manoeuvre or cough.

The chest wall consists of skin and subcutaneous tissues, muscle, bone, numerous medium-sized arteries and veins, numerous medium-sized peripheral nerves and a myriad of tiny nerve tendrils. The ribs hinge posteriorly on the transverse processes of the vertebral bodies by 'rotating' and 'gliding' joints with minuscule synovial capsules enveloped with a lattice of fine ligaments [15] (Fig. 1a). The sternum hinges at the manubriosternal symphysis and articulates with the cartilaginous distal ends of ribs 2–6 via synovial plane joints reinforced by sternocostal ligaments (Fig. 1b). The costal cartilage of ribs 7–10 articulate with each other also via plane synovial joints [15]. The chest wall has natural elastic recoil that returns the thoracic cavity to its resting state when the muscles of respiration relax.

Blunt force to the chest wall creates contusions and hematomas, tears subcutaneous tissue and intercostal muscle, bruises and lacerates intercostal vessels, injures nerve tissue and fractures the ribs, sternum, clavicle and scapula. Ribs fracture by compression deformation, both direct, e.g. during a side-impact motor vehicle crash (MVC), and indirect, e.g. during a frontal-impact MVC or cardiopulmonary resuscitation (CPR) [16–18]. The area most vulnerable to direct compression is the lateral ribs 60° from the sternum [16] (Fig. 2). Ribs 4–9 are the most commonly fractured [19]. During a frontal impact or CPR, indirect anterior lateral and lateral rib fractures begin to occur at 20% of sternal deflection [17].

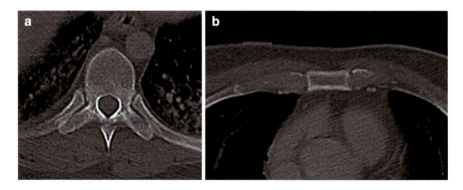

Fig. 1 (**a**) The rib heads articulate with the transverse processes and the vertebral bodies via 'rotating' and 'gliding' joints. (**b**) The cartilaginous ends of ribs 2–6 articulate with the sternum via synovial plane joints

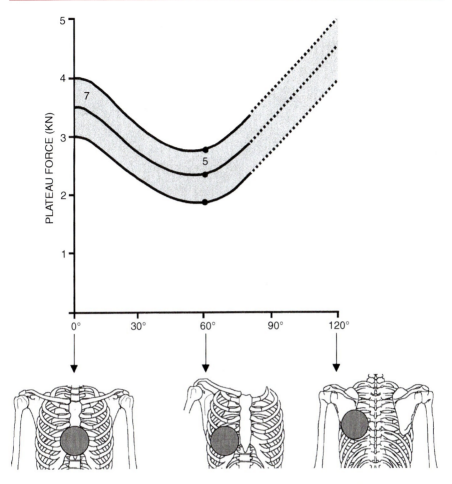

Fig. 2 The ribs are most vulnerable to fracture 60° from the sternum. (Reproduced with permission from Viano D, Lau I, Asbury C, King A, Bergman P. Biomechanics of the human chest, abdomen, and pelvis in lateral impact. Accid Anal & Prev 1989;21:553–74)

During an MVC, chest restraints commonly abrade and bruise the chest wall significantly, i.e. 'seatbelt sign', and fracture the left upper and right lower ribs along their path [20]. The addition of a frontal airbag significantly reduces the percentage of MVC victims who suffer rib fractures [20]. The ipsilateral clavicle and/or the scapula are also often fractured during high-energy blunt trauma [21, 22]. The combination of ipsilateral clavicle fracture and flail chest can lead to significant chest wall deformity [23]. The 'chest wall implosion syndrome' occurs when blunt force trauma centres on the scapula thereby forcing the underlying ribs inward and creating a posterior flail chest [24].

There is significant functional reserve in a healthy individual should one hemithorax become dysfunctional due to injury. Although most patients with significant flail chest, especially with underlying pulmonary contusion, are at risk for

Fig. 3 This young woman with severe blunt force trauma focused to the left chest did not seek medical attention for several days in spite of a nearly nonfunctional left hemithorax

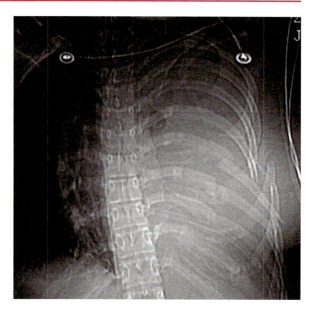

progressive respiratory failure, many can compensate (Fig. 3). This is likewise true for those with smaller amounts of unilateral chest wall tissue loss, i.e. 'open pneumothorax.' Victims of significant chest wall tissue loss, however, are at high risk of respiratory failure and death.

Children's ribs are resistant to fractures because of their elasticity. Thus an infant or toddler with rib fractures, especially posteriorly, for which a simple mechanism is reported may be a victim of abuse [25, 26]. Rib fractures in older children and adolescents are an indication of significant chest wall deflection and portend a much higher risk of cardiopulmonary and visceral injury [27, 28]. With age, ribs become less elastic and more prone to fracture. Osteoporotic individuals are especially prone. It is not unusual for an elderly or osteoporotic patient to sustain multiple rib fractures from a low energy mechanism such as a same level fall or coughing [2, 29].

Stress rib fractures, including the first rib, can result from throwing, rowing, volleyball or tennis activities in athletes with healthy bone [30]. It has been theorized that a microfracture initially occurs which is worsened with repetitive training.

Sternal Fractures

The sternum is neither easily nor commonly fractured [31, 32]. A focused blow to the midsternum, however, e.g. striking the steering wheel during a low-speed MVC, the horizontal bar during a gymnastics manoeuvre, the weight bar during lifting or being struck by a baseball, occasionally results in a sternal fracture (authors' personal experience). Most sternal fractures are nondisplaced and clinically inconsequential [33]. Occasionally sternal fractures present completely displaced (Fig. 5) and in the most severe cases can be comminuted, include disruption of the manubrial clavicular or sternocostal joints, and present as an open fracture with tissue loss. Of consequence to patients with concomitant thoracic spine fractures, a sternal fracture can contribute to instability of the thoracic spine [34].

The associated risk of blunt cardiac injury (BCI) with sternal fracture ranges from 2 to 40% depending on the use of the 'pan CT scan' for fracture detection and the BCI definition [35–37]. Overall ISS rather than fracture displacement seems to be the most important risk factor [35, 36]. Screening for BCI among patients with sternal fracture, following the Eastern Association for the Surgery of Trauma (EAST) guidelines, should consist of electrocardiogram (ECG) and troponin I [37].

Chest Wall Trauma Scoring Systems

Four main rib fracture scoring systems have been developed. All encompass the different aspects of chest trauma: clinical, radiological and anatomical. None consider all aspects together nor have been definitively validated. The main concern regarding the different scoring systems is the heterogeneity they introduce in describing the fracture pattern, the non-prognostic value in fixation necessity and the scarce relation to outcomes.

Organ Injury Scale

The Organ Injury Scale (OIS) was developed by the American Association for the Surgery for Trauma (AAST) [38]. It describes the anatomy of the lesions and stratifies the different patterns according to the anatomical severity.

Rib Fracture Score

The Rib Fracture Score involves three variables: the number of fractures, patient age and the presence of bilateral fractures [39]. The calculation derives from the following: (breaks × sides) + age factor (50–60 years = 1 point, 61–70 years = 2 points, 71–80 years = 3 points, and >80 years = 4 points). The primary ideation was intended to have a tool to triage older patients. Subsequent trials validating this score, however, have given scarce results linked to clinical activity [40].

Chest Trauma Score

The Chest Trauma Score incorporates four parameters: patient age (1–3 points), pulmonary contusion (0–3 points), number of rib fractures (1–3 points) and bilateral fractures (2 points) [41]. Validation attempts show the Chest Trauma Score doesn't differ significantly from the Chest Wall OIS and Rib Fracture Score [42].

Rib Score

The Rib Score was developed with the intention to create a total radiographic score [43]. Six radiographic variables are considered: ≥6 total fractures; ≥3 fractures with bi-cortical displacement; radiographic flail segment; at least one fracture in each anatomic region, anterior, lateral, and posterior, defined by anterior and posterior axillary lines; first rib fracture; and bilateral rib fractures. To each parameter is assigned 1 point; the score ranges from 0 to 6.

Clinical Rib Score

The Clinical Rib Score includes eight parameters: paradoxical respiration, increased depth of respiration, dullness to percussion, rib crunching, tachypnoea, chest tenderness and subcutaneous emphysema [44]. According to the likelihood ratio (LR) of degree of association with mortality, a score was given to each parameter (LR 1–2 was assigned 1 point, LR 2–3 was assigned 2 points, and LR > 3 was assigned 3 points). This score has yet to be validated.

Surgical Management

Over the last few decades, conservative management has been considered standard of care for rib fracture management. Pain control, respiration exercises (incentive spirometer) and pulmonary toilet have had good to excellent results in the majority of patients.

Rib fractures, with or without respiratory dysfunction, lung contusion, pneumonia, chronic chest wall deformities or chronic pain, can diminishment in quality of life or impact work status. Surgical stabilization of rib fractures (SSRF) is controversial, but the primary management goal is to prevent or minimize associated complications. SSRF may, in selected patients, improve clinical outcomes [45]. Published reports present evidence that suggest advantages of SSRF compared to conservative management for flail chest, multiple severe rib fractures, chest wall deformities, lung herniation and chronic nonunion [45]. SSRF, however, is not uniformly performed, due to lack of scientific evidence, clear indications and surgeon skill. Currently three randomized trials of flail chest SSRF published between 2002 and 2013 have concluded that SSRF is superior to non-operative management in terms of mortality, dependence on mechanical ventilation, ICU length of stay, tracheostomy need, pneumonia, and cost savings [46–48]. SSRF within 72 h may result in the best outcomes [49, 50].

In 2017, Kasotakis et al. reviewed the literature to propose guidelines from Eastern Association for the Surgery of Trauma [51]. Two different questions were postulated: The first question is whether operative fixation was better than non-operative management in adult patients with fail chest after blunt trauma regarding mortality, ventilator, ICU LOS and hospital LOS, incidence of pneumonia and need for tracheostomy, and pain control. The second question was postulated with the same outcomes in adult patients with multiple ribs fracture (nonflail). The authors concluded that operative management was superior for flail chest in adults but did not recommend surgical stabilization in patients affected by multiple rib fractures without flail chest. Pieracci et al. in 2018 showed how outcomes could be improved if patients underwent surgery within first 72 h; this strategy is based on anticipating or preventing the worst evolution of thoracic injuries [49]. As described above, surgical techniques are variable worldwide and await technological improvements. No single technique is considered superior to others.

There are four main concepts of successful SSRF: anatomic reduction, stable fixation, blood supply preservation, and early patient mobilization. Considering the anatomy and physiology of chest wall and respiration, it is widely agreed that surgery should be performed for fixation of broken ribs between the 3rd and the 10th. The last two pairs do not participate in breathing (11th and 12th) or are challenging to expose [50]. In the presence of 'flail segments' or floating segments (two fractures on the same rib), it would be best to fix both fractures. However, if the fixation of both fractures is not possible, the second suboptimal option would be to fix at least one of them and transform the flail chest in a mono-focal fracture that impairs less the ventilator dynamic. Those fractures for which fixation is not possible without increasing risks of undue morbidity and not substantially enhance the stability may not require surgical fixation.

Two main relative contraindications to rib fixation are described: pulmonary contusion and traumatic brain injury. The exact role of pulmonary contusion in the indications for SSRF is not well defined. In fact discordant results are reported. Regarding traumatic brain injuries, no indication can be given because of the dominating role of the severe brain trauma in the ultimate outcome.

Patient Positioning and Incision

Three different patient positions are described for access to chest wall: prone position, lateral decubitus and supine position. The position in which patients should be operated depends mainly on the fracture pattern and associated lesions. Lateral decubitus is a traditional position in thoracic surgery; it allows good exposure of lateral aspect of the thoracic wall and usually gains access to anterolateral segment of ribs. Generally, the incision with this positioning is the usual thoracotomy incision following the costal disposition. Supine position is often used for fixation of third, fourth and fifth ribs in anterior and anterolateral fractures patterns. The patient is usually flat on the back with the ipsilateral arm abducted to 90°. A bump can assist in exposing more anterolateral fractures. Skin incision is made over the inframammillary line, which results especially in female patients with better aesthetic results. Moreover this incision can be easily extended across the sternal midline or to the axilla as needed.

Prone position is chosen when ribs injured are posterior or infrascapular. In this position lateral and superior rotation of the scapula may help in improving exposure. Skin incision is calibrated over the 'auscultatory triangle'; it is formed by superior border of *latissimus dorsi*, infero-lateral border of *trapezius* and inferomedial borders of *scapula* and *rhomboid major*; as physicians use it for auscultation of the lung, surgeon use its borders to access to ribs avoiding major sections of posterolateral muscles of the thoracic wall. This positioning technique is well suited for posterior and posterolateral fractures.

Exposition and Fracture Reduction

All fractures require a minimum of 3 cm of exposure on either side of the fracture lines (both the inner and outer table of the fracture line should be considered in preparing the bones to be reconstructed). General agreement exists regarding muscle-sparing philosophy, compared to the traditional routes of access during pulmonary surgery, and fixation of rib fractures requires calibrated incisions on the fracture site, also aimed at minimizing surgical invasiveness in a population of patients already severely affected [52].

The main rule to consider whatever device is used for ORIF is to keep at least 2–2.5 cm from the costo-condral and costo-vertebral junctions. Cartilage is not effective for plate and screw fixation and is dangerous in terms of post-operative morbidity or failure. Providing the correct incision is used, fracture reduction is usually easier the earlier the intervention. Each individual fracture site should be realigned. It is important is to keep in mind that the anterior and the posterior cortical fracture lines are not always at the same level. A good exposure allows the surgeon to visualize both sides of the fracture.

A thoracoscopic, mini-invasive approach is recently postulated as a good alternative, thanks to its better view of fracture's foci (especially in posterior and/or subscapular fractures), hemothorax and/or under-vision drain placement or intercostal local anaesthesia [53].

Once realigned fixation devices should be placed in and secured to the ribs (Fig. 4). Independently from the fixation system utilized, the important part of this phase of intervention is the stabilization of hardware before proceeding to permanently fix it to the bones. Stabilizing devices before fixing them is vital to preserve the fracture reduced in line and to preserve the blood supply to the ends of the fracture. If plate and screws are used, attention should be posed to the length of the screw. A rib thickness measurement should be performed on the CT scan. Too-long screws in fact will pass through the ribs and will damage the lung; too short as a counterpart will not fix the plates. Bi-cortical screws would be the best option whenever possible. Particular attention should be posed when operating on older patients as ribs change in thickness along their course and tend to be more brittle.

Chest wall soft tissues should be sutured by layers, trying to not leave empty spaces that may favour collections. In reducing seroma risk, drain positioning may

Fig. 4 Thoracic wall fixation in a patient kept in spontaneous breathing for cervical spine (C2) fracture; fixation was done with a combination of sedation and loco-regional anaesthesia

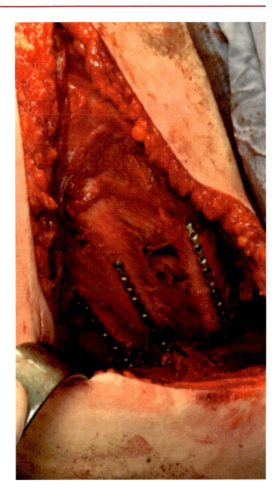

help. The layer-by-layer suturing may help in restoring blood supply to the dissected tissues.

Post-operative complications after ribs fixation are difficult to be evaluated, because patients are already affected or at risk of worse evolution from the trauma itself. One of the most important complications is the infection of the fixation systems or the failure in stabilizing the chest wall because of technical mistakes in positioning.

Sternal Fracture ORIF

The vast majority of simple and most displaced sternal fractures heal without complication. Indications for surgical stabilization include persistent painful displacement, concern about chronic sternal deformity, comminuted fractures, open fractures, associated vertebral column fracture and nonunions [54–58] (Fig. 5).

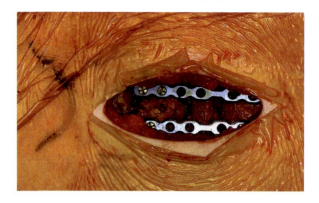

Fig. 5 Typical appearance of reduced sternomanubrial fracture fixated with locking bicortical titanium plates

Morbidly obese patients pose a potential risk for plate failure since they may be unable to mobilize from a recumbent to a standing position without placing extreme stress on their sternum from bearing their weight on their arms and shoulders during the change in position (author personal experience).

Rib and Sternal Fracture Nonunions

The risk of development of nonunions or malunions of rib and sternal fractures is believed to occur at the same rate as bony nonunions elsewhere, i.e. 2–9%, depending on injury severity and patient comorbidities [59–63]. Injury severity factors include displacement, comminution, extensive soft tissue damage, bone loss, contamination and infection [62–64]. Comorbid risk factors include smoking, advanced age, malnutrition, diabetes mellitus, peripheral vascular disease, rheumatoid arthritis and vitamin D deficiency [64, 65]. Nonsteroidal anti-inflammatory agents (NSAIDs) may impede fracture healing, although in our practices, we allow for short-term use [65]. Rib and sternal fracture nonunion stabilization is occasionally indicated for select patients with persistent pain, instability and/or deformities.

Chest Wall Injury Reconstruction

Thoracic wall reconstruction is not uncommonly performed electively for oncological disease of the thorax (i.e. thoracic wall cancer, chest wall invasion from lung cancers, congenital aplasia or trauma) [66]. Recently technological improvements permit surgeons to perform chest wall reconstruction using prosthetic materials either synthetic either biological. Biological prostheses could be a valid alternative other than anatomical flaps in thoracic wall reconstruction in contaminated or potential contaminated fields [67] (Fig. 6).

Fig. 6 Thoracic wall reconstruction with bio-prosthesis in infected field with bony necrosis

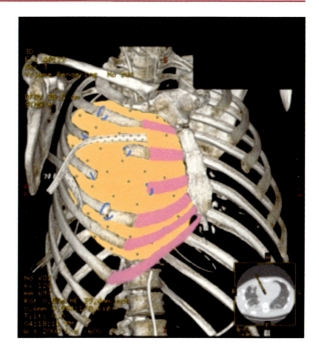

References

1. Ziegler DW, Agarwal NN. The morbidity and mortality of rib fractures. J Trauma. 1994;37(6):975–9.
2. Hanak V, Hartman TE, Ryu JH. Cough-induced rib fractures. Mayo Clin Proc. 2005;80(7):879–82.
3. Moore RS. Fracture of the first rib: an uncommon throwing injury. Injury. 1991;22(2):149–50.
4. Miles JW, Barrett GR. Rib fractures in athletes. Sports Med. 1991;12(1):66–9.
5. Flagel BT, Luchette FA, Reed RL, et al. Half-a-dozen ribs: the breakpoint for mortality. Surgery. 2005;138(4):717–23.
6. Bulger EM, Arneson MA, Mock CN, Jurkovich GJ. Rib fractures in the elderly. J Trauma. 2000;48(6):1040–6.
7. Rostas JW, Lively TB, Brevard SB, Simmons JD, Frotan MA, Gonzalez RP. Rib fractures and their association with solid organ injury: higher rib fractures have greater significance for solid organ injury screening. Am J Surg. 2017;213(4):791–7.
8. Majercik S, Cannon Q, Granger SR, VanBoerum DH, White TW. Long-term patient outcomes after surgical stabilization of rib fractures. Am J Surg. 2014;208(1):88–92.
9. Battle CE, Hutchings H, James K, Evans PA. The risk factors for the development of complications during the recovery phase following blunt chest wall trauma: a retrospective study. Injury. 2013;44(9):1171–6.
10. Shulzhenko NO, Zens TJ, Beems MV, et al. Number of rib fractures thresholds independently predict worse outcomes in older patients with blunt trauma. Surgery. 2017;161(4):1083–9.
11. Brasel KJ, Guse CE, Layde P, Weigelt JA. Rib fractures: relationship with pneumonia and mortality. Crit Care Med. 2006;34(6):1642–6.

12. Dhillon TS, Galante JM, Salcedo ES, Utter GH. Characteristics of chest wall injuries that predict postrecovery pulmonary symptoms: a secondary analysis of data from a randomized trial. J Trauma Acute Care Surg. 2015;79(2):179–86.
13. Battle CE, Hutchings H, Evans PA. Risk factors that predict mortality in patients with blunt chest wall trauma: a systematic review and meta-analysis. Injury. 2012;43(1): 8–17.
14. Holcomb JB, McMullin NR, Kozar RA, Lygas MH, Moore FA. Morbidity from rib fractures increases after age 45. J Am Coll Surg. 2003;196(4):549–55.
15. Moore K, Dalley A, Agur A, editors. 'Thorax'. Clinically orientated anatomy. 8th ed. Philadelphia: Wolters Kluwer; 2018. p. 290–318.
16. Viano D, Lau I, Asbury C, King A, Bergman P. Biomechanics of the human chest, abdomen, and pelvis in lateral impact. Accid Anal Prev. 1989;21:553–74.
17. Kent R, Bass C, Woods W, Sherwood C, et al. Muscle tetanus and loading condition effects on the elastic and viscous characteristics of the thorax. Traffic Inj Prev. 2003;4:297–314.
18. Kashigawa Y, Sasakawa T, Tampo A, et al. Computed tomography findings of complications resulting from cardiopulmonary resuscitation. Resuscitation. 2015;88:86–91.
19. Livingston D, Shogan B, John P, Lavery R. CT diagnosis of rib fractures and the prediction of acute respiratory failure. J Trauma. 2008;64:905–11.
20. Crandall J, Kent R, Patrie J, Fertile J, Martin P. Rib fracture patterns and radiologic detection – a restraint-based comparison. 44th Annual Proceedings, Association for the Advancement of Automotive Medicine, 2000. p 235–59.
21. Stahl D, Ellington M, Brennan K, Brennan M. Association of ipsilateral rib fractures with displacement of midshaft clavicle fractures. J Orthop Trauma. 2017;31:225–8.
22. Chysou K, Halat G, Hoksch B, Schmid R, Kocher G. Lessons from a large trauma center: impact of blunt chest trauma in polytrauma patients – still a relevant problem? Scan J Trauma Resusc Emerg Med. 2017;25:42–7.
23. Langenbach A, Pinther M, Krinner S, Grupp S, Ekkernkamp A, Hennig F, Schulz-Drost S. Surgical stabilization of costoclavicular injuries – a combination of flail chest injuries and a clavicula fracture. Chirurgia. 2017;112:595–606.
24. Solberg B, Moon C, Nissim A, Wilson M, Margulies D. Treatment of chest wall implosion injuries without thoracotomy: technique and clinical outcomes. J Trauma. 2009;67: 8–13.
25. Kleinman P, Schlesinger A. Mechanical factors associated with posterior rib fractures: laboratory and case studies. Pediatr Radiol. 1997;27:87–91.
26. Ouyang J, Zhao W, Xu Y, Chen W, Zhong S. Thoracic impact testing of pediatric cadaveric subjects. J Trauma. 2006;61:1492–500.
27. Kessel B, Dagan J, Swaid F, et al. Rib fractures: comparison of associated injuries between pediatric and adult population. Am J Surg. 2014;208:831–4.
28. Rosenberg G, Bryant A, Davis K, Schuster K. No breakpoint for mortality in pediatric rib fractures. J Trauma Acute Care Surg. 2016;80:427–32.
29. Vana P, Mayberry J, Luchette F. Management and complications of rib fractures in older adults. Curr Geriatr Rep. 2016;5:25–30.
30. Talbot B, Gange C, Chaturvedi A, Klionsky N, Hobbs S, Chaturvedi A. Traumatic rib injury: imaging pitfalls, complications, and treatment. Radiographics. 2017;37:628–51.
31. von Garrel T, Ince A, Junge A, Schnabel M, Bahrs C. The sternal fracture: radiographic analysis of 200 fractures with special reference to concomitant injuries. J Trauma. 2004;57: 837–44.
32. Yeh D, Hwabejire J, DeMoya M, Alam H, King D, Velmahos G. Sternal fracture – an analysis of the National Trauma Data Bank. J Surg Res. 2014;186:39–43.
33. Perez M, Rodriguez R, Baumann B, et al. Sternal fracture in the age of pan-scan. Injury. 2015;46:1324–7.
34. Watkins R, Watkins R, Williams L, et al. Stability provided by the sternum and rib cage in the thoracic spine. Spine. 2005;30:1238–86.
35. Heidelberg L, Uhlich R, Bosarge P, Kerby J, Hu P. The depth of sternal fracture displacement is not associated with blunt cardiac injury. J Surg Res. 2019;235:322–8.

36. Odell D, Peleg K, Givon A, et al. Sternal fracture: isolated lesion versus polytrauma from associated extrasternal injuries – analysis of 1,867 cases. J Trauma Acute Care Surg. 2013;75:448–52.
37. Clancy K, Velopulos C, Bilaniuk J, et al. Screening for blunt cardiac injury: an Eastern Association for the Surgery of Trauma practice management guideline. J Trauma Acute Care Surg. 2012;73:S301–6.
38. Injury scoring scale: a resource for trauma care professionals. http://www.aast.org/library/traumatools/injuryscoringscales.aspx. Accessed Aug 2019.
39. Easter A. Management of patients with multiple rib fractures. Am J Crit Care. 2001;10(5):320–7.
40. Maxwell CA, Mion LC, Dietrich MS. Hospitalized injured older adults: clinical utility of a rib fracture scoring system. J Trauma Nurs. 2012;19(3):168–74.
41. Pressley CM, Fry WR, Philp AS, Berry SD, Smith RS. Predicting outcome of patients with chest wall injury. Am J Surg. 2012;204(6):910–3.
42. Chen J, Jeremitsky E, Philp F, Fry W, Smith RS. A chest trauma scoring system to predict outcomes. Surgery. 2014;156(4):988–93.
43. Chapman BC, Herbert B, Rodil M, et al. RibScore: a novel radiographic score based on fracture pattern that predicts pneumonia, respiratory failure, and tracheostomy. J Trauma Acute Care Surg. 2016;80(1):95–101.
44. Manay P, Satoskar R, Karthik V, Prajapati R. Studying morbidity and predicting mortality in patients with blunt chest trauma using a novel clinical score. J Emerg Trauma Shock. 2017;10(3):128–33.
45. Pharaon KS, Marasco S, Mayberry J. Rib fractures, flail chest, and pulmonary contusion. Curr Trauma Rep. 2015;4:237–42.
46. Tanaka H, Yukioka T, Yamaguti Y, Shimizu S, Goto H, Matsuda H, Shimazaki S. Surgical stabilization of internal pneumatic stabilization? A prospective randomized study of management of severe flail chest patients. J Trauma. 2002;52(4):727–32; discussion 732.
47. Granetzny A, Abd El-Aal M, Emam E, Shalaby A, Boseila A. Surgical versus conservative treatment of flail chest. Evaluation of the pulmonary status. Interact Cardiovasc Thorac Surg. 2005;4(6):583–7.
48. Marasco SF, Davies AR, Cooper J, Varma D, Bennett V, Nevill R, Lee G, Bailey M, Fitzgerald M. Prospective randomized controlled trial of operative rib fixation in traumatic flail chest. J Am Coll Surg. 2013;216(5):924–32.
49. Pieracci FM, Coleman J, Ali-Osman F, Mangram A, Majercik S, White TW, Jeremitsky E, Doben AR. A multicenter evaluation of the optimal timing of surgical stabilization of rib fractures. J Trauma Acute Care Surg. 2018;84(1):1–10.
50. de Campos JRM, White TW. Chest wall stabilization in trauma patients: why, when, and how? J Thorac Dis. 2018;10(Suppl 8):S951–62. https://doi.org/10.21037/jtd.2018.04.69.
51. Kasotakis G, Hasenboehler EA, Streib EW, Patel N, Patel MB, Alarcon L, Bosarge PL, Love J, Haut ER, Como JJ. Operative fixation of rib fractures after blunt trauma: a practice management guideline from the Eastern Association for the Surgery of Trauma. J Trauma Acute Care Surg. 2017;82(3):618–26.
52. Greiffenstein P, Tran MQ, Campeau L. Three common exposures of the chest wall for rib fixation: anatomical considerations. J Thorac Dis. 2019;11(Suppl 8):S1034–43. https://doi.org/10.21037/jtd.2019.03.33.
53. Pieracci FM. Completely thoracoscopic surgical stabilization of rib fractures: can it be done and is it worth it? J Thorac Dis. 2019;11(Suppl 8):S1061–9. https://doi.org/10.21037/jtd.2019.01.70.
54. Mayberry J, Ham L, Schipper P, Ellis T, Mullins R. Surveyed opinion of American trauma, orthopedic, and thoracic surgeons on rib and sternal fracture repair. J Trauma. 2009;66:875–9.
55. Divisi D, Di Leonardo G, Crisci R. Surgical management of traumatic isolated sternal fracture and manubriosternal dislocation. J Trauma Acute Care Surg. 2013;75:824–9.
56. Schulz-Drost S, Mauerer A, Grupp S, Hennig F, Blanke M. Surgical fixation of sternal fractures: locked plate fixation by low-profile titanium plates – surgical safety through depth limited drilling. Int Orthop. 2014;38:133–9.

57. Zhao Y, Yang Y, Gao Z, Wu W, He W, Zhao T. Treatment of traumatic sternal fractures with titanium plate internal fixation: a retrospective study. J Cardiothorac Surg. 2017;12:22–6.
58. Krinner S, Grupp S, Oppel P, Langenbach A, Hennig F, Schulz-Drost S. Do low profile implants provide reliable stability in fixing the sternal fractures as a "fourth vertebral column" in sternovertebral injuries? J Thorac Dis. 2017; https://doi.org/10.21037/jtd.2017.03.37.
59. Mills L, Aitken S, Simpson A. The risk of non-union per fracture: current myths and revised figures from a population of over 4 million adults. Acta Orthop. 2017;88:343–9.
60. Fabricant L, Ham B, Mullins RJ, Mayberry J. Prospective clinical trial of resection of painful rib fracture nonunions. Am Surg. 2014;80:580–6.
61. Severson E, Thompson C, Resig S, Swiontkowski M. Transverse sternal nonunion, repair and revision: a case report and review of the literature. J Trauma. 2009;66:1485–8.
62. McKee R, Whelan D, Schemitsch E, McKee M. Operative versus nonoperative care of displaced midshaft clavicular fractures: a meta-analysis of randomized clinical trials. J Bone Joint Surg Am. 2012;94:675–84.
63. Kardalani A, Granhed H, Karrholm J, Styf J. The influence of fracture etiology and type on fracture healing: a review of 104 consecutive tibial fractures. Arch Orthop Trauma Surg. 2001;121:325–8.
64. Pharaon S, Schoch S, Marchand L, Mirza A, Mayberry J. Orthopaedic traumatology: fundamental principles and current controversies for the acute care surgeon. Trauma Surg Acute Care Open. 2018;3:1–8.
65. Jeffcoach D, Sams V, Lawson C, et al. Nonsteroidal anti-inflammatory drugs' impact on nonunion and infection rates in long-bone fractures. J Trauma Acute Care Surg. 2014;76:779–83.
66. Zardo P, Zhang R, Wiegmann B, Haverich A, Fischer S. Biological materials for diaphragmatic repair: initial experiences with the PeriGuard Repair Patch®. Thorac Cardiovasc Surg. 2011;59(1):40–4. https://doi.org/10.1055/s-0030-1250499. Epub 2011 Jan 17.
67. Coccolini F, Lotti M, Bertoli P, Manfredi R, Piazzalunga D, Magnone S, Campanati L, Ansaloni L. Thoracic wall reconstruction with Collamend® in trauma: report of a case and review of the literature. World J Emerg Surg. 2012;7(1):39. https://doi.org/10.1186/1749-7922-7-39.

Pneumothorax and Hemothorax

R. Stephen Smith, Erin Vanzant, and Fausto Catena

Incidence and Etiology

Thoracic injury is second only to traumatic brain injury as the leading cause of death secondary to injury. Thoracic injury is responsible for at least 25% of deaths resulting from trauma, and it is a contributing factor in another 25%. Associated extra-thoracic injuries are very common when significant chest wall injury is found. Rib fractures, one of the most common manifestations of thoracic wall injury, are frequently encountered in victims of trauma. Rib fractures are frequently associated with hemothorax and pneumothorax and are a frequent cause of chronic disability. For example, 94% of severely or fatally injured restrained passengers in motor vehicle crashes are found to have rib fractures.

Spontaneous pneumothorax typically occurs in tall, slender, male cigarette smokers who are younger than 40 years of age; this condition occurs secondary to distal airway inflammation and obstruction, which produces emphysematous changes. Patients with underlying pulmonary disease such as chronic obstructive pulmonary disease, malignancy, tuberculosis, idiopathic pulmonary fibrosis, cystic fibrosis, and sarcoidosis are at increased risk for spontaneous pneumothorax. In addition, pneumothorax commonly develops after a blunt chest injury, and the risk of hemothorax following chest wall injury is directly proportional to the number of ribs fractured; patients with two or more rib fractures have an incidence of hemothorax as high as 80%. Nontraumatic hemothorax is relatively uncommon and is usually secondary to associated intrathoracic pathology, such as tumors or severe pulmonary infections, which may cause erosion of thoracic vessels. The

---

R. S. Smith (✉) · E. Vanzant
University of Florida, Gainesville, FL, USA
e-mail: Robert.Smith@surgery.ufl.edu; Erin.Vanzant@surgery.ufl.edu

F. Catena
Emergency Surgery Department, Parma University Hospital, Parma, Italy

© Springer Nature Switzerland AG 2021
J. M. Galante, R. Coimbra (eds.), *Thoracic Surgery for the Acute Care Surgeon*, Hot Topics in Acute Care Surgery and Trauma,
https://doi.org/10.1007/978-3-030-48493-4_11

development of pleural effusion is relatively common in a wide variety of infectious, inflammatory, or malignant states. Medical anticoagulation or coagulopathy makes hemothorax more likely to occur following minor injury.

Chest Wall Injury

Associated Injuries

Up to 25% of patients with chest wall injuries have one or more associated injuries. Fractures of the first and second ribs, scapula, and sternum have long been associated with significant intrathoracic injury. This association is less prominent than previously thought, but fractures of these robust boney structures indicate that a great deal of kinetic energy has been transmitted to the thorax. Underlying pulmonary contusion is frequently associated with blunt chest wall trauma, and sternal fractures may be associated with cardiac contusion. Pneumothorax and hemothorax are frequently associated injuries.

The geriatric patient tolerates chest wall injury, pneumothorax, and hemothorax poorly. Concomitant cardiorespiratory comorbidities such as COPD and reduced physiologic reserves make this population ill-equipped to handle the stress of thoracic injury. Elderly patients with relatively minor chest wall injury may develop respiratory compromise soon after injury, but very frequently develop progressive respiratory insufficiency over the initial 48–72 hour after injury. Such patients should be closely observed in a monitored area for respiratory deterioration. In the pediatric population, the rib cage is extremely pliable. Therefore, pediatric patients may have significant intrathoracic injury in the absence of rib or sternal fractures, and the severity of their intrathoracic injuries may be missed.

Physical Examination and Initial Management

Inspection of the chest wall should be carried out during the initial evaluation of an injured patient. Auscultation is a mandatory component of an initial evaluation, and pulse oximetry should be used during the evaluation of all seriously injured patients. Special attention should be paid to abrasions, contusions, lacerations, or any deformity of the chest wall; asymmetric chest wall motion during respiration, paradoxical movement of the chest wall, and splinting are indicative of flail chest. Palpation of the chest wall may reveal crepitance or point tenderness associated with either rib or sternal fractures. The presence of fractures in ribs 9 through 12 should raise the suspicion of liver or spleen injury. Respiratory decompensation associated with flail chest and pneumothorax may present in a delayed fashion, and pulmonary contusion may not be recognized until 48 hour after injury. Hemothorax may also accumulate in a delayed manner.

Patients with chest wall injuries should undergo rapid evaluation of the airway, breathing, and circulation the same as with any injured patient. Supplemental oxygen is universally beneficial to all patients with a suspected thoracic injury. If a pulmonary contusion is present, judicious volume resuscitation should be carried out; overly aggressive resuscitation with crystalloid solutions is common in trauma and will worsen the severity of pulmonary contusion.

Radiographic, Sonographic, and Laboratory Evaluation

An anteroposterior chest radiograph remains standard in the evaluation of patients with chest injury. It should be recognized, however, that a plain chest radiograph will miss significant pathology. As many as seven of ten rib fractures will not be diagnosed by a plain chest radiograph. Chest radiography frequently fails to detect a small pneumothorax or hemothorax (less than 300 mL). CT scanning is the most accurate imaging technique in the detection of pneumothorax and frequently identifies an "occult" pneumothorax that is not clinically significant. Computed tomography (CT) of the chest wall with three-dimensional reconstruction is a major advance in the evaluation of chest wall injuries. Although this study is not indicated for patients with minor injury, it is the best method of demonstrating the presence of severe chest wall deformity associated with flail chest. Additionally, a CT scan is important for the evaluation of patients with pulmonary contusion or suspected great vessel injury. Ultrasound is an effective method of detecting the presence of both pneumothorax and hemothorax. The extended FAST (EFAST) examination has become standard at many trauma centers. In addition to the standard pericardial and abdominal views, the EFAST examination adds two views (second intercostal space at the midclavicular line and the sixth intercostal space at the anterior axillary line) of the pleural interface. Absence of both "lung sliding" and comet tail artifact at the pleural interface indicates the presence of a pneumothorax. A standard 3.5 MHz abdominal transducer may be used effectively in this examination, but a higher frequency transducer (7.5 MHz) increases sensitivity and accuracy. Ultrasound is at least as accurate as conventional radiographs in the detection of pneumothorax. Additionally, ultrasound is very effective in the identification of hemothorax and pleural effusion. An anechoic area superior to the diaphragm is indicative of fluid within the pleural cavity.

Evaluation of thoracic injury includes laboratory assessment. Measurement of arterial blood gases is an important method of determining the degree of respiratory compromise. Cardiac enzymes are not routinely indicated and are not directly associated with clinically significant cardiac contusion, but electrocardiographic changes may suggest cardiac contusion. If the initial electrocardiogram is abnormal, observation and cardiac monitoring for 24–48 hour are warranted.

Specific Injuries

Open Chest Wound
An open (sucking) chest wound will cause the preferential movement of air through the chest wall as opposed to through the tracheobronchial tree at the initiation of negative intrathoracic pressure associated with inspiration. This condition is

routinely associated with pneumothorax and hemothorax and can be rapidly fatal. Initial treatment involves coverage of the wound with an impervious dressing secured on three sides. This permits the efflux of accumulated air or blood, while simultaneously preserving the ability of the patient to generate negative intrathoracic pressure. This type of dressing will make respiration possible while also serving as a flutter valve for the pleural space. Chest wall injury involving significant tissue loss must be treated operatively as quickly as possible.

Pneumothorax

Etiology and Presentation

Pneumothorax is the abnormal presence of air in the intrapleural space that results in lung collapse, and it has several etiologies. *Primary spontaneous pneumothorax* occurs in the absence of underlying lung disease and most commonly presents in young, thin males; it has a strong, dose-dependent association with smoking. *Secondary spontaneous pneumothorax* occurs in the presence of underlying lung disease and is typically seen in older patients. *Traumatic pneumothorax* occurs in the presence of injury, either by a penetrating or blunt mechanism. *Occult traumatic pneumothorax* is defined as pneumothorax seen only on CT scan and not chest radiograph, whereas *nonoccult traumatic pneumothorax* is seen on chest radiograph. Sonographic detection of pneumothorax is an easily learned skill and is a standard component of the extended FAST (EFAST) examination. *Iatrogenic pneumothorax* occurs as a complication of a procedure or therapeutic intervention, most commonly barotrauma secondary to mechanical ventilation, placement of a central venous catheter, or invasive procedures that traverse the pleural space or bronchial spaces.

The presentation of pneumothorax can range from asymptomatic to imminently life threatening; when symptoms do occur, the most common are chest pain and dyspnea, but other complaints include cough and anxiety. The most common findings on physical exam are tachycardia, tachypnea, alteration or loss of breath sounds, and hyperresonance on chest wall percussion. In the setting of *tension pneumothorax*, where the air in the pleural space is under pressure and expanding, additional findings include hypotension, jugular venous distension, and diminished cardiac output due to impaired venous inflow to the heart.

Diagnosis

The standard method of confirming the presence of a pneumothorax is chest radiograph. The most reliable views are erect posteroanterior and lateral views. Studies have shown that inspiratory and expiratory films are equally sensitive. CT scan is usually not required for diagnosis but can reveal occult pneumothorax. Recent studies have shown the effectiveness of ultrasound for diagnosis of pneumothorax, which matches the sensitivity and specificity of other imaging techniques. Loss of "lung sliding" at the pleural interface and the absence of a comet-tail or ring-down artifact confirm the diagnosis.

Management

Appropriate management of pneumothorax ranges from simple observation to surgical intervention. This algorithm is determined by size, symptoms, etiology, and number of occurrences. Observation is most often used for asymptomatic patients and patients whose pneumothorax is occult or occupies less than 20% of the pleural space on chest radiograph. Observation includes close monitoring for the onset of symptoms as well as repeat chest radiograph approximately 6 hour after the initial films. Supplemental oxygen is routinely employed to increase the rate at which pleural air is absorbed. The onset of symptoms or an increase in occupied pleural space should prompt a reevaluation for the necessity of more invasive therapy.

Beyond observation, several methods have been employed to evacuate pleural air, with resultant lung re-expansion. The least invasive of these is simple aspiration after placing an 8- to 12-Fr catheter. This technique has been described as effective in the setting of primary spontaneous pneumothorax and iatrogenic pneumothorax. It is not as reliable as conventional tube thoracostomy and is not commonly used as the primary treatment method in most centers. Smaller chest tubes utilizing a sequential dilatation over a wire technique have become increasingly popular, particularly among non-surgeons. While these devices appear to be useful in isolated pneumothorax, their utility in patients with hemothorax remains unproven.

Heimlich valves and other flutter-valve devices have been utilized in the treatment of spontaneous pneumothorax and iatrogenic pneumothorax. Such devices allow for the outpatient treatment of these conditions and are effective 85% of the time. Follow-up with repeat exam and chest X-ray is usually arranged within 48 hour.

Tube thoracostomy still remains the most widely used method of pneumothorax management. A variety of tube sizes can be employed, but a size equal to or greater than 32 Fr should be utilized for any traumatic mechanism or other mechanisms in which concern for associated hemothorax exists. Because the procedure is painful, appropriate analgesia and sedation should be employed. Tube thoracostomy carries infection risk, and therefore, every effort to provide appropriate sterile precautions should be made. The prophylactic use of antibiotics is controversial, but the literature supports the option of a perioperative prophylaxis; however, prolonged administration of antibiotics is not warranted in patients with tube thoracostomy.

Once these steps have been performed, and adequate local anesthesia of the skin, muscle, and periosteum is accomplished, a small skin incision is made at the nipple line, in the fifth intercostal space, between the anterior and midaxillary lines. Blunt dissection is then carried through the muscle, and a Pean or Kelly clamp can be used to penetrate the pleura. Tunneling to an intercostal space cephalad to the skin incision is often utilized but is not required. The tube is then directed to the apex for simple pneumothorax; if necessary, it can be directed posteriorly for hemothorax.

Digital identification of the pleural cavity, as well as condensation of water vapor in the tube, can help to confirm the proper placement of the tube, which should be secured to the skin with sturdy, nonabsorbable suture and connected to a suction drainage system. An occlusive dressing is used, and chest radiograph confirms the appropriate placement of the tube. The drainage system, typically attached to wall suction, has an in-line water-seal chamber. Complications of tube placement include infection, bleeding, empyema, malpositioning, occlusion, and iatrogenic injury of the lung.

Tension pneumothorax requires immediate decompression. This determination is made clinically; no imaging study is required or warranted. Immediate decompression may be achieved by placing a large-bore (14–16 gauge) needle or catheter in the second intercostal space at the midclavicular line or in the fifth or sixth intercostal space at the anterior axillary line. A rush of air should be appreciated. This intervention converts a tension pneumothorax to a simple pneumothorax, and standard tube thoracostomy can be performed as definitive therapy. Unfortunately, needle thoracostomy has been shown to be an unreliable method of pleural decompression and as many as 50% of attempted needle thoracostomies do not enter the pleural cavity. Therefore, it is imperative that a formal tube thoracostomy follows needle thoracostomy immediately.

Thoracostomy tube removal can be considered when the pneumothorax has resolved without suction, and tube drainage is minimal; 24-hour totals of 75–200 mL have been described as the maximum output for tube removal. Optimal methods of removal have been debated to minimize pneumothorax recurrence, and these rates appear to be equivalent when performed at end inspiration or end expiration.

Certain clinical scenarios merit the use of surgical intervention for the ultimate resolution of pneumothorax. This can be accomplished with thoracotomy or minimally invasive thoracoscopic techniques. A second episode of primary spontaneous pneumothorax doubles the recurrence rate to 50%, whereas a first episode of secondary spontaneous pneumothorax has a recurrence rate approaching 50%. Because of this, the recommendations for surgical intervention include these scenarios, as well as the failure of a pneumothorax to resolve, or persistent air leak after 4 days. Other indications for surgical intervention can include bilateral pneumothorax, patients in high-risk professions (pilots, submariners, divers, etc.), and patients with AIDS.

Thoracoscopic techniques continue to increase in prevalence and have been shown in multiple studies to be as effective and safe as thoracotomy, but with much shorter recovery times. Therefore, the minimally invasive technique is now considered the procedure of choice in this setting. Re-expansion and prevention of recurrence may be accomplished in several ways: pleurodesis involves the invocation of an inflammatory response of the pleura, either by chemical or mechanical means. The mechanical method is most often utilized surgically by abrading the pleural surfaces. Chemical pleurodesis has also been utilized most commonly with talc. Due to the availability of minimally invasive surgical techniques, the nonoperative chemical methods are used much less frequently, as these are painful procedures with recurrence rates up to 25%.

Video-assisted thoracoscopic surgery (VATS) requires appropriate training and experience. With general anesthesia and single-lung ventilation, the patient is positioned in the lateral decubitus position. A single trocar is inserted inferior to the scapular tip at roughly the sixth intercostal space. After visual inspection, two additional ports are placed under direct vision in a triangulated fashion. Mechanical abrasion is then achieved. If a bleb is responsible for the pneumothorax, an endoscopic linear stapler is utilized for resection. Saline injection into the cavity with subsequent ventilation can reveal any further parenchymal leak, and chest tube placement completes the procedure, with lung re-expansion. Thoracoscopy is contraindicated in unstable patients or patients that are not candidates for single-lung ventilation.

Hemothorax

Etiology and Presentation

Hemothorax is defined as the presence of blood in the pleural cavity. The most likely mechanism is penetrating or blunt trauma. Other less common sources can be seen, such as infections, tumors, rupture of blebs, pancreatitis, and ruptured aneurysm. Hemothorax can present in a wide clinical spectrum from small, asymptomatic collections to massive hemothorax in an unstable patient. The diagnosis of hemothorax by physical exam can be difficult, with findings that include diminished breath sounds, dullness to percussion, and hemodynamic changes. Unilateral opacification of a hemithorax may be appreciated on chest radiograph, but CT is more sensitive in revealing a small or moderate hemothorax, and ultrasound will reliably identify fluid in the pleural space.

Management

The initial management of a suspected hemothorax is tube thoracostomy. It is important to remember to do this in the context of the standard resuscitation scheme of injured patients, to include airway control, ventilatory assistance, and circulatory resuscitation. Indications for immediate thoracotomy include an initial output greater than 1500 mL or an output greater than 200 mL/h over 4 hour. Close monitoring of patients who do not reach these thresholds is also important, as clotting of the thoracostomy tube may obscure continued bleeding, and hemodynamic changes or ventilatory difficulty may warrant more immediate surgical intervention.

If thoracotomy is required, it is best achieved in the lateral decubitus position through a posterolateral approach under general anesthesia. Hemodynamically unstable patients are best approached through an anterolateral thoracotomy incision with the patient in a supine position. With single-lung ventilation, if tolerated, and appropriate prepping and draping, an incision at the fifth intercostal space provides the best exposure. Exposure may be improved by the removal of a rib, but this is rarely necessary.

Although the most common source of traumatic hemothorax is an injured intercostal or internal mammary artery injury, bleeding frequently results from injury to lung parenchyma or the great vessels. In this case, intercostal vessels may be suture ligated or clipped. Tractotomy or wedge resections, which may both be achieved with stapling devices, may be adequate to expose, seal, or resect the source of hemorrhage from lung parenchyma. With more significant parenchymal injury, formal lobectomy or pneumonectomy may be required. Vascular control of the hilum can be achieved by incising the inferior pulmonary ligament and grasping the hilar vessels, either with digital pressure or with a large vascular clamp (Fig. 1). Twisting the hilum of the lung 180° has been described in the literature, but this is a somewhat cumbersome maneuver. Once the hilum is controlled, the source of bleeding can be identified, and the extent of resection can be determined. Stapled pulmonary tractotomy and stapled wedge resection are very effective operative techniques to obtain hemostasis and reduce postoperative pneumothorax (Figs. 2 and 3). Once the procedure is complete, the chest wall is closed, and chest tubes are left in place to assist in lung expansion and evacuation of residual fluid.

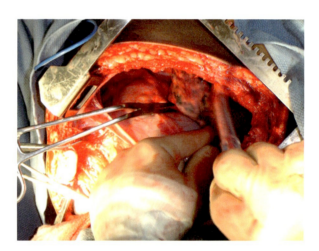

Fig. 1 Cross-clamping of the pulmonary hilum to control massive hemothorax secondary to gunshot wound

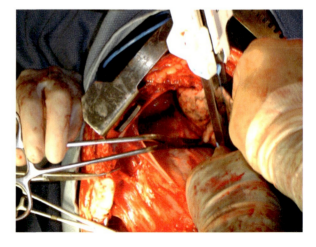

Fig. 2 Pulmonary tractotomy for control of hemorrhage secondary to penetrating injury

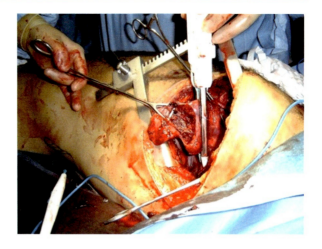

Fig. 3 Wedge resection of lower lobe to control hemorrhage and air leak secondary to a gunshot wound

In very rare instances, with an exsanguinating patient who is coagulopathic, hypothermic, and acidotic, a damage-control procedure may be required. In this setting, packing may be employed to achieve control of hemorrhage and air leak, taking care not to affect cardiac function and venous return adversely. The patient is returned to the operating room after those physiologic conditions are improved. In the stable patient with ongoing hemorrhage, the thoracoscopic approach may be considered, but the procedure must be converted to thoracotomy at any sign of instability or if adequate visualization, evacuation, or hemorrhage control is not possible.

Patients who have persistent or retained hemothorax as a result of delayed diagnosis or failure to evacuate with thoracostomy tube drainage are at risk for fibrothorax. This condition can result in chronically diminished pulmonary function, pain, and dyspnea. Avoidance of this complication requires aggressive therapy when the retained hemothorax is identified. CT scan is the most sensitive imaging study for this diagnosis, and a hemothorax that occupies more than a third of the pleural space should be evacuated. Video-assisted thoracoscopic surgery is indicated for these patients, as second chest tubes placed more than 24 hour after injury uniformly fail to drain the hemothorax in almost 50% of patients. This intervention should be performed as early as possible in the hospital course as this approach is unlikely to be successful if not performed within 72 hour. Thrombolytic agents have been used to dissolve retained hemothorax with some success. Currently, tissue plasminogen activator (TPA) is the most commonly used agent. After evacuation of the hemothorax with a standard chest tube, 50 mg of TPA in 100–200 mL of saline is instilled via the tube thoracostomy which is then clamped for approximately 1 hour. If possible, the patient's position is changed frequently to optimize distribution of the TPA solution. Caution is imperative when contemplating this technique in patients with recent episodes of bleeding. This process may be repeated daily, but should not delay needed thoracoscopic evacuation of clot.

Further Reading

Baumann MH, Strange C, Heffner JE, et al., and the AACP Pneumothorax Consensus Group. Management of spontaneous pneumothorax: an American College of Chest Physicians Delphi consensus statement. Chest. 2001;119(2):590–602.

Casos SR, Richardson JD. Role of thoracoscopy in acute management of chest injury. Curr Opin Crit Care. 2006;12(6):584–9.

Chen J, Jeremitsky E, Philp F, Fry WR, Smith RS. A chest trauma scoring system to predict outcomes. Surgery. 2014;156:988–93.

Inaba K, Karamanos E, Skiada D, Grabo D, Hammer P, Martin M, Sullivan M, Eckstein M, Demetriades D. Cadaveric comparison of the optimal site for needle decompression of tension pneumothorax by prehospital providers. J Trauma Acute Care Surg. 2015;79:1044–8.

Kent R, Woods W, Bostrom O. Fatality risk and the presence of rib fractures. Ann Adv Automot Med. 2008;52:73–92.

Knudtson JL, Dort JM, Helmer SD, Smith RS, et al. Surgeon-performed ultrasound for pneumothorax in the trauma suite. J Trauma. 2004;56(3):527–30.

Kulvatunyou N, Erickson L, Vijayasekaran A, Gries L, Joseph B, Freise RF, O'Keeffe T, Tang AL, Wynne JL, Rhee P. Randomized clinical trial of pigtail catheter versus chest tube in injured patients with uncomplicated traumatic pneumothorax. Br J Surg. 2014;101:17–22.

Smith RS. Cavitary endoscopy in trauma: 2001. Scand J Surg. 2002;91(1):67–71.

Pulmonary Contusions and ARDS

Emiliano Gamberini, Luca Bissoni, Giovanni Scognamiglio, and David H. Livingston

Definition of ARDS

The definition of ARDS has undergone many changes since it was first described 50 years ago. The most recent definition is the Berlin definition, which was proposed by a working group from the European Society of Intensive Care Medicine and endorsed and by the American Thoracic Society and the Society of Critical Care Medicine [4]. The Berlin definition overcame many of the limitations of the previous definitions, and it improved on their ability to prognosticate outcome. There are several essential features of the current definition. The first is the development of ARDS must occur within 7 days of a known clinical insult or new or worsening respiratory symptoms. It also categorizes the disease into three categories based on PaO_2/FiO_2 ratio:

- Mild ARDS ($200 < PaO_2/FiO_2 \leq 300$ mmHg)
- Moderate ARDS ($100 < PaO_2/FiO_2 \leq 200$ mmHg)
- Severe ARDS ($PaO_2/FiO_2 \leq 100$ mmHg)

These groups had different outcomes with hospital mortality increasing from 27% for mild ARDS to 32% for moderate and 45% for severe. Not surprisingly, there was increased meantime on mechanical ventilation from 5 to 7 to 9 days, respectively. Similar to older definition, the chest radiograph is required to have diffuse bilateral opacities, which are not explained by volume overload, and the respiratory failure itself cannot be explained by hydrostatic factors, heart failure, or volume overload. Given the inflammatory nature ARDS and despite much research, there is no current biomarker or set of markers that improve the sensitivity and specificity for diagnosing ARDS or classify its severity or prognosticate the outcome of the disease.

Pathophysiology

Despite decades of research, the pathophysiology and pathogenesis of ARDS remains incompletely understood. While there is clearly an inflammatory component to the disease process, as outlined above, the current Berlin definition does not include any biomarkers or measures of inflammation. The clinical scenarios of ARDS are many and quite varied. Most commonly, they include sepsis, multiple trauma, hemorrhagic shock, pneumonia, and aspiration. Other less common but consistent causes of ARDS include inhalation injury, pulmonary contusion, near drowning, pancreatitis, and transfusion of blood products.

As can be seen from the above causes, one schema to characterize ARDS would be to divide the disease into pulmonary and extrapulmonary etiologies. While this distinction may appear arbitrary in pulmonary ARDS, the insult directly affects the lung parenchyma and the alveolar epithelium is the first structure injured. In contrast, extrapulmonary ARDS is secondary to a systemic process with the endothelial cell interacting with the inflammatory cells and cytokines. With ongoing research, these factors may play a role in improving targeting therapies.

Another classic way ARDS has been pathologically and clinically characterized has been by the phase of the disease: early and late. These phases correspond to the progression of ARDS from the exudative to fibroproliferative phases [5]. There are associated alterations in lung matrix and activation of coagulation and fibrosis pathways, with cell proliferation and apoptosis.

In the early phase, there is endothelial and epithelial damage, an inflammatory cascade, and increased vascular permeability. This early phase occurs in the first few hours or days of the insult.

Neutrophils play a critical role in the pathogenesis of ARDS [6, 7]. Neutrophils accumulate in throughout the lung and are present in the pulmonary microcirculation, lung interstitium, and alveolar airspaces of patients with ARDS. ARDS is also associated with systemic neutrophil priming, decreased neutrophil apoptosis, and delayed clearance of neutrophils from the lungs. In experiment models, reducing circulating neutrophil numbers or preventing them from reaching the lung ameliorates lung injury. The abundance of neutrophils results in the release harmful mediators including cytokines, proteases, reactive oxygen species, and matrix metalloproteinases leading to further pulmonary damage. Neutrophils also synergize with other inflammatory cells and mediators that further lung damage [8]. Specific cytokines such as interleukin-1 (IL-1), IL-6, IL-8, and tumor necrosis factor (TNF) are pro-inflammatory and may exacerbate lung injury. Injury to the alveolar epithelium is a prominent feature histologically with loss of alveolar epithelial barrier integrity and extensive necrosis of alveolar epithelial type I cells. Disruption of the alveolar epithelial and endothelial barriers leads to the formation of the classic non-hydrostatic protein-rich edema in the interstitium and alveolar spaces. The loss of alveolar spaces due to edema leads to hypoxia and altered pulmonary physiology associated with early ARDS.

Coagulation cascade abnormalities are also characteristic in ARDS with an imbalance in both pro- and anticoagulation factors. The formation of microthrombi and vascular occlusion in capillary beds are common features, and the role of platelets in the pathophysiology of ARDS are increasingly recognized [9]. There is excellent crossover and similarities between coagulation and inflammation. For example, protein C concentrations are low in plasma and lung edema fluid in ARDS patients.

In the later phase of ARDS, there is disordered healing and fibroblastic proliferation, which fills the airspaces with granulation tissue containing proliferating alveolar type II cells, angiogenesis, and an extracellular matrix rich in collagen and fibrin. This phase occurs as early as 7–10 days after initial injury although some data may suggest that it coincides with inflammatory proliferative lung injury [10]. Elevated levels of N-terminal procollagen peptide III, which was thought to be a marker of collagen synthesis, has been detected in BAL fluid of patients with ARDS as soon as early as 24 h.

Given the number of inflammatory and other cells and cellular products involved in the pathophysiology of ARDS, there has been a great deal of research to identify biomarkers and pathways to develop therapeutic interventions. This work has also clearly demonstrated that while inflammation is a prominent feature of ARDS, not all inflammation is similar between patients [11].

A partial list of the biomarkers that have been identified to be involved in ARDS is shown in Table 1 [12].

Despite the identification of multiple candidate biomarkers, there has been, unfortunately, no pharmacologic therapy that has been developed to improve ARDS outcomes.

Table 1 Partial list of biomarkers involved in ARDS

Epithelial	Endothelial	Pro-inflammatory	Anti-inflammatory	Coagulation
Receptor for advanced glycation end products (RAGE)	Angiopoietin-2 (ANG-1/2)	IL-1β	IL-1RA	PAI-1
Surfactant proteins (SP)	vWF	TNFα	STNF-RI/II	
Krebs von den Lungen-6 (KL-6) protein	VEGF	IL-6	IL-10	
Club cell secretory protein 16 (CC16)		IL-8		
Keratinocyte growth factor (KGF)		IL-18		
Fibroblast growth factor (FGF)		CXCL8		
		Procalcitonin		

However, what this line of research has demonstrated is a biologic basis for the clinical heterogeneity of ARDS. Future use of advanced bioinformatics and genetic modeling will identify subtypes that could potentially lead to a more personalized targeted approach for a disease process that has significant morbidity and mortality.

Respiratory Monitoring

Compliance

In respiratory physiology, lung compliance describes the propensity of the lung to distend. It can be calculated by the following equation:

$$C = DV / DP$$

where C is compliance, DV is the change in volume, and DP is the change in pressure.

In general, airway pressure during inflation is influenced by volume, respiratory system compliance (lung + chest wall), and resistance to flow [13]. If measured at zero flow, C is defined as "static compliance" (Cstat).

Cstat is different from dynamic compliance (Cdyn), because Cstat is not influenced by the resistance of the respiratory system. In ventilated patients, DV is the tidal volume given by the ventilator and DP is defined by Pplat-PEEP (Pplat is the Pinsp measured at zero flow and PEEP is the positive end-expiratory pressure) [14].

Elastance

It is defined as the propensity of the lung to return to the original resting position. It is the inverse of compliance [13, 14]:

$$E = 1 / C$$

Transpulmonary Pressure

Transpulmonary pressure defines the pressure across the alveolar membrane:

$$PL = PAW - Ppl$$

where PL is the transpulmonary pressure, PAW is the end-inspiratory plateau pressure and Ppl is the pleural pressure. It allows the determination of the pressure that directly distends the lung, eliminating the part of it needed to distend the thoracic cage.

Esophageal pressure (Pes) is an important parameter to help guide patient ventilation because it accurately estimates pleural pressure and allows for the determination of transpulmonary pressure.

A special NGT with gastric and esophageal balloons can be used to measure pleural pressure in vivo [15] with measurement of esophageal pressure, as Pes = Ppl:

$$PL = PAW - Pes$$

It is possible to calculate PLinsp (PAW − Pes insp) by making an end-inspiratory pause on the ventilator, and PLexp (PEEP − Pes exp) with an end-expiratory pause. PLinsp and PLexp are useful in guiding the clinician to set the ventilator [16], avoiding derecuitment and overdistension.

Driving Pressure

It is defined by the compliance formula as

$$DP = Vt / Crs$$

where Vt is the tidal volume and Crs the compliance of the respiratory system.

It allows, in absence of an esophageal balloon, to set a protective ventilation, choosing a VT normalized on the Crs (i.e., globally decreased in ARDS, in relation to its severity) [17].

It can be easily calculated with the following equation:

$$DP = Pplat - PEEP$$

Mechanical Ventilation in ARDS Patients

The increasing knowledge of ARDS pathophysiology has led to suggestions that a lung-protective ventilatory strategy can ensure adequate oxygenation (PaO_2 between 60 and 80 mmHg) and minimize VILI. Unfortunately, entirely "safe" lung-protective ventilation does not exist, and the ventilatory support should be individualized according to the best compromise among respiratory mechanics, recruitability, gas exchange, and hemodynamics.

This difference is paramount because although mechanical ventilation is needed to manage both causes of acute respiratory failure, different ventilatory strategies should be implemented. Primary ARDS with prevalent contusions and consolidations have in general the worst response to recruitment with positive end-expiratory pressure (PEEP). This does not mean that PEEP plays a less important role in this type of ARDS, but PEEP may, in fact, improve gas exchange through mechanism other than lung recruitment, perhaps by acting on ventilation-perfusion ratio [5].

Many modalities of ventilation can be used to oxygenate and ventilate ARDS patients. Globally, they are referred to as "protective ventilation" strategies. The purpose of protective ventilation is to eliminate barotrauma and ventilate gently a lung that is already damaged and has a profound modification of its response to the pressure delivered by the ventilator.

It is important to describe the concept of "baby lung" [18]. It is a functional and anatomical description of modifications suffered by the lungs during ARDS, identified by CT scan examination in the early 1980s.

What had previously described as a homogeneous lung did not appear as homogeneous on CT, with the parenchymal densities concentrated primarily in the most dependent regions.

That means that the pulmonary parenchyma could grossly be divided in a minor portion that is typically aerated, equivalent to the lung of a 5–6-year-old boy (with normal compliance), and other non-aerated portions that are poorly aerated and overinflated [18]. Compressive basal atelectasis increases physiological dead space. As a result, compliance is decreased and elastance ($1/C$) is augmented. Diminished compliance will shift the lower inflection point on the pressure-volume curve to the right, flattening the initial inspiratory part of the curve with an associated rise in airway resistance. Furthermore, the transpulmonary pressure will be decreased: higher plateau pressures will be needed for alveolar opening and recruitment maneuvers (Fig. 1).

According to the "baby lung" theory, ARDS lung is not just stiff as previously thought but rather small with reduced volume.

That being said, when clinicians set the ventilator, they should be aware that the pulmonary parenchyma that will be ventilated is as big as a child's one and that it must be protected from any further additional damage.

Protective ventilation can be achieved by different strategies, using different modalities of respiratory monitoring in relation to the severity of the disease and its evolution over the days.

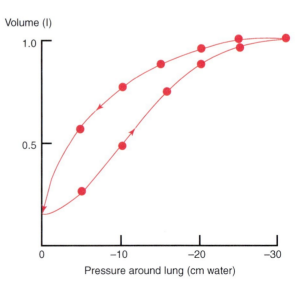

Fig. 1 Pulmonary *P/V* curve

Controlled Ventilation

Mechanical ventilation is a supportive therapy that guarantees gas exchange while reducing muscle activity [19].

A completely safe ventilatory strategy does not exist yet, and the respiratory support must be tailored to every single patient [20].

Once defined the disease (primary vs. secondary ARDS), the first step to set the ventilator is to select a proper tidal volume (Vt), the fraction of inspired oxygen (FiO_2), the positive end-expiratory pressure (PEEP), and the respiratory rate (RR).

Although mechanical ventilation is essential to manage respiratory failure, in addition to direct injury and secondary inflammatory-mediated damage, the lung is also subject to ventilator-induced lung injury (VILI).

The so-called protective ventilation is aimed to reduce the ventilator-induced damage (VILI), limiting overdistension.

As general rules, the following settings can be suggested: Vt 6 ml/kg/predicted body weight, Pplateau < 30 cmH_2O, RR aimed to the maintenance of CO_2, allowing permissive hypercarbia and mild respiratory acidosis (pH ≥ 7.2).

VT Selection

As already stated, clinicians have to deal with a 5-year-old boy's lung; thus the first step is to adjust the Vt to the size of the baby lung. A milestone study on ventilator strategies in ARDS (ARMA trial) demonstrated how using a Vt of 6 ml/kg/(predicted body weight), as compared to the old conventional setting of 12 ml/kg, could reduce mortality [21]. However, even predicted body weight is poorly related to the resting volume. In the last few years, the use of the driving pressure (DP) has recently been proposed [17] with the aim to better individualize the Vt. Recently, Amato et al. found that in patients ventilated with different combinations of tidal volumes and PEEPs, DP was the factor that was mostly associated with the outcome. Higher mortality was found when higher plateau pressure was observed, along with higher driving pressure with a cutoff of 15 cmH_2O [17]. The main limitation in setting ventilation using DP is that it does not take into account the real distending pressure of the alveoli (transpulmonary pressure, PL as stated above) but rather a global distending pressure of the respiratory system (lung and chest wall). This is important because chest wall can also be altered in ARDS patients [5], leading to elevation of the plateau pressure (and DP) without a significant PL elevation.

Remember that appropriate PEEP selection is fundamental because of its relationship with recruitment (and then with compliance) and its ability to increase the baby lung size that can be ventilated by the Vt, resulting in a DP ≤ 15 cmH_2O, even with Vt ≥ 6 ml/kg.

PEEP Selection

Clinical experience and meta-analysis strongly suggest that PEEP level should range from 5 to even 15–20 cmH_2O, depending on the severity of ARDS [22]. Every time we set a PEEP level, hemodynamics must be reassessed. Sometimes, the increase in oxygenation is not secondary to the alveolar recruitment but rather to a decreased cardiac output (secondary to increased intrathoracic pressures) with a reduction of right to left shunt. In the case of hemodynamic deterioration, PEEP should be reduced.

PEEP is set to keep the lung open, preventing intra-tidal collapse and de-collapse. The amount of lung parenchyma that could undergo this phenomenon is proportional to the severity of ARDS, and it is correlated to its recruitability. Before setting a PEEP level, it is therefore important to assess the lung recruitability (CT scan, thoracic echo) and reevaluate again, every time a recruitment maneuver or a modification of PEEP level is performed. Successful lung recruitment can be assessed by either a new CT scan, where increased aeration of previously collapsed lung regions (anatomical lung recruitment) will be visible or by recalculating mechanical parameters such as compliance, driving pressure, or transpulmonary pressure to appraise their improvements (physiological recruitment) [23].

The use of the esophageal balloon to evaluate PL can be useful to set the right PEEP level [24]. The use of pleural pressure measurements can help to find the PEEP level that prevents lung injury due to cyclic alveolar collapse or overdistension. The goals are to reach an end-expiratory transpulmonary pressure closed to 0 or slightly above and an end-inspiratory transpulmonary pressure < 25 cmH_2O, to prevent overdistension.

To simplify the choice of the PEEP level, it is also possible to use the ARDSnet recommendations, with a defined FiO_2/PEEP ratio: a proper PEEP level will be chosen according to the FiO_2%, for a $SatO_2$ goal of 88–95%. Indeed, this is the $SatO_2$ value that roughly corresponds to $PaO_2 \geq 60$ mmHg: taking a glance at the hemoglobin dissociation curve, 60 mmHg is the threshold at which the plateau begins and the curve tends to infinite. At pressures ≥ 60 mmHg, the standard dissociation curve is relatively flat, which means that the oxygen content of the blood does not change significantly even with large increases in the oxygen partial pressure. Below this value, the hemoglobin-O_2 dissociation is way faster and affinity for O_2 decreases dramatically: this is the point where huge desaturation occurs even with little drops in PaO_2 (Fig. 2).

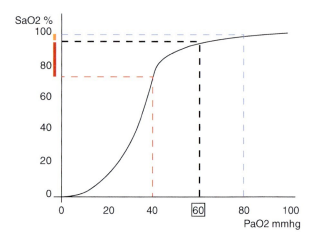

Fig. 2 Hemoglobin saturation curve

Recruitment Maneuvers

A recruitment maneuver is defined as a technique in which sustained high pressures are applied to the patient's airway in order to diminish the number of collapsed of alveoli, during mechanical ventilation.

The purposes of recruitment are:

- To improve oxygenation
- To reduce atelectrauma by preventing opening and closure of distal airways and alveoli
- To reduce overdistension (stress) by applying PEEP to a "bigger" baby lung (same Vt in a wider volume with increased compliance) and ventilating a more homogeneous parenchyma

There are different kinds of recruitment techniques. The key point is to administer high pressures (40–45 cmH_2O) to reopen the collapsed parenchyma that would not open otherwise with protective ventilation (as a result of an increased opening pressure) and keep it open with a titrated PEEP that maximizes compliance, avoiding overdistension.

In relation to ARDS type, be it primary or secondary, the patient could be classified as a responder or a not responder.

According to clinical experience and literature, the following can be endorsed as recruitment maneuvers:

- High-level continuous positive airway pressure: CPAP 40 cmH_2O for 40 s
- Intermitted sighs: maintain the ongoing lung protective strategy, introducing sighs with a plateau pressure of 40–45 cmH_2O [25]
- Stepwise progressive recruitment maneuver in pressure control mode, maintaining DP at a steady 15 cmH_2O, with 5 cmH_2O increments in PEEP until a peak pressure is achieved (35–45 cmH_2O), with a pre-established maximum PEEP (15–20 cmH_2O).

The last one is the recommended technique in terms of safety and efficacy [26].

As for PEEP selection, a bedside measurement of both compliance and PL or a CT control could be used to asses if more parenchyma is being recruited and ventilated.

Complications of hereby advocated maneuvers are hemodynamic impairment (with risk of extreme bradycardia and possible cardiac arrest), lung parenchyma rupture with PNX, and transient deterioration of gas exchange.

Pronation

A recent multicenter prospective controlled trial (the PROSEVA study) showed that prone positioning decreased 28- and 90-day mortality, increased ventilator-free days, and decreased time to extubation [27].

CT scans of pronated ARDS patients (in late 1980s) revealed an unexpected finding: the disappearance of the postero-basal densities after prone positioning had been obtained and their redistribution to the new dependent lung regions. These findings changed the concept of the baby lung as an anatomically confined entity into a functional matter, leading to the development of a pathophysiological model known as "sponge lung" model [20, 28, 29].

Edema increases the lung weight and squeezes the gas out of the dependent lung regions producing alveolar collapse and increasing CT densities in dependent regions (compression atelectasis). The size of open and patent airways and the amount of gas decreases along the vertical axis.

Hence in supine position, the dependent regions collapse because of the gravity distribution of edema and superimposed pressure of the lung and mediastinum and because of the different shape of both the lung and the chest wall that results in nonhomogeneous expansion of alveolar units. Indeed, the isolated lung has normally a conical shape with the dependent part being bigger than the nondependent one. On the other hand, chest wall has a cylindrical shape. Given that, the two structures share both the same volume, the lung must expand its upper regions more than the lower ones, resulting in a greater expansion of the nondependent alveolar units.

After the pronation of the patient, the shunt lessens and the oxygenation improves following the recruitment of the dorsal areas that overcomes the de-recruitment of the ventral regions.

Moreover, transpulmonary pressure decreases along the ventral to the dorsal axis and the sizes of alveolar units decrease toward the dependent areas. After pronation, the intrapleural pressure becomes less negative in nondependent and less positive in dependent regions, by virtue of thoracic-lung shape modifications [30]. Thereafter, PL and the regional inflation distribution become more homogeneous throughout the lung. Human and animal studies have shown that from supine to prone position, pulmonary blood flow in dorsal regions is maintained unmodified and prevalent in the dorsal areas [24]. That said, turning the patient to the prone position will result in a better *V/Q* ratio of the dorsal region of the lung, along with a dorsal recruitment being greater than concurrent ventral de-recruitment [28, 31, 32].

In conclusion, prone position can grant:

An improvement in oxygenation
A better CO_2 clearance
A reduction of overdistension
A better and homogeneous ventilation of the lung (less stress and strain)
Better hemodynamic parameters by enhanced right ventricular function
Better clearance of secretions

Potential complications are:

Pressure sores
Endotracheal tube dislocation
Difficulty in airway suctioning
Worsening of gas exchange
Unintentional removal of vascular catheters
Enteral nutrition intolerance
Need for increased sedation and muscle paralysis
Reduced venous return in ECMO [28]

Assisted Ventilation

From a physiological point of view, spontaneous breathing during mechanical ventilation provides various beneficial effects, including better gas exchange and prevention of diaphragmatic dysfunction [33, 34].

The transpulmonary pressure is the pressure needed to inflate the lung:

$$PL = Paw - Ppl$$

During muscular paralysis, PL depends mainly on the pressure delivered by the ventilator. During spontaneous effort instead, negative changes in Ppl may be coupled with positive pressure changes from the ventilator, magnifying PL [34].

Moreover, the change in Ppl generated by inspiratory muscle contractions in ARDS lung is not uniformly transmitted across the lung surface but rather it is concentrated in dependent lung regions [34, 35]. The consequent elevation in PL causes a local overstretch, making the air shift from nondependent to dependent regions (pendelluft).

Inspiratory PL and the effect of the pendelluft rise as spontaneous effort increases. Thus, mild spontaneous efforts may be beneficial to recruit the collapsed lung while excessive ones could cause local overstretch [34, 36].

In severe ARDS, the local increase in PL is higher than in mild ones:

1. The pressure needed to overcome the lower compliance is higher.
2. Demand of spontaneous effort is much higher and difficult to control even with sedation (that is the reason why neuromuscular paralysis is needed during the first 48 h).

Excessive muscular contraction could lead to an unacceptable increase or risk of VILI (stress and strain).

In conclusion, in the early stage of severe ARDS, assisted ventilation should be avoided. In less severe forms, and after 48–72 h of muscular paralysis in the severe ones, spontaneous efforts should be encouraged avoiding excessive contractions and consequently uncontrolled increase in PL [34].

Extracorporeal Membrane Oxygenation (ECMO)

ECMO is a temporary extracorporeal respiratory support used for the treatment of respiratory failure refractory to conventional therapies. If a hemodynamic failure coexists, it could also serve as a temporary circulatory support.

In ARDS patients, it could be used in different settings to support gas exchange (veno-venous ECMO), to support circulatory failure (veno-arterial ECMO), or both (veno-artero-venous ECMO). When the ECMO circuit is connected, venous blood is withdrawn by a pump. Then it passes through the oxygenator, where gas exchanges take place, and it is reinfused into the venous or arterial system.

According to the Extracorporeal Life Support Organization (ELSO) guidelines, the use of ECMO should be considered when the PaO_2/FiO_2 ratio is ≤ 150, whereas ECMO is indicated when the ratio is ≤ 80. A $PaCO_2 \geq 80$ mmHg or a Pplat ≥ 30 cmH$_2$O are also considered as an indication for ECMO.

The main limitation in the ARDS traumatized patients is the need for anticoagulation and the risk of bleeding. ECMO is however been used successfully in adult trauma patients, and it can offer an additional treatment to the most severe forms [37].

Pulmonary Contusion

Lung contusion is the most frequently diagnosed intrathoracic injury after blunt trauma [38]. In the early phase, the impairment of oxygenation correlates well with the area of involved lung tissue [39]. Respiratory relief could be achieved in spontaneous breathing patients in many ways:

- Oxygen therapy (facial mask, high-flow nasal cannula (HFNC))
- Continuous positive airway pressure (CPAP)
- Noninvasive mechanical ventilation with facial mask (NIV)
- Adequate pain management to permit cough and pulmonary drainage by intravenous or regional techniques
- Fluid restriction to avoid worsening of pulmonary edema

As previously seen, a pulmonary contusion can evolve in ARDS during the days and breathing efforts will likely lead to volutrauma and barotrauma [34].

In severe cases, invasive mechanical ventilation is essential.

Unfortunately, a general optimal ventilatory strategy that is applicable to all patients does not exist and ventilatory settings have to be tailored to each patient.

Chest trauma can lead to disproportionate or unilateral lung trauma. In these circumstances, it is difficult to set a protective ventilation strategy because what is beneficial for a lung part could be actually harmful for another one. After CT scan and bedside evaluation of mechanical properties of the respiratory system (compliance, DP, weight, IAP), clinicians set the ventilator and control over time gas exchange and patient global status.

In cases of deterioration, there are two other options:

- Independent lung ventilation (selective ventilatory management according to the different mechanical properties of the lungs, with two different ventilator and a double lumen tube that allows differential treatment of the lungs with tailored PEEP, VT, and RR) [40, 41].
- ECMO [37].

ARDS: Medical Management

While lung-protective mechanical ventilation strategies still remain the cornerstone of treatment, other medical options should as well be implemented while dealing with ARDS, including fluid management, neuromuscular blocking agents, corticosteroids, and inhaled pulmonary vasodilating agents (prostacyclins and nitric oxide). The absence of specific pharmacological therapy for ARDS, despite decades of research, might relate to its complex pathophysiology. Although specific medical treatments are still missing, the recent advances in our understanding of alveolar injury have identified key processes and mediators that represent promising targets for future therapies. Unfortunately, evidence-based recommendations establishing a standard-of-care approach beyond lung-protective ventilation are lacking.

Fluid Balance and Administration

The accumulation of interstitial and alveolar fluid in the lungs plays a pivotal role in the pathogenesis of ARDS. The increased permeability of the alveolar-capillary membrane due to dysregulated, tissue-destructive inflammation will determine alveolar edema. The quantity of pulmonary edema fluid, related to extravascular lung water, can increase several times before a significant decrease in arterial oxygenation occurs so that the detrimental effect of alveolar edema may not be immediately detectable. Clinically, this manifests as hypoxemia, with bilateral opacities on chest radiography, decreased lung compliance, and augmentation of physiological dead space. In most patients, ARDS occurs after a generalized process of systemic inflammation resulting from conditions such as severe sepsis, burn injury, major trauma, hemorrhagic shock, and necrotizing pancreatitis that are responsible for hemodynamic shock. In this phase, early and adequate fluid administration is essential to prevent the development of multiorgan dysfunction, which can impact mortality [42, 43]. As inflammation breaks through, fluids will leave the vessels to the extravascular space; as a result, the patient is now "empty" inside (the heart), but he is "filled up" outside (the interstitium), and probably this condition will span about 72 h. As the inflammatory state resolves, the excessive fluid can have a detrimental impact on patient outcome.

These three treatment phases, typical for all patients with hemodynamic derangement, can be addressed as follows:

1. Resuscitation
2. Maintenance
3. De-resuscitation

Hypertonic saline (3% and 7.4% NaCl), human albumin solution, and packed red blood cells (PRBC) are probably the best "fluid challenges" during phase 1, but it is difficult to postulate which one is the best option. Blood products can be preferred over crystalloids to ameliorate perfusion without worsening tissue edema even if Hb is >10 g/dL. Administration of albumin to raise oncotic pressure and promote the water movement from the interstitium to the intravascular space has been suggested as a method to reduce edema [44].

In critically ill patients, invasive hemodynamic monitoring can be beneficial in assessing intravascular volume status and optimizing patient resuscitation. Traditional pressure-based parameters such as central venous pressure may be misleading in the presence of elevated intrathoracic and intra-abdominal pressure and can lead to erroneous clinical decisions regarding fluid status. Therefore, cardiac index (CI), stroke volume variation (SVV%, strictly related to Δ-Ups and Δ-Downs in invasive blood pressure waveform), right ventricular end-diastolic volume index (RVEDI), and arterial lactate have proven themselves to be the most reliable variables during the resuscitation phase. The general approach in this patient population is to avoid excessive fluid overload in all of the phases. The Fluid and Catheter Treatment Trial (FACTT) by the ARDSNet group [45] conducted in the post-resuscitative period demonstrated significantly fewer ventilator days in a group of critically ill patients that received fewer crystalloids. A bedside fast echocardiography is the first step to correctly evaluate a patient's volemic state: it is noninvasive and replicable and any intensivist should be able to perform it. Facing a "prevalent" respiratory failure, transpulmonary thermodilution (TPTD) can be useful in managing capillary leak by providing the extravascular lung water index value (ELWI) [46], with a less invasive method than a Swan Ganz catheter. The normal value for EVLWI is reported to be approximately 7 mL/kg and results from the equilibrium between fluid leakage and lymphatic drainage. Values of the EVLWI exceeding 20 mL/kg have been reported during severe pulmonary edema and should be avoided. Nonetheless, TPTD can have accuracy limits in patients with left ventricle ejection fraction ≤40% or in severe depression of arterial vascular tone since cardiovascular parameters are just calculated (and not directly measured) on the basis of invasive arterial waveform.

A Swan Ganz catheter with in-continuous cardiac output and SvO_2 monitoring can be a good choice to assess volemic status of patients, but it is a far more invasive technique than TPTD.

As stated above, any intensivist should be able to perform a rapid bedside echo exam to assess fluid status, whereas the best way to improve fluid balance is by weighing patients every day: ICU beds with weighing scales are commercially available.

Once the patient is hemodynamically stable and vasopressors are being weaned or discontinued, any effort should be made to reduce fluid administration during the maintenance phase and be aggressive with fluid removal during the de-resuscitative phase.

This fluid administration dilemma forces the clinician to modify the early goal-directed resuscitation approach and consider "permissive hypovolemia." Whether this approach is optimal for ARDS patients is unclear [47].

A good starting point to reduce fluid administration is to pay attention to medication and daily fluid volume: high-protein/high-calorie EN nutrition and IV medications can be a good choice as they can reduce enteral feeding volume [48].

During maintenance and de-resuscitative phases, negative fluid balance can be obtained using either diuretics or renal replacement therapy. Renal replacement therapy, even in the absence of severe acute kidney injury, is helpful in avoiding weight gain over the first 72 h, while some fluid is inevitably given, such as nutritional support and drugs. Continuous renal replacement therapies help revert acidosis and can have a role in cytokine absorption and washout.

Pain Management and Muscle Paralysis

The first step in the management of respiratory failure is to ensure adequate analgesia and, if necessary, sedation and muscle paralysis: anxiety, pain, and endotracheal tube intolerance will all determine ventilation asynchrony, triggering a vicious cycle with detrimental stress/strain damage. First-choice sedative in this scenario should be ketamine because of no inhibitory effect on spontaneous respiratory activity, its indirect bronchodilation effect, and very limited cardiovascular depressant effect [49]. IV infusion ketamine can be used in place of opioids when there is the need to sedate the patient or to improve synchrony with mechanical ventilation.

When dealing with trauma-related ARDS, pain management is paramount. The new paradigm is multimodal analgesia which can be considered as a more rational approach to pain management [50]: by using different ways of administration and different drugs, it is possible to reduce the need for sedation, opioids, and side effects. The combined use of different analgesics (opioids, NSAIDs, local anesthetics) produces synergistic analgesia and enables clinicians to use lower total doses [51]. Pain management and low sedative administration are useful for ensuring spontaneous and assisted ventilation, diminishing the risk of VAP (ventilator-induced pneumonia). Multimodal means also different ways of administration: epidural catheters in trauma patients with local anesthetic continuous infusion (e.g., ropivacaine 0.2–0.3%, along with adjuvants, clonidine or morphine) can reduce patient's pain. Regional anesthesia can also help reducing rehabilitation time.

For decades, the leading pharmacological supportive therapy for ARDS has been neuromuscular blockade, which facilitates lung-protective ventilation by minimizing patient-ventilator asynchrony [52]. Indeed, in addition to direct injury and secondary inflammatory-mediated damage, the lung is also subject to ventilator-induced lung injury (VILI). That said, NMBAs can reduce the stress/strain generated in the lung by lowering the negative increase in pleural pressure during spontaneous efforts, avoiding the generation of a harmful transpulmonary pressure. A major control over inspiratory volumes and pressures reduces volutrauma, whereas a better control of expiratory volumes and pressures reduces atelectrauma: these all will lead to less pulmonary and systemic inflammation [53, 54]. However, NMBAs can increase the risk of ICU-acquired weakness and diaphragmatic dysfunction, prolonging the duration of mechanical ventilation.

Cis-atracurium or rocuronium (IV bolus + IV continuous infusion) are commonly used for muscle paralysis.

Steroids

Corticosteroids have theoretical therapeutic potential in ARDS due to their powerful anti-inflammatory action. Steroids have positive immunomodulatory effects reducing edema, surfactant depletion, hyaline membrane formation, and alveolar capillary membrane damage. High-dose and short-duration therapies (methylprednisolone up to 30 mg/kg/day) have demonstrated no improvement in mortality and an increased risk of infection [55]. On the other hand, following Meduri's studies, several case series and uncontrolled trials have reported clinical improvement and reductions in inflammatory cytokines after administration of prolonged, low-dose glucocorticoid use in early, severe ARDS [56]. These improvements tend to occur after at least 2–3 days, so corticosteroids are not a therapy that will provide immediate benefits in a patient with refractory hypoxemia. If corticosteroids are given, it would be reasonable to follow 2007 Meduri protocol (MP 2 mg/kg once, then 0.5 mg/kg every 6 h for 14 days, then a taper over 18 days). After a few days, it would be advisable to taper off if no clinical response is shown, assuming there is no other indication for corticosteroids [57]. Indeed, low-dose steroids are also indicated in septic shock to revert tissue unresponsiveness to amines; as septic shock is among the major causes of secondary ARDS, Meduri MP can have a double role in this scenario.

Critical illness polyneuropathy and myopathy are concerns with prolonged corticosteroid courses, although this has not been definitively linked to these regimens [58]. Nonetheless, the role of corticosteroids in ARDS remains controversial despite a large number of clinical trial and meta-analyses, because improvements have been observed to be delayed and inconsistent.

Vasodilating Agents

Inhaled nitric oxide (iNO) and prostacyclins act as selective pulmonary vasodilators through vascular muscle relaxation [59]. As it is administered by inhalation (20–40 ppm), iNO serves as a local vasodilator of capillary vessels in well-aerated alveoli, improving the V/Q match and reducing pulmonary vascular resistance: as a result, right ventricular performance enhances and amelioration in arterial oxygenation will be observed. However, the beneficial effect on arterial oxygenation lasts for the first 24–48 h after initiation, without any apparent effects on long-term outcomes including mortality [60]. Improved oxygenation is not associated with increased survival rates because the temporary improvement of oxygenation does not indicate improved lung function, reduction of lung injury, or resolution of the underlying cause of ARDS.

Most of the data on inhaled prostacyclin use in patients with ARDS comes from either prospective nonrandomized or observational cohort studies using inhaled epoprostenol (iEPO), alprostadil, or iloprost: effects on oxygenation appear to be similar when comparing iNO to iEPO, but iNO is far more expensive than iEPO [61, 62].

B2 Agonists

B2 agonists can increase sodium transport by activating β2 receptors on alveolar type I and type II cells, accelerating resolution of pulmonary edema. This hypothesis was tested in a single-center, phase 2 RCT demonstrating that a 7-day infusion of salbutamol significantly reduced extravascular lung water. A subsequent multicenter RCT of 7 days of intravenous salbutamol was stopped early due to increased 28-day mortality in the salbutamol group [63, 64]. This lack of efficacy is consistent with two other RCTs using inhaled salbutamol. Neither nebulized nor intravenous β2-agonist therapy improved outcomes in ARDS in multicenter clinical trials, with studies reporting an associated increase in cardiac arrhythmia and 28-day mortality [65].

Vitamins and Statins

Vitamin C is an essential nutrient for the repair and maintenance of the pulmonary microvasculature. High-dose ascorbic acid (vitamin C) has proposed to be a useful adjunct in minimizing the effects of free radical injury since it attenuates post-burn lipid peroxidation [66]: daily dose is 1–2 g by parenteral infusion. The evidence has prompted Cochrane Reviews to recommend vitamin C supplementation in the management of patients with pneumonia, although its independent impact on ARDS has not yet been established.

Vitamin D is well known for its role in calcium homeostasis. As nearly all immune cells express vitamin D receptors (VDR), this vitamin could also have a role in immune signaling: patients with vitamin D deficiency are more likely to be admitted to ICU and have worse outcomes [67, 68].

Statins can reduce inflammation and progression of lung injury in experimental models and were shown to be safe and to reduce non-pulmonary organ dysfunction in a phase 2 RCT. Two large multicenter RCTs were conducted to examine the effect of statins in patients with ARDS: there was no significant difference in 60-day in-hospital mortality. Meta-analysis suggests that statins neither provide benefit for lowering the morbidity of ALI/ARDS in high-risk patients nor improve the clinical outcomes of ALI/ARDS patients. Hence, it may not be appropriate to advocate statin use for the prevention and treatment of ALI/ARDS [69, 70].

Aspirin

The effects of aspirin in preventing the occurrence of ARDS among adult patients are controversial. Aspirin is a nonselective inhibitor of cyclooxygenase (COX) which is widely used in primary and secondary prevention of cardiovascular disease. Evidence showed that platelets play an essential role in both the onset and progress of lung injury by modulating immune function. Observational studies have demonstrated that patients are less likely to develop ARDS and organ dysfunction if they were taking long-term aspirin therapy before admission to hospital. According to a recent meta-analysis, the preventive administration of aspirin could reduce the rate of ARDS but not the mortality in patients at risk [71].

Summary

ARDS, be it primary or secondary, stills remains a major cause of mortality. Although much research has been performed during the last four decades, protective ventilation continues to be the cornerstone of treatment, while reliable medical therapies are still lacking.

While there are many ventilatory modalities available, any ventilator parameter should be tailor set to the patient: Vt, PEEP, and RR should be chosen wisely after evaluating a patient's specific characteristics. Prone positioning and ECMO are rescue treatments for refractory hypoxemia.

As for medical treatment, fluid management is paramount as alveolar edema is the prominent aspect of ARDS. Pain management can be advocated when dealing with trauma-related hypoxemia, whereas muscle paralysis can be mandatory to reduce stress and strain damage. Other therapies, such as steroids, statins, and inhaled vasodilators, have been suggested over the years as brand new magic bullets, but none has been successful in demonstrating modifications of mortality or outcome.

References

1. Ware LB, Matthay MA. The acute respiratory distress syndrome. N Engl J Med. 2000;342:1334–49.
2. Bernard GR. Acute respiratory distress syndrome: a historical perspective. Am J Respir Crit Care Med. 2005;172:798–806.
3. Brun-Buisson C, Minelli C, Bertolini G, et al. Epidemiology and outcome of acute lung injury in European intensive care units: results from the ALIVE study. Intensive Care Med. 2004;30:51–6.
4. Ranieri VM, Rubenfeld GD, Thompson BT, Ferguson ND, Caldwell E, Fan E, et al. Acute respiratory distress syndrome: the Berlin Definition. JAMA. 2012;307(23):2526–33.
5. Spadaro S, Park M, Turrini C, Tunstall T, Thwaites R, Mauri T, Ragazzi R, Ruggeri P, Hansel TT, Caramori G, Volta CA. Biomarkers for acute respiratory distress syndrome and prospects for personalised medicine. J Inflamm (Lond). 2019;16:1.
6. Zemans RL, Matthay MA. What drives neutrophils to the alveoli in ARDS? Thorax. 2017;72(1):1–3.
7. Vassallo A, Wood AJ, Subburayalu J, Summers C, Chilvers ER. The counter-intuitive role of the neutrophil in the acute respiratory distress syndrome. Br Med Bull. 2019;131(1):43–55.
8. Williams AE, José RJ, Mercer PF, Brealey D, Parekh D, Thickett DR, O'Kane C, McAuley DF, Chambers RC. Evidence for chemokine synergy during neutrophil migration in ARDS. Thorax. 2017;72(1):66–73.
9. Yadav H, Kor DJ. Platelets in the pathogenesis of acute respiratory distress syndrome. Am J Physiol Lung Cell Mol Physiol. 2015;309(9):L915–23.
10. Marshall RP, Bellingan G, Webb S, Puddicombe A, Goldsack N, McAnulty RJ, Laurent GJ. Fibroproliferation occurs simultaneously with inflammatory lung injury early in the

acute respiratory distress syndrome and impacts on outcome. Am J Respir Crit Care Med. 2000;162:1783–8.
11. Calfee CS, Delucchi K, Parsons PE, Thompson BT, Ware LB, Matthay MA, Thompson T, Ware LB, Matthay MA. Subphenotypes in acute respiratory distress syndrome: latent class analysis of data from two randomized controlled trials. Lancet Respir Med. 2014;2:611–20.
12. Murray DD, Itenov TS, Sivapalan P, Eklöf JV, Holm FS, Schuetz P, Jensen JU. Biomarkers of acute lung injury the individualized approach: for phenotyping, risk stratification and treatment surveillance. J Clin Med. 2019;8(8):1163.
13. Grinnan DC, et al. Clinical review: Respiratory mechanics in spontaneous and assisted ventilation. Crit Care. 2005;9:472–84.
14. Lumb AB. Nunn's applied respiratory physiology. Edinburgh: Churchill-Livingstone. Elsevier; 2012.
15. Yoshida T, et al. Esophageal manometry and regional transpulmonary pressure in lung injury. Am J Respir Crit Care Med. 2018;197(8):1018–26.
16. Yoshida T, et al. Guiding ventilation with transpulmonary pressure. Intensive Care Med. 2018;45(4):535–8.
17. Amato MB, et al. Driving pressure and survival in the acute respiratory distress syndrome. N Engl J Med. 2015;372:747–55.
18. Gattinoni L, et al. The concept of "baby lung". Intensive Care Med. 2005;31:776–84.
19. Gattinoni L, et al. Ultra protective ventilation and hypoxemia. Crit Care. 2016;20:130.
20. Umbrello M, et al. Current concepts of ARDS: a narrative review. Int J Mol Sci. 2017;18:64.
21. The Acute Respiratory Distress Syndrome Network, et al. Ventilation with lower tidal volumes as compared with traditional tidal volumes for acute lung injury and the acute respiratory distress syndrome. N Engl J Med. 2000;342:1301–8.
22. Gattinoni L, et al. Friday night ventilation: a safety starting tool kit for mechanically ventilated patients. Minerva Anestesiol. 2014;80:1046–57.
23. Gattinoni L, et al. Lung recruitment in patients with the acute respiratory distress syndrome. N Engl J Med. 2006;354:1775–86.
24. Talmor D, et al. Mechanical ventilation guided by esophageal pressure in acute lung injury. N Engl J Med. 2008;359:2095–104.
25. Barbas CSV, et al. Lung recruitment maneuvers in acute respiratory distress syndrome. Respir Care Clin. 2003;9:401–18.
26. Garcia-Fernandez J, et al. Recruitment manoeuvres in anesthesia: how many more excuses are there not to use them ? Rev Esp Anestesiol Reanim. 2018;65(4):209–17.
27. The PROSEVA Study Group. Prone positioning in severe acute respiratory distress syndrome. N Engl J Med. 2013;358:2159–68.
28. Koulouras V, et al. Efficacy of prone position in acute respiratory distress syndrome patients: a pathophysiology-based review. World J Crit Care Med. 2016;5(2):121–6.
29. Gattinoni L, et al. Body position changes redistribute lung computed-tomographic density in patients with acute respiratory failure. Anesthesiology. 1991;74:15–23.
30. Guerin C, et al. Mechanism of the effects of prone positioning in acute respiratory distress syndrome. Intensive Care Med. 2014;40:1634–42.
31. Nyren S, et al. Pulmonary perfusion is more uniform in the prone than in the supine position: scintigraphy in healthy humans. J Appl Physiol. 1985;86:1135–41.
32. Kallet RH, et al. A comprehensive review of prone position in ARDS. Respir Care. 2015;60(11):1660–87.
33. Putensen C, et al. Long-term effects of spontaneous breathing during ventilatory support in patients with acute lung injury. Am J Respir Care Med. 2001;164:43–9.
34. Yoshida T, et al. The role of spontaneous effort during mechanical ventilation: normal lung versus injured lung. J Intensive Care. 2015;3:18.
35. Yoshida T, et al. Spontaneous effort causes occult pendelluft during mechanical ventilation. Am J Respir Crit Care. 2013;188:1420–7.
36. Hraiech S, et al. Balancing neuromuscular blockade versus preserved muscle activity. Curr Opin Crit Care. 2015;21:26–33.

37. Cordell-Smith JA, et al. Traumatic lung injury treated by extracorporeal membrane oxygenation (ECMO). Injury. 2006;37(1):29–32.
38. Ritcher T, et al. Ventilation in chest trauma. J Emerg Trauma Shock. 2011;4(2):251–9.
39. Mizushima Y, et al. Changes in contused lung volume and oxygenation in patients with pulmonary parenchymal injury after blunt chest trauma. Am J Emerg Med. 2000;18:385–9.
40. Katsaragakis S, et al. Independent lung ventilation for asymmetrical chest trauma: effect on ventilatory and haemodynamic parameters. Injury. 2005;36:501–4.
41. Anantham D, et al. Critical review: Independent lung ventilation in critical care. Crit Care. 2005;9:594–600.
42. Boyd JH, Forbes J, Nakada TA, et al. Fluid resuscitation in septic shock: a positive fluid balance and elevated central venous pressure are associated with increased mortality. Crit Care Med. 2011;39(2):259–65.
43. Sakr Y, Rubatto Birri PN, Kotfis K, et al. Higher fluid balance increases the risk of death from sepsis: results from a large international audit. Crit Care Med. 2017;45(3):386–94.
44. Mangialardi RJ, Martin GS, Bernard GR, et al. Hypoproteinemia predicts acute respiratory distress syndrome development, weight gain, and death in patients with sepsis. Ibuprofen in Sepsis Study Group. Crit Care Med. 2000;28:3137–45.
45. Wiedemann HP, Wheeler AP, Bernard GR, et al., National Heart, Lung, and Blood Institute Acute Respiratory Distress Syndrome (ARDS) Clinical Trials Network. Comparison of two fluid management strategies in acute lung injury. N Engl J Med. 2006;354(24):2564–75.
46. Jozwiak M, Teboul J-L, Monnet X. Extravascular lung water in critical care: recent advances and clinical applications. Ann Intensive Care. 2015;5:38.
47. Grissom CK, Hirshberg EL, Dickerson JB, et al. Fluid management with a simplified conservative protocol for the acute respiratory distress syndrome. Crit Care Med. 2015;43(2):288–95.
48. Rice TW, Wheeler AP, Thompson BT, et al., National Heart, Lung, and Blood Institute Acute Respiratory Distress Syndrome (ARDS) Clinical Trials Network. Initial trophic vs full enteral feeding in patients with acute lung injury: the EDEN randomized trial. JAMA. 2012;307(8):795–803.
49. Oddo M, Crippa IA, Mehta S, Menon D, Payen J-F, Taccone FS, Citerio G. Optimizing sedation in patients with acute brain injury. Crit Care. 2016;20:128.
50. Devlin JW, Skrobik Y, Gélinas C, Needham DM, Slooter AJC, Pandhari-Pande PP, et al. Clinical practice guidelines for the prevention and management of pain, agitation/sedation, delirium, immobility, and sleep disruption in adult patients in the ICU. Crit Care Med. 2018;46(9):e825–73.
51. Faust AC, Rajan P, Sheperd LA, Alvarez CA, McCorstin P, Doebele RL, et al. Impact of an analgesia-based sedation protocol on mechanically ventilated patients in a medical intensive care unit. Anesth Analg. 2016;123(4):903–9.
52. Murray MJ, Cowen J, DeBlock H, Erstad B, Gray AW, Tescher AN, et al. Clinical practice guidelines for sustained neuromuscular blockade in the adult critically ill patient. Crit Care Med. 2002;30:142–56.
53. Grawe ES, Bennett S, Hurford WE. Early paralysis for the management of ARDS. Respir Care. 2016;61(6):830–8.
54. Papazian L, Forel JM, Gacouin A, Penot-Ragon C, Perrin G, Loundou A. Neuromuscular blockers in early acute respiratory distress syndrome. N Engl J Med. 2010;363(12):1107–16.
55. Peter JV, John P, Graham PL, Moran JL, George IA, Bersten A. Corticosteroids in the prevention and treatment of acute respiratory distress syndrome (ARDS) in adults: meta-analysis. BMJ. 2008;336(7651):1006–9.
56. Meduri GU, Bridges L, Shih MC, Marik PE, Siemieniuk RA, Kocak M. Prolonged glucocorticoid treatment is associated with improved ARDS outcomes: analysis of individual patients' data from four randomized trials and trial-level meta-analysis of the updated literature. Intensive Care Med. 2016;42(5):829–40.
57. Thompson BT, Ranieri VM. Steroids are part of rescue therapy in ARDS patients with refractory hypoxemia: no. Intensive Care Med. 2016;42(5):921–3.

58. Annane D, Pastores SM, Rochwerg B, et al. Guidelines for the diagnosis and management of critical illness-related corticosteroid insufficiency (CIRCI) in critically ill patients (Part I): Society of Critical Care Medicine (SCCM) and European Society of Intensive Care Medicine (ESICM) 2017. Crit Care Med. 2017;45(12):2078–88.
59. Dellinger RP, Zimmerman JL, Taylor RW, et al. Effects of inhaled nitric oxide in patients with acute respiratory distress syndrome: results of a randomized phase II trial. Inhaled nitric oxide in ARDS Study Group. Crit Care Med. 1998;26(1):15–23.
60. Adhikari NK, Dellinger RP, Lundin S, et al. Inhaled nitric oxide does not reduce mortality in patients with acute respiratory distress syndrome regardless of severity: systematic review and meta-analysis. Crit Care Med. 2014;42(2):404–12.
61. Fuller BM, Mohr NM, Skrupky L, et al. The use of inhaled prostaglandins in patients with ARDS: a systematic review and meta-analysis. Chest. 2015;147(6):1510–22.
62. Torbic H, Szumita PM, Anger KE, et al. Inhaled epoprostenol vs inhaled nitric oxide for refractory hypoxemia in critically ill patients. J Crit Care. 2013;28(5):844–8.
63. Perkins GD, McAuley DF, Thickett DR, et al. The beta-agonist lung injury trial (BALTI): a randomized placebo-controlled clinical trial. Am J Respir Crit Care Med. 2006;173:281–7.
64. Matthay MA, Brower RG, Carson S, et al. Randomized, placebo-controlled clinical trial of an aerosolized β-agonist for treatment of acute lung injury. Am J Respir Crit Care Med. 2011;184(5):561–8.
65. Gao Smith F, Perkins GD, Gates S, et al. Effect of intravenous β-2 agonist treatment on clinical outcomes in acute respiratory distress syndrome (BALTI-2): a multicentre, randomised controlled trial. Lancet. 2012;279(9812):229–35.
66. Kremer T, Harenberg P, Hernekamp F, et al. High-dose vitamin C treatment reduces capillary leakage after burn plasma transfer in rats. J Burn Care Res. 2010;31(3):470–9.
67. Zhang Y, Leung DY, Richers BN, et al. Vitamin D inhibits monocyte/macrophage pro-inflammatory cytokine production by targeting MAPK phosphatase-1. J Immunol. 2012;188(5):2127–35.
68. Dancer RC, Parekh D, Lax S, et al. Vitamin D deficiency contributes directly to the acute respiratory distress syndrome (ARDS). Thorax. 2015;70(7):617–24.
69. Calfee CS, Delucchi KL, Sinha P, et al. Acute respiratory distress syndrome subphenotypes and differential response to simvastatin: secondary analysis of a randomised controlled trial. Lancet Respir Med. 2018;6:691–8.
70. Nagendran M, McAuley DF, Kruger PS, et al. Statin therapy for acute respiratory distress syndrome: an individual patient data meta-analysis of randomised clinical trials. Intensive Care Med. 2017;45(5):663–71.
71. Yu H, Ni YN, Liang ZA, Liang BM, Wang Y. The effect of aspirin in preventing the acute respiratory distress syndrome/acute lung injury: a meta-analysis. Am J Emerg Med. 2018;36(8):1486–91.

Tracheal and Bronchial Injury

Preston Miller and Walter L. Biffl

Epidemiology

Tracheal and bronchial injuries are uncommon yet they are often lethal regardless of mechanism. Asensio in a literature review of patients with penetrating neck trauma found that 331 of 4193 (8%) had a laryngotracheal injury [1]. By comparison, in a series by Graham, less than 1% of patients (4 of 666) with penetrating chest trauma had a tracheobronchial injury [2]. Those with blunt mechanisms severe enough to cause tracheobronchial injury are likely to have serious concomitant trauma. Due to the high probability of on-scene death, the true incidence of injury is difficult to establish and autopsy reports have provided a great deal of information on the subject. Bertelsen and Howitz reviewed 1178 autopsies of blunt trauma deaths and reported that 33 patients had tracheobronchial injuries for a rate of 2.8%. Traffic accidents were the most common cause of injury and the majority of cases were thoracic rather than cervical. A reported 82% of patients died immediately [3]. Campbell reviewed 15,136 surviving and deceased patients with blunt chest trauma. The reported rate of tracheobronchial trauma was low (0.3%) with a high mortality rate of 67% [4]. More recently, Kummer published a series of 104 patients with traumatic airway injuries (pharynx, larynx, and tracheobronchial tree) who survived until hospital arrival. The incidence of traumatic airway injury was 0.4% for blunt mechanisms and 4.5% for penetrating. Mortality was 36% for blunt and 16% for penetrating [5].

The morphology of tracheobronchial injuries varies based on mechanism. Penetrating injuries consist of a hole or laceration in the tracheobronchial tree usually caused by a knife or bullet. Knife wounds almost always occur in the cervical trachea, whereas gunshot wounds can occur anywhere along the tracheobronchial tree. Gunshot wounds generally create larger defects with some degree of tissue loss depending on bullet caliber and velocity. In contrast to penetrating injuries, there are variable mechanisms by which blunt injuries occur. A direct blow to the neck may cause a "clothesline"-type injury whereby the cervical trachea is crushed against the vertebral bodies. Other mechanisms of blunt tracheobronchial disruption are relatively complex and consist of three components working in conjunction as described by Kirsh [6]:

1. Sudden anteroposterior compression of the thoracic cage with simultaneous widening of the transverse diameter. This lateral widening separates the lungs, pulling the main bronchi apart and placing traction on the carina. Rupture occurs when the force of traction exceeds the elasticity of the tracheobronchial tree.
2. Glottic closure during impact. This results in a rigid, pressurized tracheobronchial tree which can lead to perforation along the membranous surface of the trachea.
3. Rapid deceleration causing shearing stress on the cricoid and carina which are points of fixation along the tracheobronchial tree.

In a review of 265 patients with blunt tracheobronchial trauma, Kiser found that injury occurred within 2 cm of the carina in 76% of patients and within the first 2 cm of the right main bronchus in 46% of patients [7]. This finding is consistent with other reports and is predicted by the Law of LaPlace which states that wall stress is proportional to vessel diameter. Therefore, perforation is most likely to occur where the trachea and bronchus are largest. In terms of injury morphology, Symbas reviewed the literature for 183 cases and found that 74% of ruptures were transverse, 18% were longitudinal and 8% were complex [8].

Clinical Presentation

The clinical presentation of tracheobronchial trauma varies depending on the mechanism, location, and severity of injury. In patients with cervical trauma, signs suggestive of laryngotracheal injury include dysphagia, hemoptysis, subcutaneous emphysema, respiratory distress, and stridor. Air escaping from a penetrating neck wound is highly indicative of tracheal injury [9]. Thoracic tracheobronchial injuries commonly present with respiratory distress, subcutaneous emphysema, pneumothorax, and pneumomediastinum [10]. A rupture that is confined to the mediastinum will present with pneumomediastinum and occasionally pneumopericardium. An injury that decompresses into the pleural space will typically cause a pneumothorax. Tension physiology may result, especially if the patient is receiving positive pressure ventilation. A continuous air leak with persistent pneumothorax after adequate tube thoracostomy suggests a tracheobronchial injury with a bronchopleural fistula. Respiratory distress may worsen after chest tube placement due to loss of tidal volume through the tube.

Because of the high-energy required for blunt thoracic tracheobronchial rupture, patients nearly always have additional traumatic injuries. Chest wall trauma such as rib fractures may be the presumed source of a pneumothorax. Thus, tracheobronchial injury can be masked by other trauma, which leads to a delay in diagnosis. Glazer reviewed multiple case series and found that 50% of tracheobronchial injuries are not diagnosed during the first 24–48 h of hospitalization [11]. Furthermore, up to 10% of cases will have a complete absence of clinical or radiographic signs and are only recognized months later after a bronchial stricture develops [12]. One explanation is that peribronchial connective tissues remain intact around the injury and allow for continued ventilation of the affected lung. As the injury heals, ingrowth of granulation tissue leads to bronchial stenosis with distal atelectasis and in some cases pneumonia.

Patterns of concomitant injury vary widely. Trauma to the cervical trachea often involves the esophagus, recurrent laryngeal nerves, spine, carotid arteries, and jugular veins. With blunt trauma severe enough to produce a thoracic tracheobronchial rupture, multiple regions may be involved including head, chest, abdomen, spine, and extremities. It is important to note that concomitant trauma is often severe and may be the primary determinant of outcome [13]. Any severe injury to the chest, especially those with transmediastinal penetration, should alert one to the possibility of tracheobronchial injury. Maintaining a high index of suspicion is critical to diagnose these injuries promptly and appropriately.

Diagnostic Evaluation

The patient presenting with obvious signs of tracheobronchial injury will generally require airway control. If there is time and equipment is available, fiber-optic intubation is recommended in order to (a) confirm the diagnosis, (b) ensure the endotracheal tube is placed distal to the site of injury, and (c) avoid the pitfall of having the endotracheal tube exit the airway through a laceration [14]. For those injuries that are not immediately clinically apparent, the diagnostic evaluation may include some combination of imaging studies, bronchoscopy, or surgical exploration.

Imaging

Tracheobronchial injuries are typically associated with escape of air into the surrounding soft tissues. Consequently, subcutaneous emphysema or pneumomediastinum are usually seen on imaging and are the hallmarks of tracheobronchial injury. Indeed, the absence of either finding is felt to essentially rule out significant tracheobronchial injury—particularly when high-resolution CT scan is used. As noted above, there may be some cases of occult injury with intact peribronchial tissues which will require a high index of suspicion. In the absence of subcutaneous or mediastinal air, hemoptysis, a voice change, or irregularity of the airways on imaging, further workup is not routinely indicated.

While subcutaneous emphysema or pneumomediastinum are cardinal signs of tracheobronchial injury, they are not by any means pathognomonic. Pneumomediastinum is found in as many as 5% of chest CT scans after trauma, and only about 10% of such patients will have significant aerodigestive injuries [15, 16]. Consequently, confirmatory bronchoscopy is recommended.

Bronchoscopy

Bronchoscopy is critical in the diagnosis and management of tracheobronchial injuries [13]. It will readily confirm an injury and localize it to facilitate appropriate airway placement and plan repair. Flexible fiber-optic bronchoscopy is the technique most commonly employed. It is imperative that the airway be cleared of blood and secretions and a circumferential view be obtained. In the intubated patient, the endotracheal tube may have been inserted distal to the area of injury. In order to visualize and confirm injury, the tube will need to be carefully withdrawn using the bronchoscope as a guide. Once the examination is complete, the tube is advanced under direct visualization.

A large majority of blunt tracheobronchial injuries occur within 2 cm of the carina, so examination of the right and left mainstem bronchi and segmental airways is mandatory.

Exploration

Some airway injuries will be discovered at the time of surgical exploration, usually in a patient with penetrating trauma and indications for immediate surgery. It is important to expose the trachea adequately, including circumferential assessment to detect transtracheal injuries. Intraoperative bronchoscopy can be a useful adjunct in this regard, in the setting of cervical as well as thoracic injuries.

Management

Airway Control

Airway control is critical in any trauma patient, and especially in the patient with airway injury. Hypoxia and hypoventilation may occur due to loss of tidal volume, and airway occlusion may occur due to tracheobronchial crush injury, laceration, or endotracheal tube malposition as described above. Orotracheal or nasotracheal intubation may be performed; fiber-optic intubation is recommended if there is suspicion of airway injury. In the case of a cervical laceration that involves the trachea, direct intubation of the trachea is expedient and safe.

Once a secure airway is in place, diagnosis and management can occur in an unhurried manner. Complete bronchoscopic evaluation is performed first. Very small or partial thickness injuries may be managed nonoperatively, and carefully selected patients may be best served by endobronchial stenting [17]. However, the majority of significant traumatic injuries should be repaired.

Exposure

The proximal half of the trachea may be exposed in the neck. A standard cervical sternocleidomastoid incision is generally employed for neck exploration. If isolated tracheal injury is present or bilateral cervical exploration is planned, a collar incision is more appropriate. The trachea is exposed directly and may be mobilized by performing blunt dissecting along its anterior aspect.

The distal trachea, right mainstem bronchus, and proximal left mainstem bronchus are most readily exposed via a right posterolateral thoracotomy incision. The distal left mainstem bronchus is approached via left posterolateral thoracotomy [18].

Repair

Simple tracheal lacerations can be repaired primarily with interrupted absorbable sutures. More extensive lacerations may require debridement, or even segmental resection of the trachea. Temporary placement of an endotracheal tube in the operative field may be necessary to allow resection and mobilization of the trachea; once sutures are placed and the trachea is reapproximated, the endotracheal tube may be replaced and positioned.

For injuries in the bronchi, single-lung ventilation will allow repair.

Concomitant esophageal or vascular injury repairs should be separated from tracheal repairs by an interposed muscle flap. The strap muscles or sternocleidomastoid are used in the neck, and intercostal muscle in the chest.

Tracheostomy

Tracheostomy is not routinely necessary following tracheobronchial repair. It has been recommended in the setting of a tracheal laceration involving more than one-third the circumference of the trachea, an injury with a significant airway crush component, or cervical spinal cord injury with tetraplegia and the need for mechanical ventilator support [19].

Conclusions

Tracheobronchial injuries are uncommon. Their presence is usually manifest by subcutaneous emphysema, pneumomediastinum, or persistent air leak from tube thoracostomy. Bronchoscopy is key to diagnosis and planning management.

Surgical repair is mandatory for significant injuries, but select patient may be managed nonoperatively or with tracheobronchial stenting.

References

1. Asensio JA, Valenziano CP, Falcone RE, Grosh JD. Management of penetrating neck injuries. The controversy surrounding zone II injuries. Surg Clin North Am. 1991;71:267–96.
2. Graham JM, Mattox KL, Beall AC. Penetrating trauma of the lung. J Trauma. 1979;19:665–9.
3. Bertelsen S, Howitz P. Injuries of the trachea and bronchi. Thorax. 1972;27:188–94.
4. Campbell DB. Trauma to the chest wall, lung, and major airways. Semin Thorac Cardiovasc Surg. 1992;4:234–40.
5. Kummer C, Netto FS, Rizoli S, Yee D. A review of traumatic airway injuries: potential implications for airway assessment and management. Injury. 2007;38:27–33.
6. Kirsh MM, Orringer MB, Behrendt DM, Sloan H. Management of tracheobronchial disruption secondary to nonpenetrating trauma. Ann Thorac Surg. 1976;22:93–101.
7. Kiser AC, O'Brien SM, Detterbeck FC. Blunt tracheobronchial injuries: treatment and outcomes. Ann Thorac Surg. 2001;71:2059–65.
8. Symbas PN, Justicz AG, Ricketts RR. Rupture of the airways from blunt trauma: treatment of complex injuries. Ann Thorac Surg. 1992;54:177–83.
9. Symbas PN, Hatcher CR, Vlasis SE. Bullet wounds of the trachea. J Thorac Cardiovasc Surg. 1982;83:235–8.
10. Welter S. Repair of tracheobronchial injuries. Thorac Surg Clin. 2014;24:41–50.
11. Glazer ES, Meyerson SL. Delayed presentation and treatment of tracheobronchial injuries due to blunt trauma. J Surg Educ. 2008;65:302–8.
12. Dowd NP, Clarkson K, Walsh MA, Cunningham AJ. Delayed bronchial stenosis after blunt chest trauma. Anesth Analg. 1996;82:1078–81.
13. Karmy-Jones R, Wood DE. Traumatic injury to the trachea and bronchus. Thorac Surg Clin. 2007;17:35–46.
14. Schaefer SD. Management of acute blunt and penetrating external laryngeal trauma. Laryngoscope. 2014;124:233–44.
15. Dissanaike S, Shalhub S, Jurkovich GJ. The evaluation of pneumomediastinum in blunt trauma patients. J Trauma. 2008;65:1340–5.
16. Macleod JB, Tibbs BM, Freiberger DJ, Rozycki GS, Lewis F, Feliciano DV. Pneumomediastinum in the injured patient: inconsequential or predictive? Am Surg. 2009;75:375–7.
17. Grewal HS, Dangayach NS, Ahmad U, Ghosh S, Gildea T, Mehta AC. Treatment of tracheobronchial injuries: a contemporary review. Chest. 2019;155:595–604.
18. Koletsis E, Prokakis C, Baltayiannis N, Apostolakis E, Chatzimichalis A, Dougenis D. Surgical decision making in tracheobronchial injuries on the basis of clinical evidences and the injury's anatomic setting: a retrospective analysis. Injury. 2012;43:1437–41.
19. Levy RD, Degiannis E, Hatzitheophilou C, et al. Management of penetrating injuries of the cervical trachea. Ann R Coll Surg Engl. 1997;79:195–200.

Lung Injury

Samuel P. Carmichael II, Yoram Kluger,
and J. Wayne Meredith

Introduction

Trauma is the leading cause of death among persons up to 45 years of age and the fourth leading cause of death for all ages, resulting in over 150,000 deaths and >3 million non-fatal injuries annually [1]. Among injured patients admitted in the United States, roughly 1/3 will have trauma to the chest with underlying lung injury in the majority [2]. Injury to the thorax is present following both blunt and penetrating trauma and is the major contributing factor in approximately 75% of trauma mortality [3].

While the majority of thoracic trauma may be managed with supportive measures and/or tube thoracostomy, roughly 20–40% of patients following penetrating mechanism and 15–20% after blunt mechanism will require resectional intervention to the traumatized lung if thoracotomy is needed [3]. Of these, anatomic resection is uncommon (0.5%) and the majority are adequately managed with either tractotomy or nonanatomic stapled resection of the injured lung [4, 5].

Though the chest may be entered in an emergent fashion (i.e., resuscitative thoracotomy) with secondary discovery of lung injury, operative indications for the acutely injured lung may take on one of two forms: hemorrhage or massive air leak. Traditionally, surgeons have considered 1500 mL chest tube output upon insertion and/or 200–300 mL/h of ongoing drainage to be indications for thoracotomy on the basis of mortality benefit [6, 7]. Significant caveats to this include (1) time to presentation (i.e., duration of pleural blood accumulation), (2) diffuse lung

---

S. P. Carmichael II (✉) · J. W. Meredith
Department of Surgery, Wake Forest University, Winston-Salem, NC, USA
e-mail: scarmich@wakhealth.edu; merediw@wakehealth.edu

Y. Kluger
Department of General Surgery, Rambam Health Care Campus, Haifa, Israel
e-mail: y_kluger@rambam.health.gov.il

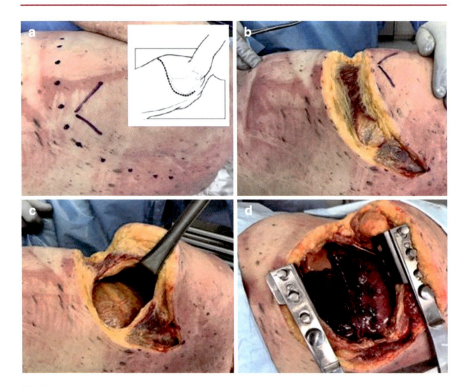

Fig. 1 Left posterolateral incision with arrow indicating tip of scapula. (**a**) Exposure of latissimus dorsi laterally and trapezius medially, revealing the auscultatory triangle. (**b**) Development of the sub-serratus plane with exposure of the chest wall through the auscultatory triangle. (**c**) Exposure of the chest via the fifth intercostal interspace

parenchymal bleeding, and (3) coagulopathy. In practice, however, the decision to enter the chest should be based on patient physiology rather than an absolute or persisting volume of effluent from thoracostomy [8].

The incision most favorable for exposure of the lung is a fifth intercostal space posterolateral thoracotomy on the affected side (Fig. 1). Additional exposures pertinent to injuries by lung region are listed in Table 1. In the majority of cases, simple suture repair of laceration or stapled wedge resection are the therapeutic options of choice [3]. Huh et al. retrospectively reviewed 15 years of operative lung injury from a single urban trauma center ($n = 397$), revealing repair rates of 58% pneumonorraphy, 21% wedge resection or lobectomy, 11% tractotomy, 8% pneumonectomy, and 2% evacuation of hematoma [9].

Blunt Injury

Blunt trauma to the lung, most commonly caused by motor vehicle accidents and falls, is the most common pulmonary injury overall [10]. Of these, pulmonary contusion (Fig. 2) is the most common type in all-comers (30–75%), given its presence

Table 1 Surgical approaches for traumatic injuries to the lung and associated structures

Site	Sternotomy	Right thoracotomy	Left thoracotomy
Main PA	+++	0	++
Right PA	++	+++	0
Left PA	++	0	+++
Right UL	++	+++	0
Right ML	++	+++	0
Right LL	+	+++	0
Left UL	+	0	+++
Left LL	0	0	+++
Right hilum	++	+++	0
Left hilum	++	0	+++

Table modified from Meredith JW, Hoth JJ. Thoracic trauma: when and how to intervene. Surg Clin North Am. 2007;87(1):95–118. https://doi.org/10.1016/j.suc.2006.09.014
PA pulmonary artery, *UL* upper lobe, *ML* middle lobe, *LL* lower lobe

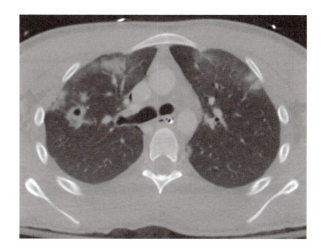

Fig. 2 Pulmonary contusions bilaterally with traumatic pneumatocele of the right lung

with both blunt and penetrating mechanisms [2]. The contused lung is thought to result from laceration with adjacent hemorrhage versus injury to the alveolar capillary wall. Wagner and colleagues elaborate four types of contusion: compression with rupture (I), compression with shearing across the vertebral bodies (II), laceration associated with rib fracture (III), and lateral compression (IV) [11].

In comparison to penetrating trauma, blunt mechanism causes a more profound and diffuse lung injury. As such, caution should be considered prior to operation for parenchymal injury to the lung, particularly in the coagulopathic patient. Since the pulmonary circulation is a low-pressure system, thoracostomy drainage, lung re-expansion, and correction of coagulopathy may satisfactorily tamponade hemorrhage and determine subsequent need for operation. Immediate surgical intervention in this setting risks further exacerbation of bleeding.

Of note, primary blast lung injury (PBLI—Fig. 3) is a particular type of blunt trauma defined as both clinical and radiographic evidence of lung injury within a short time (12 h) of exposure and not related to secondary causality. PBLI accounts

Fig. 3 Demonstration of blast injury to the chest and abdominal wall

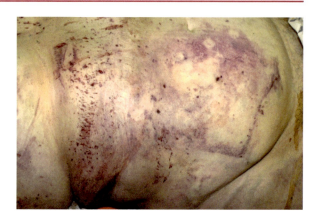

for 6–11% of military casualties in recent conflicts and is created when a shock wave at high pressure (up to 250,000 atm) travels supersonically away from an explosion [12]. This mechanism, most common after closed-space detonations, creates a diffuse parenchymal injury, lung laceration, pneumatocele, and alveolar rupture.

Evaluation

Physical exam of the injured patient may reveal dyspnea, tachypnea, cyanosis, hemoptysis, and variably coarsened or disparate breath sounds depending upon the magnitude of injury. Other signs on the secondary exam include the presence of paradoxical chest wall motion from segmental rib fracture and subcutaneous emphysema. Blunt injury to the lung may or may not result in hemodynamic instability, often depending upon presence or absence of tension physiology. Oxygenation and ventilation are most likely affected proportional to the area of lung incorporated into the injury.

Chest radiography may reveal patchy infiltration traversing lung segmental boundaries, consistent with alveolar hemorrhage [2]. Computed tomography (Fig. 2) increases the sensitivity and specificity for detection of blunt pulmonary injury beyond that of plain radiography. Unique to blast lung injury may be noted a pattern of bilateral peri-hilar infiltrates ("batswing" or "butterfly wing" pattern), consistent with central areas of contusion [13]. Point of care chest ultrasonography (FAST – Focused Assessment with Sonography for Trauma) should be considered as an adjunct to diagnosis of blunt lung injury (sensitivity 94.6%, specificity 96.1%), potentially assisting with diagnosis in austere environments without the aid of computed tomography [14].

Management

The majority of treatment to the bluntly injured lung is nonoperative and consists of supportive therapy to optimize pulmonary mechanics while the affected segments are allowed to heal. This strategy is summarized in a threefold approach:

multimodal pain management (oral, intravenous, epidural), balanced volume resuscitation, and pulmonary toilet (incentive spirometry, chest physiotherapy, bronchodilators, mobility). Patients with severe blunt chest trauma requiring mechanical ventilation are at risk for the complications of lung injury (acute respiratory distress syndrome and ventilator associated pneumonia) [15, 16]. Though approximately 80% of blast lung injuries will ultimately require mechanical ventilation, adequate spontaneous breathing at 2 h after incident are unlikely to require intubation and may be safely discharged to close observation after 6 h [12].

While endovascular management for injuries to the thorax is best described for aortic and thoracic outlet injury, embolization of bleeding vessels within the pulmonary circulation may be an alternative to surgery at institutions with interventional radiology support [17].

Operative Intervention

Blunt trauma results in severe diffuse lung injury and is more difficult to treat surgically with worse outcomes compared to penetrating injury [18]. Where tractotomy and wedge resection are more common in penetrating mechanisms, anatomic lobectomy and pneumonectomy are more commonly performed if resection is required in association with blunt trauma [3].

Hilar control should be the initial maneuver performed if significant bleeding is encountered upon entry into the chest. This can be accomplished via placement of a large clamp (Fig. 4) or incising the inferior pulmonary ligament to the inferior pulmonary vein with subsequent 180 degree rotation (hilar twist maneuver). If exsanguinating injury to the pulmonary vein and artery is identified, pneumonectomy should be expeditiously considered. Trauma pneumonectomy is extremely morbid with high mortality (54% in blunt mechanism, 34% in penetrating mechanism) and should only be performed for the patient in extremis, having quickly exhausted other attempts at hemostasis [19, 20]. Distal to the clamp, the hilar structures may

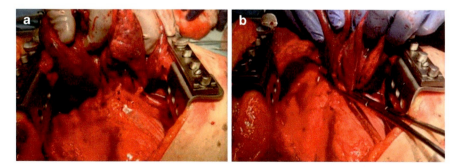

Fig. 4 Preparation for pneumonectomy via posterolateral incision. Demonstration of view following division of inferior pulmonary ligament from diaphragm (**a**) and subsequent hilar clamp placement (**b**)

be stapled (separate loads for vascular and bronchial structures) or sharply divided and oversewn with 3–0 polypropylene suture. In comparison, there is no difference in survival between stapled versus suture ligation in pneumonectomy. Advantages of stapled resection include a significant reduction in operative time with no difference in burst pressure of the bronchus or pulmonary artery [21]. Acute right heart strain and right heart failure are the major immediate mortality risks in this setting. Venoarterial extracorporeal membrane oxygenation may therefore be an appropriate treatment consideration.

Damage control thoracotomy is an alternative and/or adjunct to resectional procedure should diffuse parenchymal injury be encountered in the physiologically exhausted patient, as indicated by acidemia, hypothermia, and coagulopathy. Temporary packing of lung, bone, venous, or chest wall bleeding is a valid and reasonable option in this scenario. The technical aspects of this operation include (1) direct placement of laparotomy pads for parenchymal packing, (2) insertion of thoracostomy tubes for pleural drainage, and (3) temporary wound closure with vacuum-assisted sponge dressing. If needed, rib spaces may be re-approximated with interrupted absorbable suture, passing immediately superior to the cephalad rib and including the intercostal muscle at the inferior rib to protect the neurovascular bundle. In review of a single-center experience, O'Connor et al. describe application of this procedure to both blunt and penetrating mechanisms, +/− partial lung resection, and definitive closure on a mean of 3 days. It is important to note that fewer packs should be utilized for hemostasis in the chest, given the possibility of compromised oxygenation/ventilation or tamponade physiology [22, 23].

Penetrating Injury

The majority of trauma to the thorax requiring operative intervention is penetrating in nature. Mechanistically, single-projectile gunshot wounds are the most common, followed by stab wounds and shotgun blasts [24]. However, similar to blunt injury, penetrating injury is most usually managed by tube thoracostomy. When operation is required, tractotomy or nonanatomic wedge resection is typically therapeutic.

Evaluation

Following primary survey, standard secondary exam of the patient with penetrating injury to the chest should include demarcation of any ballistic trauma, detailing trajectory of the weapon (i.e., bullet, knife, etc.). This approach may be aided by radio-opaque adhesive markers that can be applied to the skin and are visible by chest radiography. This quick estimation of the projectile path may inform the surgeon's intervention and/or incision of choice, particularly in the setting of hemodynamic instability (i.e., transmediastinal gunshot wound). In the absence of hemodynamic instability, further evaluation with diagnostic multi-detector computed tomography can further delineate injury pattern prior to intervention.

Chest ultrasonography (FAST ultrasound) may aid in the diagnosis and/or exclusion of cardiac injury by identification of pericardial effusion with a sensitivity of 79% and specificity of 95.6% [25]. Chest radiography is useful for diagnosis of associated hemo-pneumothorax. Computed tomography details the tract of penetrating injury and status of the pleural space. CT has a negative predictive value of 99% in the hemodynamically stable patient, effectively ruling out the need for operative intervention with nonsignificant imaging [26].

Management

Hemo-pneumothoraces often require immediate drainage for symptoms or hemodynamic instability in the resuscitation bay. As such, tube thoracostomy placement is both therapeutic and diagnostic, identifying massive air leak and ongoing bleeding as indications for the operating room [24]. Though placement of thoracostomy is a commonly performed procedure, it carries a 19% complication rate (52% malposition) [27]. Evaluation by interventional radiology for catheter-based therapy is a consideration in the hemodynamically stable patient with identifiable parenchymal hemorrhage following thoracostomy drainage.

Operative Intervention

Lung-sparing operative techniques (suture pneumonorrhaphy, tractotomy, and nonanatomic resection) satisfactorily manage approximately 85% of penetrating pulmonary trauma [24].

Suture pneumonorrhaphy is accomplished following selective ligation of bleeding vessels within the wound bed and a running-locking absorbable suture to reapproximate the wound edges. Stapled tractotomy (Fig. 5) is intended to open a tunnel created by the missile or penetrating object for individual suture ligation of bleeding vessels or bronchi. Failure of hemostasis with tractotomy may result in need for lobectomy in deep lobar injuries or nonanatomic stapled resection to the periphery of the lung. The authors recommend 3–0 pledgeted polypropylene suture in horizontal mattress for this purpose and/or consideration of continuous nonpledgeted 3–0 polypropylene running/locking for reapproximation of stapled edges. Oversewing of entrance and exit wounds in this setting may be successful in stopping hemorrhage into the pleural space, but runs the risk of creating parenchymal hematoma or forcing blood into the tracheobronchial tree with subsequent exacerbation of respiratory dysfunction. It is important, at the conclusion of the case, to visualize reinflation of the lung for identification and treatment of air leaks prior to closure with thoracostomy.

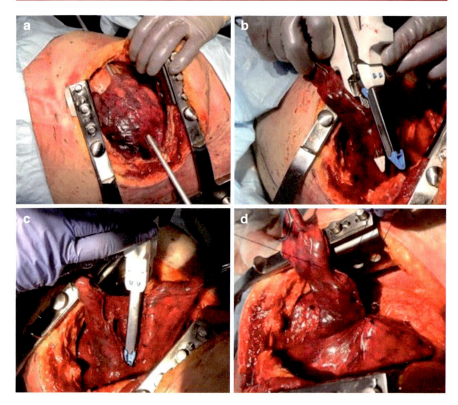

Fig. 5 Tractotomy for non-hilar injury. Demonstration of missile tract. (**a**) Stapled opening of tract. (**b**) Division of posterior lung. (**c**) Running reapproximation of stapled edges with PDS suture

While the majority of these interventions are performed via thoracotomy, video-assisted thoracoscopic surgery (VATS) is an option for the appropriate hemodynamically stable patient. Though typically reserved for evacuation of blood from the pleural space following failed thoracostomy evacuation, VATS is a consideration for excellent visualization of the lung parenchyma, mediastinum, and diaphragm for evaluation of injury and possible pneumonorrhaphy [24].

References

1. The American Association for the Surgery of Trauma. Trauma Facts—The American Association for the Surgery of Trauma. The American Association for the Surgery of Trauma. http://www.aast.org/trauma-facts. Published 2017. Accessed 14 Apr 2019.
2. Miller DL, Mansour KA. Blunt traumatic lung injuries. Thorac Surg Clin. 2007;17(1):57–61. https://doi.org/10.1016/J.THORSURG.2007.03.017.
3. Meredith JW, Hoth JJ. Thoracic trauma: when and how to intervene. Surg Clin North Am. 2007;87(1):95–118. https://doi.org/10.1016/j.suc.2006.09.014.

4. Karmy-Jones R, Jurkovich GJ, Shatz DV, et al. Management of traumatic lung injury: a western trauma association multicenter review. J Trauma. 2001;51(6):1049–53. https://doi.org/10.1097/00005373-200112000-00004.
5. Demetriades D, Velmahos GC. Penetrating injuries of the chest: indications for operation. Scand J Surg. 2002;91(1):41–5. https://doi.org/10.1177/145749690209100107.
6. Karmy-Jones R, Jurkovich GJ, Nathens AB, et al. Timing of urgent thoracotomy for hemorrhage after trauma. Arch Surg. 2003;136(5):513. https://doi.org/10.1001/archsurg.136.5.513.
7. McNamara JJ, Messersmith JK, Dunn RA, Molot MD, Stremple JF. Thoracic injuries in combat casualties in Vietnam. Ann Thorac Surg. 1970;10(5):389–401. https://doi.org/10.1016/S0003-4975(10)65367-2.
8. Mowery NT, Gunter OL, Collier BR, et al. Practice management guidelines for management of hemothorax and occult pneumothorax. J Trauma Inj Infect Crit Care. 2011;70(2):510–8. https://doi.org/10.1097/TA.0b013e31820b5c31.
9. Huh J, Wall MJ, Estrera AL, Soltero ER, Mattox KL. Surgical management of traumatic pulmonary injury. Am J Surg. 2003;186(6):620–4. https://doi.org/10.1016/J.AMJSURG.2003.08.013.
10. Mowery NT, Meredith JW. Thoracic trauma. In: Grippi MA, Elias JA, Fishman JA, et al., editors. Fishman's pulmonary diseases and disorders. 5th ed. New York, NY: McGraw-Hill Education; 2015. http://accessmedicine.mhmedical.com/content.aspx?aid=1122366711.
11. Wagner RB, Crawford WO, Schimpf PP. Classification of parenchymal injuries of the lung. Radiology. 1988;167(1):77–82. https://doi.org/10.1148/radiology.167.1.3347751.
12. Scott TE, Kirkman E, Haque M, Gibb IE, Mahoney P, Hardman JG. Primary blast lung injury—a review. Br J Anaesth. 2017;118(3):311–6. https://doi.org/10.1093/bja/aew385.
13. Avidan V, Hersch M, Armon Y, et al. Blast lung injury: clinical manifestations, treatment, and outcome. Am J Surg. 2005;190(6):945–50. https://doi.org/10.1016/j.amjsurg.2005.08.020.
14. Soldati G, Testa A, Silva FR, Carbone L, Portale G, Silveri NG. Chest ultrasonography in lung contusion. Chest. 2006;130(2):533–8. https://doi.org/10.1378/CHEST.130.2.533.
15. Watkins TR, Nathens AB, Cooke CR, et al. Acute respiratory distress syndrome after trauma: development and validation of a predictive model. Crit Care Med. 2012;40(8):2295–303. https://doi.org/10.1097/CCM.0b013e3182544f6a.
16. Miller PR, Croce MA, Bee TK, et al. ARDS after pulmonary contusion: accurate measurement of contusion volume identifies high-risk patients. J Trauma. 2001;51(2):223–8; discussion 229–30. http://www.ncbi.nlm.nih.gov/pubmed/11493778. Accessed 30 Jun 2019.
17. Arthurs ZM, Sohn VY, Starnes BW. Vascular trauma: endovascular management and techniques. Surg Clin North Am. 2007;87(5):1179–92. https://doi.org/10.1016/j.suc.2007.07.006.
18. Stewart KC, Urschel JD, Nakai SS, Gelfand ET, Hamilton SM. Pulmonary resection for lung trauma. Ann Thorac Surg. 1997;63(6):1587–8. https://doi.org/10.1016/S0003-4975(97)00442-6.
19. Phillips B, Turco L, Mirzaie M, Fernandez C. Trauma pneumonectomy: a narrative review. Int J Surg. 2017;46:71–4. https://doi.org/10.1016/J.IJSU.2017.08.570.
20. Matsushima K, Aiolfi A, Park C, et al. Surgical outcomes after trauma pneumonectomy: revisited. J Trauma Acute Care Surg. 2017;82(5):927–32. https://doi.org/10.1097/TA.0000000000001416.
21. Wagner JW, Obeid FN, Karmy-Jones RC, Casey GD, Sorensen VJ, Horst HM. Trauma pneumonectomy revisited: the role of simultaneously stapled pneumonectomy. J Trauma. 1996;40(4):590–4. http://www.ncbi.nlm.nih.gov/pubmed/8614038. Accessed 22 Apr 2019.
22. O'Connor JV, DuBose JJ, Scalea TM. Damage-control thoracic surgery. J Trauma Acute Care Surg. 2014;77(5):660–5. https://doi.org/10.1097/TA.0000000000000451.
23. Mackowski MJ, Barnett RE, Harbrecht BG, et al. Damage control for thoracic trauma. Am Surg. 2014;80(9):910–3. http://www.ncbi.nlm.nih.gov/pubmed/25197880. Accessed 17 May 2019.
24. Petrone P, Asensio JA. Surgical management of penetrating pulmonary injuries. Scand J Trauma Resusc Emerg Med. 2009;17:8. https://doi.org/10.1186/1757-7241-17-8.

25. Rozycki GS, Ochsner MG, Jaffin JH, Champion HR. Prospective evaluation of surgeons' use of ultrasound in the evaluation of trauma patients. J Trauma. 1993;34(4):516–26; discussion 526–7. http://www.ncbi.nlm.nih.gov/pubmed/8487337. Accessed 11 Jun 2019.
26. Strumwasser A, Chong V, Chu E, Victorino GP. Thoracic computed tomography is an effective screening modality in patients with penetrating injuries to the chest. Injury. 2016;47(9):2000–5. https://doi.org/10.1016/J.INJURY.2016.05.040.
27. Hernandez MC, El Khatib M, Prokop L, Zielinski MD, Aho JM. Complications in tube thoracostomy. J Trauma Acute Care Surg. 2018;85(2):410–6. https://doi.org/10.1097/TA.0000000000001840.

Cardiac Injury

Kristina J. Nicholson, Ravi K. Ghanta, Matthew J. Wall Jr, and Andrew B. Peitzman

> "The surgeon who should attempt to suture a wound of the heart would lose the respect of his colleagues."
> —Theodore Billroth, 1885

History

Documentation of cardiac injury can be found from 3000 BC in the Edwin Smith Papyrus [1]. Homer graphically describes penetrating injury to the heart in the Iliad [2]. In one of the first descriptions of treatment of cardiac injury in 1829, Baron Larrey successfully drained a hemopericardium resulting from a stab wound [3]. However, the first known successful repair of a penetrating cardiac wound was in Germany by Ludwig Rehn in 1896 [4]. In 1902, Luther Hill repaired a stab wound to the heart of a 13-year-old boy on a kitchen table in Alabama [5]. During World War II, the initial treatment for suspected cardiac injury was pericardiocentesis,

---

K. J. Nicholson
Department of Surgery, University of Pittsburgh, Pittsburgh, PA, USA
e-mail: nicholsonkj@upmc.edu

R. K. Ghanta
Division of Cardiothoracic Surgery, Baylor College of Medicine, Houston, TX, USA
e-mail: ravi.ghanta@bcm.edu

M. J. Wall Jr
Michael E. DeBakey Department of Surgery, Baylor College of Medicine, Ben Taub General Hospital, Houston, TX, USA
e-mail: mwall@bcm.edu

A. B. Peitzman (✉)
University of Pittsburgh School of Medicine, F-1281, UPMC-Presbyterian, Pittsburgh, PA, USA
e-mail: peitzmanab@upmc.edu

with a repeat attempt with recurrence. Only with the second recurrence was cardiorrhaphy advocated [6].

As diagnosis and management of traumatic injury have evolved significantly over the past decades, with the advent of ultrasonography, computed tomography, and damage control interventions, so have diagnosis and management of cardiac injury. Prior to the ready availability of current imaging techniques, the diagnosis of hemopericardium suggestive of cardiac injury required significantly more invasive and time-consuming means, including pericardiocentesis or pericardial window. With the introduction of point-of-care ultrasound in the 1980s and 1990s, surgeons could diagnose hemopericardium by noninvasive means, facilitating triage to compartments of the body for hemorrhage control and reducing the number of invasive diagnostic procedures.

Increased diagnostic accuracy in traumatic cardiac injury has also led to a more sophisticated understanding of the causes and injury patterns associated with cardiac trauma (Table 1). While patients with a mechanism suspicious for blunt cardiac

Table 1 American Association for the Surgery of Trauma Organ Injury Scale for the heart

Grade I
1. Blunt cardiac injury with minor EKG abnormality (nonspecific ST or T wave changes, premature atrial or ventricular contractions, or persistent sinus tachycardia
2. Blunt or penetrating pericardial wound without cardiac injury, tamponade, or cardiac herniation

Grade II
1. Blunt cardiac injury with heart block or ischemic changes without cardiac failure
2. Penetrating tangential cardiac wound, up to but not extending through endocardium, without tamponade

Grade III
1. Blunt cardiac injury with sustained or multifocal ventricular contractions
2. Blunt or penetrating cardiac injury with septal rupture, pulmonary or tricuspid incompetence, papillary muscle dysfunction, or distal coronary artery occlusion without cardiac failure
3. Blunt pericardial laceration with cardiac herniation
4. Blunt cardiac injury with cardiac failure

Grade IV
1. Penetrating tangential myocardial wound, up to but not through endocardium, with tamponade
2. Blunt or penetrating cardiac injury with septal rupture, pulmonary or tricuspid incompetence, papillary muscle dysfunction, or distal coronary artery occlusion producing cardiac failure
3. Blunt or penetrating cardiac injury with aortic or mitral incompetence
4. Blunt or penetrating cardiac injury of the right ventricle, right or left atrium
5. Blunt or penetrating cardiac injury with proximal coronary artery occlusion
6. Blunt or penetrating left ventricular perforation
7. Stellate injuries, less than 50% tissue loss of the right ventricle, right or left atrium

Grade V
1. Blunt avulsion of the heart
2. Penetrating wound producing more than 50% tissue loss of a chamber

injury (BCI) were admitted previously for days of observation, data now support the use of simple diagnostic testing which may exclude significant BCI and allow early discharge in the absence of other significant injuries.

Demographics and Etiology

Cardiac injury occurs in two categories which have distinct etiologies, injury patterns, and morbidity profiles. The majority of patients with penetrating or major blunt cardiac injury (blunt chamber or valvular rupture) die at the scene. Survivorship is more likely with a palpable pulse, narrow complex electrocardiogram (EKG), or signs of life at the scene [7]. With both blunt and penetrating cardiac injury, injuries occur most commonly to the anterior surface of the heart; vulnerable to the anterior stab wound or the heart and sternum striking the steering wheel in a high-speed motor vehicle crash. Chamber involvement is right ventricle > left ventricle > right atrium > left atrium [8]. Over 80% of penetrating cardiac injuries are ventricular injuries [8]. Penetrating cardiac injury (PCI) is injury to the heart which occurs as a result of direct violation of the myocardium by an object, typically the result of stab or gunshot wound. PCI occurs primarily in young males and may lead to emergency department thoracotomy in up to 25%, and death in up to 30% of those who survive to hospital care [8].

Patients with PCI frequently present with hemodynamic instability, with approximately one-half demonstrating signs of cardiac tamponade and the other half experiencing instability related to blood loss via a defect in the pericardium. The presence of all signs of *Beck's triad*—muffled heart tones, jugular venous distension, and hypotension—is the exception, not the rule. Cardiac tamponade physiology results from the acute accumulation of blood under pressure within the pericardium, which compresses the cardiac chambers and prevents diastolic filling of the ventricles. As the pericardium is not distensible acutely, as little as 75–100 mL of pericardial blood may impede cardiac function. Once tamponade physiology begins, minor increases in pericardial volume result in disproportionate increases in pressure with rapid clinical deterioration (Fig. 1) [9]. However, multiple series have demonstrated cardiac tamponade on presentation as a protective effect for patient survival, with some reporting up to sixfold higher survival with cardiac tamponade (although a few papers describe contrary results) [7, 8, 10]. This is perhaps due to a limitation of blood loss by the tamponade effect. Recent data also suggest that in some regions, the proportion of PCI surviving to the hospital evaluation due to stabbing may be decreasing, while that attributable to firearms is on the rise [8]. The change in weapons and less predictable injury pattern have generated the proposal to expand what has traditionally been the "cardiac box" to be more reflective of current injury patterns from gunshot wounds (Fig. 2) [11–13].

Blunt cardiac injury (BCI) is distinct from PCI in etiology and injury pattern. It occurs as the result of rapid deceleration or blunt force transmitted through the thoracic wall to the heart. Diagnosis and description of the epidemiology of BCI remain

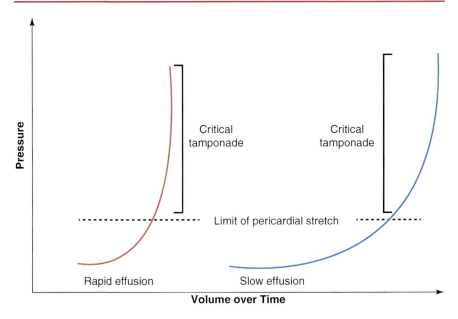

Fig. 1 Cardiac tamponade. Pericardial pressure-volume curves are shown when pericardial volume rises rapidly (left) or slowly (right). Rapidly increasing intrapericardial volume reaches the limit of pericardial volume (flat segment) and then quickly exceeds the limit of parietal pericardial stretch with further disproportionate rise in pressure for small changes in pericardial volume. The curve on the right shows a gradual increase in pericardial fluid which allows time for the pericardium to stretch (From Spodick DH. Acute pericardial tamponade. NEJM. 2003;349(7):684–690 [9])

difficult, as no clear definition has been accepted. BCI occurs most commonly in cases of motor vehicle collision (MVC) or cases of pedestrians struck by motor vehicles and contributes to 20% of MVC-related deaths [14, 15]. BCI is also associated with other significant blunt force mechanisms such as blasts, sports injuries, and falls. Patients are most frequently male, although with less predominance than in PCI, and slightly older than the PCI population, with mean age in the fifth decade [15]. BCI can range in severity from minor cardiac contusion to fatal cardiac rupture (Table 1) [16]. *Commotio cordis*, arrhythmia caused by direct blow to the precordial area, is often seen after sports injuries and may also be fatal.

The exact incidence of cardiac injury in the trauma patient is unknown and may vary widely depending on the definition of BCI. Studies of the National Trauma Data Bank (NTDB) have reported cardiac injury in less than 10% of trauma admissions, with a 0.3% rate of BCI [17, 18]. Other smaller, single-institution studies, however, have reported rates of 16–76% of cardiac contusion, highlighting the variability in the literature and difficulty in estimating the incidence of BCI [19]. Regardless of the actual frequency of cardiac injury in trauma patients, trauma patients with cardiac injury incur higher mortality than in those without.

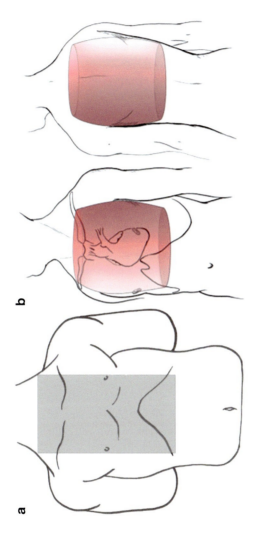

Fig. 2 (**a**) The traditional cardiac box (From Peitzman AB, Fabian TC, Rhodes M, Schwab CW, Yealy DM. The trauma manual, 4th ed. Wolters-Kluwer, Philadelphia, 2013, page 329 [11]) (**b**) The expanded cardiac box based on current injury patterns (From Bellister SA, Dennis BM, Guillamondegui OD. Blunt and penetrating cardiac trauma. Surg Clin N Am. 2017;97:1065–1076 [12])

Prehospital Issues

In recent decades, prehospital trauma care has improved significantly. Trauma systems and organization have improved, better triaging patients to appropriate care. Prehospital resuscitation strategies have also evolved, especially with the recent advent of prehospital blood product administration [20]. These improvements in prehospital trauma care have led to increasing numbers of patients with severe injuries surviving to hospital care and is likely a contributing factor to reported increases in proportions of GSWs and in-hospital deaths after PCI [8]. The prehospital care of cardiac injury is primarily recognition and rapid transport. Any other treatment is supportive and provided en route, addressing other injuries which may be amenable to field interventions, such as attending to extremity bleeding or decompressing a tension pneumothorax. Cardiac tamponade is a "load and go" scenario for prehospital providers. Thus, it is important to recognize injury patterns associated with the different etiologies of cardiac injury.

Penetrating cardiac injury related to stab wounds is likely to be associated with injuries of immediately adjacent structures such as lungs and great vessels, or contents of adjacent compartments, including the lower neck and upper abdomen. As previously stated, attention to the possibility of associated tension pneumothorax is important, as is hemostatic treatment of significant blood loss from superficial bleeding or injury to neck vessels. Other sites of stab wounds leading to significant blood loss should also be identified and addressed in the prehospital setting.

Injuries associated with firearms are related to the number, trajectory, and type of bullets. This information is often unobtainable in the chaotic prehospital setting. While adjacent structures to the heart are clearly at increased risk, gunshot wounds are associated with multicavity injuries, with higher associated mortality than stab wounds to the heart [8].

In the case of BCI, unless an isolated significant blunt force is applied directly over the heart, patients are likely to have multisystem injury [21]. Locally, patients with BCI may have sternal or rib fractures, particularly in elderly patients. Children, however, may sustain significant force to the thorax causing BCI without bony injuries due to increased compliance of the ribs; a higher index of suspicion is required to avoid missed cardiac injury. As motor vehicle collision is the most common cause of BCI, other associated injuries may include fractures of the extremities, spine, and pelvis, injury to the abdominal viscera, chest wall injury, associated hemothorax, thoracic aortic injury, and intracranial hemorrhage [17].

Emergency Center Presentation and Management

The evaluation of the patient with potential cardiac injury follows the Advanced Trauma Life Support (ATLS) protocols. Thoughtful communication with Emergency Medical Services to determine patterns of injury can help drive the diagnostic approach. For patients in extremis, a brief timeline of events, rhythm strips, and duration of external cardiac compressions can be helpful but are often difficult to quantitate.

For penetrating trauma, categorizing each wound can help suggest possible injuries. Stab wounds that occur over the anterior mediastinum may suggest the pursuit of subtle signs of developing tamponade. Particularly for multiple gunshot wounds, an attempt to predict possible pathways of projectile is made; however, this can be highly unreliable. The surgeon examining the patient documents the wounds and attempts to recreate in his/her mind a three-dimensional anatomic reconstruction to determine if cardiac or major vascular structures are at risk. Diagnostic modalities include chest radiographs, EKG, and pericardial FAST examination. Chest X-rays are examined for any signs of chest injury including pneumothorax/hemothorax, as well as to help document and predict potential penetrating injury patterns. Recognize that hemopericardium does not routinely present as an enlarged cardiac silhouette on the chest film, but with an appropriate injury pattern, cardiac injury may present with hemothorax. Ultrasound examination of the pericardium is an essential tool to detect potential cardiac injury. The purpose of this examination is primarily to identify the presence of fluid in the pericardium, rather than a detailed evaluation of valvular function or wall motion. When performed by trained individuals, it is highly sensitive and specific [22]. It also has the advantage that it can be repeated, allowing serial evaluation. It is not uncommon in an urban environment, with rapid transport times, that the initial examination of the pericardium is negative. However, with time, fluid accumulates, and the FAST can become positive.

Echocardiography

Full echocardiography is seldom needed acutely for penetrating cardiac injuries. It may have efficacy in the multiply injured patient with suspicion for blunt cardiac injury or the patient who has preexisting cardiac disease to characterize cardiac function and volume status. Echocardiography can be used in the subacute setting to document valvular or septal injury [23].

Electrocardiogram

Electrocardiogram (EKG) can be useful in patients when screening for blunt cardiac injury. The presence of arrhythmia, conduction defects, or ST segment changes suggests a myocardial contusion [24]. For penetrating cardiac injury, a simple rhythm strip showing the basic rhythm and the presence of wide or narrow complexes gives a sense of their status in patients who present in extremis.

Subxiphoid Window

Subxiphoid window is much less commonly performed due to the sensitivity of the FAST exam [25]. This is sometimes performed in patients where the FAST is equivocal, and there is high suspicion for injury. This is typically done during laparotomy, as a transdiaphragmatic exploration of the pericardium to exclude cardiac injury in a patient with abdominal injury. Decades ago, pericardiocentesis was recommended when the majority of penetrating cardiac injuries were created by small punctures. A clotted hemopericardium, however, is not amenable to acute evacuation via pericardiocentesis. While pericardiocentesis has been supplanted by the FAST exam, it is sometimes used in unstable patients when no other measures are available, although pericardiocentesis has a significant complication profile [26].

Emergency Department Thoracotomy

For a patient in extremis with signs of life and an injury pattern consistent with a cardiac injury, emergency department (ED) thoracotomy may be required. Common indications for ED thoracotomy are patients who suffer a potentially salvageable cardiac arrest with a high likelihood of cardiac injury or patients with severe post-injury hypotension due to cardiac tamponade, thoracic hemorrhage, cardiac herniation, or air embolism [27]. For cardiac injury, salvageable patients often present with cardiac tamponade, so relief of tamponade is the initial goal. The chest is opened via a left anterolateral thoracotomy in the fourth interspace following the rib (Fig. 3). The chest is examined to detect whether there is a large hemothorax, tamponade, or both, as each has different prognoses. The pericardium is opened anterior to the phrenic nerve and the tamponade released. This may result in improvement in hemodynamic parameters, enabling the patient to be moved to the operating room.

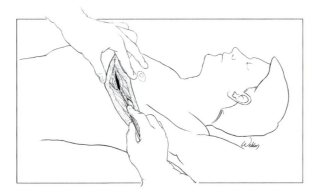

Fig. 3 Emergency center left anterior thoracotomy (Reproduced with permission from tfm publishing Ltd. Hirshberg A, Mattox KL. TOP KNIFE: the art & craft of trauma surgery. Shrewsbury, UK: tfm publishing Ltd.; Chapter 11: pp. 160. Copyright © 2005, Asher Hirshberg MD & Kenneth L Mattox MD; Illustrations © 2005, Baylor College of Medicine)

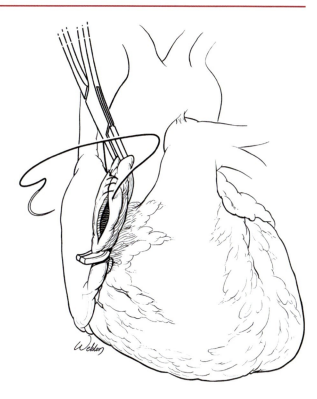

Fig. 4 Use of partial occluding clamp to temporize bleeding and allow cardiorrhaphy (Reproduced with permission from tfm publishing Ltd. Hirshberg A, Mattox KL. TOP KNIFE: the art & craft of trauma surgery. Shrewsbury, UK: tfm publishing Ltd.; Chapter 13: pp. 183. Copyright © 2005, Asher Hirshberg MD & Kenneth L Mattox MD; Illustrations © 2005, Baylor College of Medicine)

If hemodynamics do not improve, the descending thoracic aorta is cross-clamped, increasing perfusion to the coronary arteries and brain. The primary goals of the ED thoracotomy are to release tamponade, temporize hemorrhage, and improve hemodynamics for transport to definitive care in the operating room. Temporizing measures start with placing a finger on the injury. Simple cardiac lacerations can be oversewn with simple, continuous 3-0 or 4-0 polypropylene sutures on a large needle. Lacerations to the thinner atria can be temporarily controlled with a partial occluding clamp (Fig. 4). Lacerations of the thicker ventricle can be temporarily occluded with a Foley catheter balloon (Fig. 5). Avoid pulling up too hard on the catheter, as this may tear the myocardium, making cardiorrhaphy far more difficult. In addition, a skin stapler can be used to temporarily close cardiac lacerations; definitive repair is then performed in the operating room (Fig. 6). The pattern of injury that most benefits from emergency department thoracotomy is a single stab wound to the anterior chest that presents in tamponade.

Operative Approach

The operative approach to cardiac trauma depends on the hemodynamic status and pattern of injury. Patients in extremis or with anticipated multiple injuries are often managed with bilateral anterolateral thoracotomy with trans-sternal extension, or

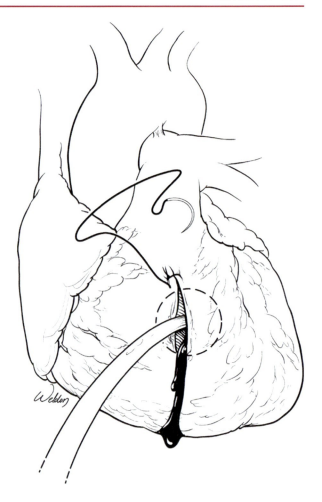

Fig. 5 A Foley catheter balloon can be used to control ventricular bleeding (Reproduced with permission from tfm publishing Ltd. Hirshberg A, Mattox KL. TOP KNIFE: the art & craft of trauma surgery. Shrewsbury, UK: tfm publishing Ltd.; Chapter 13: pp. 183. Copyright © 2005, Asher Hirshberg MD & Kenneth L Mattox MD; Illustrations © 2005, Baylor College of Medicine)

clamshell incision. The initial left anterolateral thoracotomy allows relief of tamponade, cross-clamping of the descending thoracic aorta, and resuscitation. It can then be extended into the clamshell thoracotomy to address other injuries. This is the most versatile incision when a true exploratory thoracotomy is performed on the patient in extremis. In scenarios with more time to plan incisions, either left anterolateral thoracotomy or median sternotomy is commonly used for cardiac injury. It is important to understand the limitations of each.

Left anterolateral thoracotomy is easily performed with minimal instrumentation. This is performed in the fourth intercostal space following the curvature of the rib. A generous incision from the sternum to the posterior-axillary line is performed. Intercostal muscles are divided in one area to minimize injury to the lung and then this is extended with cautery or scissors. Anterolateral thoracotomy has the advantages that it can be performed either in the ED or the operating room, is very versatile, and allows relief of tamponade and cross-clamping the descending thoracic

Fig. 6 Use of skin stapler to temporarily close a cardiac laceration (Reproduced with permission from tfm publishing Ltd. Hirshberg A, Mattox KL. TOP KNIFE: the art & craft of trauma surgery. Shrewsbury, UK: tfm publishing Ltd.; Chapter 13: pp. 183. Copyright © 2005, Asher Hirshberg MD & Kenneth L Mattox MD; Illustrations © 2005, Baylor College of Medicine)

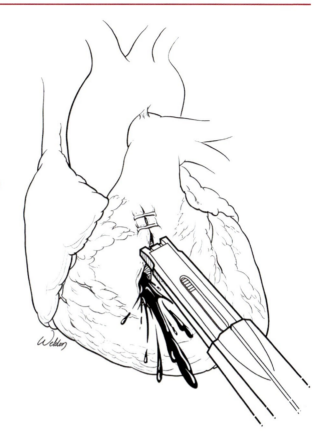

aorta. It also has the advantage of better access to posterior parts of the heart and facilitates management of these injuries with less lifting of the irritable heart. For injuries to the right heart, a trans-sternal extension is often required.

Median sternotomy is commonly used for elective cardiac surgery and is also useful for trauma. It provides good exposure to the anterior surfaces of the heart. Significant manipulation of the heart is required, however, to expose posterior structures, and cross-clamping the descending thoracic aorta is more difficult. It is also a good incision for anterior thoracic vascular trauma and for the rare patient who requires cardiopulmonary bypass for repairs. Median sternotomy does require instruments to divide the sternum. Both incisions are used in many busy centers. In our practice, we tend to address cardiac trauma through a left anterolateral thoracotomy due to ease of performance and versatility. We reserve median sternotomy for stab wounds to the anterior chest where the injury is likely to be on the anterior surface of the heart.

The heart is then examined. It is manipulated gently as it is often cold and irritable. A series of 711 penetrating cardiac injuries noted 40% of injuries were to the right ventricle, 40% to the left ventricle, 24% to the right atrium, and 3% to the posterior left atrium [28]. Bleeding is temporized with finger pressure, partially occluding clamps, a Foley catheter balloon, or skin staples. A strategy for repair is then developed. When manipulating the heart, it is important to gently lift rather than compress it as the heart fills passively. Warm saline is poured on the heart to prevent hypothermia. When suturing muscle, it is important to note it can be very friable, particularly in the older population. Simple sutures, either continuous or interrupted 3-0 or 4-0 polypropylene suture on a large needle, are routinely used. The key maneuver is to tie these down carefully as they can be easily avulsed through the muscle. As a surgeon often holds the heart while suturing, a skilled assistant can be employed to tie the sutures down. In older patients or those with friable muscle, these suture lines may need to be reinforced with interrupted pledgeted sutures. Temporary clamping of the vena cavae (inflow occlusion) may help to decrease bleeding during repair and temporarily decrease wall tension in friable tissues while the repair sutures are tied down. Injuries immediately adjacent to coronary arteries are addressed by placing deep mattress sutures traversing the injury but under the coronary artery (Fig. 7). Thus, when tied down, these sutures control the injury underneath the coronary artery without narrowing or occluding the coronary artery.

The majority of cardiac injuries that survive transport to the hospital are simple lacerations. Less than 10% of cardiac injuries are complex injuries involving the coronary arteries, cardiac septae, or cardiac valves. Coronary injuries that occur in the distal segments or to minor coronary arteries are managed with simple ligation. Acute coronary bypass is seldom needed and is usually indicated for injury to high

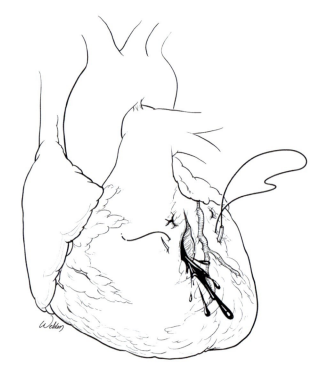

Fig. 7 Deep mattress sutures to repair a cardiac laceration near a coronary artery. Sutures should pass deep to the artery to prevent narrowing of the coronary vessel (Reproduced with permission from tfm publishing Ltd. Hirshberg A, Mattox KL. TOP KNIFE: the art & craft of trauma surgery. Shrewsbury, UK: tfm publishing Ltd.; Chapter 13: pp. 186. Copyright © 2005, Asher Hirshberg MD & Kenneth L Mattox MD; Illustrations © 2005, Baylor College of Medicine)

proximal left anterior descending or right coronary arteries in patients with otherwise survivable injuries. Thus for penetrating cardiac trauma, the need for acute coronary bypass is less than 1% [28].

For blunt cardiac injuries, the injury spectrum can range from contusion to massive rupture of the heart (Table 2). Chamber rupture that can potentially be repaired typically occurs in the atria, at the atrial appendages, or in the thinner-walled right ventricle. In fortunate scenarios, these can be identified and oversewn. Other potentially operative blunt cardiac injuries include avulsion of the heart at points of fixation such as the inferior vena cava-right atrial junction, superior vena cava-right atrial junction, and pulmonary vein-atrial junctions [29–31]. Some of these can be repaired with oversewing of the defect. In an unusual situation with a complex disruption in a patient with otherwise survivable injuries, cardiopulmonary bypass may be required.

Cardiac valvular injury is rare (Table 3). Aortic valve injuries are probably more common, but more likely to be lethal on scene. Valvular injuries may be identified postoperatively on patients with penetrating injuries who undergo cardiorrhaphy

Table 2 Types of blunt cardiac injury

Myocardial contusion
Myocardial rupture
Septal injury
Valvular injury
Pericardial rupture
Commotio cordis

Table 3 Overview of blunt valvular injuries

Blunt cardiac valvular injury		
Valve	Signs and symptoms	Treatment
Tricuspid valve	Late onset	Afterload reduction
	Pansystolic murmur, increased with inspiration	Diuresis
	Third heart sound	Intra-aortic balloon pump
	Right ventricular dysfunction	Surgical repair
Pulmonic valve	Late onset	Often no treatment necessary
	Diastolic decrescendo murmur	
	Right ventricular dilatation	
Mitral valve	Acute or late onset	Afterload reduction
	Holosystolic, high-pitched murmur	Diuresis
	Loud P2, third heart sound	Intra-aortic balloon pump
	Pulmonary edema	Surgical repair
	Cardiogenic shock	
Aortic valve	Acute onset	Medical treatment often unsuccessful
	Widened pulse pressure	Emergent surgical repair
	Decrescendo diastolic murmur	
	Pulmonary edema	
	Cardiogenic shock	

(From Huis in't Veld MA, Craft CA, Hood RE. Blunt cardiac trauma review. Cardiol Clin. 2018;36:183–191 [43])

and are found to have a murmur postoperatively. These valvular injuries may require repair in a subacute manner days after the initial repair. Cardiac septal injuries are equally uncommon with an incidence of 1.9% among cardiac injuries [28]. These also are typically diagnosed days after the initial repair when a murmur on physical exam is noticed. The management of these septal injuries depends on symptoms and the size of the intracardiac shunt.

Pericardial Injury

Pericardial injury occurs secondary to penetrating or blunt mechanism. This may result in a confusing picture as the patient may present with exsanguination into a hemithorax as opposed to tamponade. Blunt pericardial rupture is rare, with an overwhelming majority of these cases diagnosed either intraoperatively or on autopsy [32]. The heart may herniate through the pericardial defect, preventing filling, or the heart may rotate into the right chest, obstructing venous return. This can mimic cardiac tamponade with low cardiac output. Positional hypotension has been noted to be a suggestive physical examination finding of cardiac herniation due to pericardial rupture. It is extremely difficult to diagnose, and a high index of suspicion helps [32, 33].

Postoperative Care

The care of patients after repair of cardiac injury can differ from the care of the usual trauma patient in that the pump has been injured. Thus, appropriate monitoring of volume status, contractility, and afterload is considered, as these patients may have an element of cardiac dysfunction. Hemodynamic instability may necessitate the need for more invasive monitoring to guide resuscitation. Physical exam can reveal a murmur, suggesting valvular injury or septal injury and should be pursued with a formal echocardiogram guiding therapy. Some centers suggest a routine postoperative echocardiogram in patients with significant operative cardiac injury [23].

Screening for Blunt Cardiac Injury

BCI represents a spectrum of injury ranging from mild cardiac contusion to blunt cardiac laceration and rupture, which is almost uniformly fatal (see Table 2) [19]. Thoughtful screening for BCI is critical to avoid unnecessary admissions and diagnostic interventions, while still recognizing clinically significant injury. This is made more difficult by the fact that most patients with BCI are either asymptomatic or simply complain of chest pain which may be attributable to other injuries. While sternal fracture was previously thought to be associated with BCI, recent data suggest otherwise and a consistent injury pattern associated with BCI has not been identified [34–36]. On the other hand, BCI which requires treatment is uniformly in the multiply injured patient, generally in the intensive care unit [17]. Thus, screening is based primarily upon clinical suspicion and mechanism of injury, with those resulting in blunt anterior chest trauma being of particular concern. Physical exam findings may include, but are not limited to, chest wall deformity, seat-belt sign, and subcutaneous emphysema [12]. Additionally, definitions of BCI vary widely and consensus diagnostic criteria have not been established to date. While diagnostic thresholds differ across institutions, most definitions include some combination of clinical data, troponin values, hemodynamic parameters, and imaging findings. To provide a standard framework for discussion of BCI severity, the American Association for the Surgery of Trauma (AAST) has published its organ injury scale for the heart (Table 1) [16].

Electrocardiogram

In patients with significant blunt thoracic trauma, or in whom suspicion of BCI is high for other reasons, EKG is an inexpensive and effective screening tool and is the only Level 1 recommendation in the 2012 BCI Screening Guidelines of the Eastern Association for the Surgery of Trauma (Fig. 8) [24, 37]. EKG findings suggestive of BCI include new arrhythmia, ST segment changes, and heart block and warrant admission to a monitored floor at a minimum. The most frequently identified arrhythmias in BCI include sinus tachycardia and atrial fibrillation; however, the presence of other dysrhythmias may also be indicative of BCI. Right bundle branch block, ST-T changes, or Q-waves also suggest BCI. When available, the EKG should be compared to prior studies to determine whether abnormalities are new [24].

Troponin

While troponin I level alone does not have high sensitivity (23%) and specificity for BCI, in combination with EKG, negative predictive value approaches 100% in a thoracic trauma population [12, 38]. In fact, in the absence of other injuries requiring admission, patients with normal admission EKG and 8-h troponin I level can be safely discharged with low suspicion of missed BCI. Those with elevated troponin I levels and normal EKG, however, need to be admitted with continuous cardiac monitoring as the elevated troponin I level may indicate significant cardiac injury. High-sensitivity troponin T levels have also been studied in a small cohort of patients with suspected BCI and found to have low sensitivity (54.8%) and specificity (69.1%) alone or in combination with EKG changes (64.5% and 53.3%, respectively) [39]. This poor diagnostic accuracy is partially attributable to cross-reactivity with abnormal skeletal muscle [40], and measurement of troponin T is not commonly used in the diagnosis of BCI [41].

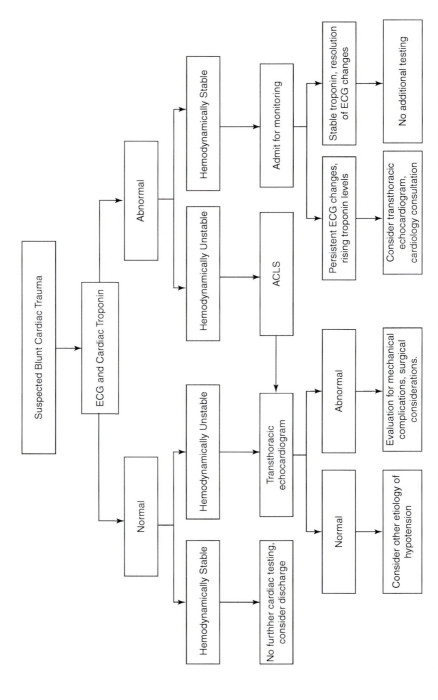

Fig. 8 Evaluation for blunt cardiac injury (Modified from Bock JS, Benitez RM. Blunt cardiac injury. Cardiol Clin. 2012;30:545–555 [37])

Echocardiography

Echocardiography should be used selectively in patients suspected of BCI based on EKG and troponin I levels. While those ruled out for BCI with negative troponin I and normal EKG do not require further workup with echocardiogram, patients with hemodynamic instability not attributable to hemorrhage or with persistent arrhythmias require further evaluation of cardiac function and structure via echocardiogram [24]. While transesophageal echocardiogram provides higher-quality evaluation of cardiac function, transthoracic echocardiogram is more readily available outside of the operating room and is an adequate next step in patients requiring further evaluation. Transthoracic echocardiogram may, however, be difficult in patients with significant blunt trauma to the chest due to pain from other injuries, and thus transesophageal echocardiogram should be considered for these patients [12].

Other Studies

Chest X-ray is routinely performed during the trauma evaluation and may reveal other injuries to the thorax, such as rib fractures or more severe sternal fractures. However, chest X-ray is unlikely to reveal any findings specific for BCI. Chest X-ray findings suspicious for significant cardiac injury may include an enlarged cardiac silhouette and pneumopericardium. More recently, computed tomography and magnetic resonance imaging have been found to be useful for BCI after the acute resuscitation and management of the unstable patient. They can characterize the extent of myocardial injury and identify whether abnormal EKG tracings, elevated troponins, or abnormal echocardiogram findings are due to BCI or acute myocardial infarction, thus guiding decisions regarding further diagnostic workup and interventions [42]. Nuclear medicine imaging studies have also been considered in the evaluation of BCI; however they are expensive and time-consuming and add little information not readily obtained on echocardiography [24].

Patient Management in BCI

Patients sustaining BCI are likely to have multisystem trauma and may have comorbid medical conditions. Thus, the approach is to provide comprehensive care while attending to injuries requiring urgent intervention. In general, even patients who are hemodynamically unstable related to BCI may undergo urgent interventions for other traumatic injuries with appropriate monitoring and resuscitation.

In the case of cardiac contusion, which is likely the most common type of BCI, care is supportive. Unlike an acute myocardial infarction, ischemia is usually not present with BCI, and the myocardium recovers fully. Management of more severe BCI is dependent upon the location and degree of injury within the heart or pericardium [43].

Summary

Cardiac injury is a rare but potentially serious component of the trauma complex in an injured patient. Evaluation starts with basic ATLS principles regardless of mechanism, but further workup and treatment differ depending on severity of patient illness and mechanism of injury. EKG and troponin I levels are useful initial tests in patients with suspected BCI and when negative can exclude clinically significant injury.

References

1. Breasted JH. The Edwin Smith surgical papyrus: published in facsimile and heiroglyphic transliteration with translation and commentary in two volumes. Chicago, IL: University of Chicago Press; 1930.
2. Homer. The Iliad with an English Translation by A.T. Murray, Ph.D. in two volumes. Cambridge, MA: Harvard University Press; 1924.
3. Larrey D. Chirurgie. 1829;2:303.
4. Rehn L. Ueber Penetrerende Herzwunden und Herznaht. Arch Klin Chir. 1897;55:315.
5. Hill LL. A report of a case of successful suturing of the heart, and table of 37 other cases of suturing by different operators with various terminations and conclusions drawn. Med Rec. 1902;2:846.
6. Blalock A, Ravitch MM. A consideration of the nonoperative treatment of cardiac tamonade resulting from wounds of the heart. Surgery. 1943;14:157–62.
7. Mina MJ, Jhunjhunwala R, Gelbard RB, et al. Factors affecting mortality after penetrating cardiac injuries: 10-year experience at urban level I trauma center. Am J Surg. 2017;213:1109–15.
8. Morse BC, Mina MJ, Carr JS, et al. Penetrating cardiac injuries: a 36-year perspective at an urban, level I trauma center. J Trauma Acute Care Surg. 2016;81:623–31.
9. Spodick DH. Acute cardiac tamponade. N Engl J Med. 2003;349:684–90.
10. Moreno C, Moore EE, Majure JA, Hopeman AR. Pericardial tamponade: a critical determinant for survival following penetrating cardiac wounds. J Trauma. 1986;26:821–5.
11. Peitzman AB, Fabian TC, Rhodes M, Schwab CW, Yealy DM. The trauma manual. 4th ed. Philadelphia: Wolters-Kluwer; 2013.
12. Bellister SA, Dennis BM, Guillamondegui OD. Blunt and penetrating cardiac trauma. Surg Clin North Am. 2017;97:1065–76.
13. Jhunjhunwala R, Mina MJ, Roger EI, et al. Reassessing the cardiac box: a comprehensive evaluation of the relationship between thoracic gunshot wounds and cardiac injury. J Trauma Acute Care Surg. 2017;83:349–55.
14. Schultz JM, Trunkey DD. Blunt cardiac injury. Crit Care Clin. 2004;20:57–70.
15. Teixeira PG, Georgiou C, Inaba K, et al. Blunt cardiac trauma: lessons learned from the medical examiner. J Trauma. 2009;67:1259–64.
16. Ottosen J, Guo WA. Blunt cardiac injury. Chicago, IL: Website of the American Association for the Surgery of Trauma; 2012.
17. Grigorian A, Milliken J, Livingston JK, et al. National risk factors for blunt cardiac injury: hemopneumothorax is the strongest predictor. Am J Surg. 2019;217:639–42.
18. Yousef R, Carr JA. Blunt cardiac trauma: a review of the current knowledge and management. Ann Thorac Surg. 2014;98:1134–40.
19. Shorr RM, Crittenden M, Indeck M, Hartunian SL, Rodriguez A. Blunt thoracic trauma. Ann Surg. 1987;206:200–5.
20. Smith IM, James RH, Dretzke J, Midwinter MJ. Prehospital blood product resuscitation for trauma: a systematic review. Shock. 2016;46:3–16.

21. Leite L, Goncalves L, Nuno VD. Cardiac injuries caused by trauma: review and case reports. J Forensic Leg Med. 2017;52:30–4.
22. Rozycki GS, Feliciano DV, Schmidt JA, et al. The role of surgeon-performed ultrasound in patients with possible cardiac wounds. Ann Surg. 1996;223:737–46.
23. Mattox KL, Limacher MC, Feliciano DV, et al. Cardiac evaluation following heart injury. J Trauma. 1985;25:758–65.
24. Clancy K, Velopulos C, Bilaniuk JW, et al. Screening for blunt cardiac injury: an Eastern Association for the Surgery of trauma practice management guideline. J Trauma Acute Care Surg. 2012;73:S301–6.
25. Meyer DM, Jessen ME, Grayburn PA. Use of echocardiography to detect occult cadiac injury after penetrating thoracic trauma: a prospective study. J Trauma. 1995;39:907–9.
26. Ivatury RR, Simon R, Rohman M. Cardiac complications. In: Mattox KL, editor. Complications of trauma. New York: Churchill Livingstone; 1994. p. 409–28.
27. Biffl WL, Moore EE, Johnson JL. Emergency department thoracotomy. In: Moore M, Feliciano DV, Mattox KL, editors. Trauma. New York: McGraw-Hill; 2004.
28. Wall MJJ, Mattox KL, Chen CD, Baldwin JC. Acute management of complex cardiac injuries. J Trauma. 1997;42:905–12.
29. Bakaeen FG, Wall MJ Jr, Mattox KL. Successful repair of an avulsion of the superior vena cava from the right atrium inflicted by blunt trauma. J Trauma. 2005;59:1486–8.
30. Wall MJ Jr. Commentary: blunt rupture of two cardiac chambers following a motor vehicle collision. J Trauma Acute Care Surg. 2019;87(3):737.
31. Miner J, Kirkland J, Hardman C, Bini JK. Blunt rupture of two cardiac chambers following a motor vehicle collision. J Trauma Acute Care Surg. 2019;87(3):736.
32. Wall MJ Jr, Mattox KL, Wolf DA. The cardiac pendulum: blunt rupture of the pericardium with strangulation of the heart. J Trauma. 2005;59:136–41; discussion 41-2.
33. Galindo Gallego M, Lopez-Cambra MJ, Fernandez-Acenero MJ, et al. Traumatic rupture of the pericardium. Case report and literature review. J Cardiovasc Surg (Torino). 1996;37:187–91.
34. Heidelberg L, Uhlich R, Bosarge P, Kerby J, Hu P. The depth of sternal fracture displacement is not associated with blunt cardiac injury. J Surg Res. 2019;235:322–8.
35. Yilmaz EN, Van Heek NT, Van Der Spoel JI, Bakker FC, Patka P, Haarman HJTM. Myocardial contusion as a result of isolated sternal fractures: fact or myth? Eur J Emerg Med. 1999;6:293–5.
36. Roy-Shapira A, Levi I, Khoda J. Sternal fractures: a red flag or a red herring? J Trauma. 1994;37:59–61.
37. Bock JS, Benitez RM. Blunt cardiac injury. Cardiol Clin. 2012;30:545–55.
38. Velmahos GC, Karaiskakis M, Salim A, et al. Normal electrocardiography and serum troponin I levels preclude the presence of clinically significant blunt cardiac injury. J Trauma. 2003;54:45–50; discussion −1.
39. Pfortmueller CA, Lindner G, Leichtle AB, Fiedler GM, Exadaktylos AK. Diagnostic significance of high sensitivity troponin in diagnosis of blunt cardiac injury. Intensive Care Med. 2014;40:623–4.
40. Jaffe AS, Vasile VC, Milone M, Saenger AK, Olson KN, Apple FS. Diseased skeletal muscle: a noncardiac source of increased circulating concentrations of cardiac troponin T. J Am Coll Cardiol. 2011;58:1819–24.
41. Bertinchant JP, Polge A, Mohty D, et al. Evaluation of incidence, clinical significance, and prognostic value of circulating cardiac troponin I and T elevation in hemodynamically stable platients with suspected myocardiac contusion after blunt chest trauma. J Trauma. 2000;48:924–31.
42. Baxi AJ, Restrepo C, Mumbower A, McCarthy M, Rashmi K. Cardiac injuries: a review of multidetector computed tomography findings. Trauma Mon. 2015;20:e19086.
43. Huis In't Veld MA, Craft CA, Hood RE. Blunt cardiac trauma review. Cardiol Clin. 2018;36:183–91.

Blunt Thoracic Aortic Injury in Thoracic Surgery for the Acute Care Surgeon

Anna Romagnoli, Pedro Teixeira, Viktor Reva, and Joseph DuBose

Introduction

Blunt traumatic aortic injury (BTAI) after trauma is an uncommon but lethal entity, with incidence of <1% [1, 2]. Information recovered at autopsy suggests that these injuries are actually the second-most frequent cause of mortality after blunt trauma [3, 4] with the majority of patients expiring prior to arrival at the emergency department [5]. Blunt thoracic aortic injury is imparted by significant blunt force trauma and is associated with an 85% prehospital mortality [6]. A more recent autopsy study of trauma victims identified these injuries as the primary cause of death in 1/3 of automobile collision mortalities, with 80% of these deaths occurring prior to arrival to an emergency department [5]. Motor vehicle collisions (>70%) appear to comprise the majority of mechanisms contributing to this specific injury, followed by motorcycle collisions, struck pedestrians, and falls [7, 8].

Numerous pathophysiologic mechanisms have been proposed as causative with regard to BTAI—including shear, torsion, pinch, stretch, and hydrostatic forces. A combination of such mechanical forces, however, is likely at play in the types of deceleration injury observed [4]. The location of the injury is consistent anatomically. More than 60% of blunt aortic injuries occur at the aortic isthmus where the

A. Romagnoli · J. DuBose (✉)
R Adams Cowley Shock Trauma Center, University of Maryland Medical System, Baltimore, MD, USA

P. Teixeira
Department of Surgery and Perioperative Care, Dell Medical School,
University of Texas at Austin, Austin, TX, USA

V. Reva
Department of War Surgery, Kirov Military Medical Academy,
Saint-Petersburg, Russian Federation

Department of Polytrauma, Dzhanelidze Research Institute of Emergency Medicine,
Saint-Petersburg, Russian Federation

fixed descending thoracic aorta meets the relatively mobile aortic arch [5]. This results in significant strain in the setting of abrupt deceleration. Blunt thoracic aortic injuries less commonly occur at other locations: the ascending aorta (8–27%), aortic arch (8–18%), and distal descending aorta (11–21%) [5, 6, 9–12].

Historically, the American Association of Surgery for Trauma (AAST) classified thoracic vascular injuries based on the type of artery and the extent of arterial circumference involved [13], but this system fails to adequately characterize these heterogeneous lesions. The current most commonly utilized grading system—proposed by Azzizadeh et al. [14] and later adopted by the Society for Vascular Surgery (SVS) in its clinical practice guidelines for BTAI management [15]—describes BTAI as a spectrum of lesions based on the anatomical layers of the aorta involved. These include intimal tear (grade I), intramural hematoma (grade II), pseudoaneurysm (III), and full-thickness injury resulting in frank rupture (IV) [14, 15].

The treatment of BTAI patients who survive to reach care has evolved considerably over the past several decades. Traditionally, early open repair was the mainstay of intervention. In recent years, however, initial medical management with delayed thoracic endovascular aortic repair (TEVAR) has emerged as the preferred treatment paradigm for patients with these injuries and appropriate anatomy and physiology conducive to this modality [7, 14–28].

Presentation and Workup

BTAI patients may be asymptomatic or may experience a range of symptoms including chest pain radiating to neck, back, or shoulder. Patients may be hemodynamically normal or present in obvious shock [29]. Anteroposterior chest X-ray is the initial diagnostic test of choice. A widened or otherwise abnormal-appearing mediastinum may be seen in up to 93% of patients with BTAI [30, 31]. Pathologic widening of the mediastinum is defined as a mediastinal silhouette of >8 cm at the level of the aortic knob or a width at the same level that exceeds 25% of the total chest width [30, 31] (Fig. 1). Other suggestive radiographic findings include left

Fig. 1 Widened mediastinum on anteroposterior chest X-ray

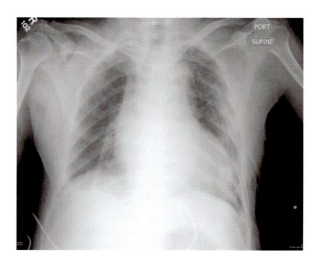

pleural effusion, first and second rib fractures, tracheal deviation, depressed left bronchus, an indistinct aortic knob, or apical capping [30, 31]. Patients with any of these abnormalities visualized on chest X-ray should undergo additional imaging, especially in the setting of a suspicious mechanism of injury. Importantly, a normal chest X-ray has a low sensitivity in the diagnosis of thoracic aortic injury and consequently should not be used to definitively exclude the diagnosis [32].

Computed tomographic angiography (CTA), with its high sensitivity (95–100%) and negative predictive value (99–100%) is the diagnostic test of choice for blunt thoracic aortic injury [9, 33–35] (Fig. 2). This imaging technology and improved trauma imaging protocols have supplanted traditional catheter-based angiography as the most efficient means of identifying BTAI. It is important to appreciate that false positives using this modality are not uncommon with low-grade injuries. There is evidence as well that CTA may have limitations—particularly in the detection of minor injuries. In one examination of patients undergoing formal angiography after CTA, Bruckner et al. found that CTA had a specificity of only 40% and a positive predictive value of only 15% [35]. This study is, however, now over a decade old; continued improvements in computed tomography imaging capabilities and trauma imaging protocols have improved the utility of modern CTA for the accurate detection and precise characterization of BTAI. Most subsequent studies have validated well the utilization of CTA after trauma due to the high sensitivity and ability to exclude BTAI with a very high negative predictive value [33–35].

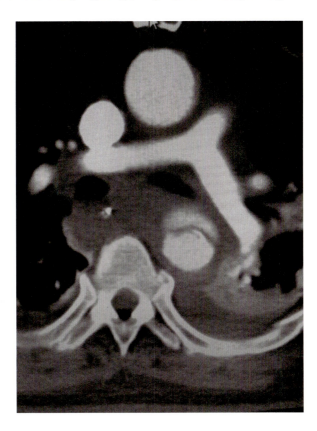

Fig. 2 Computed tomography angiography demonstrating grade III injury

If the diagnosis remains unclear after CTA, formal angiography and transesophageal echocardiogram [36] are both established methods of evaluating a patient for BTAI (Fig. 3). Intravascular ultrasound (IVUS), an emerging ultrasound capability, has also proven a reliable and sensitive tool in this setting, especially useful for the more precise characterization of minor injuries [37] (Fig. 4). While IVUS negates

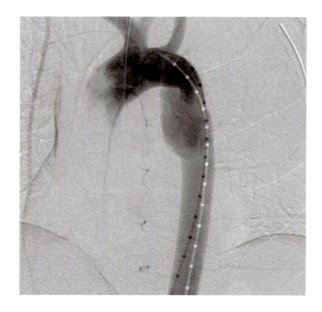

Fig. 3 Preintervention grade III BTAI demonstrated on contrast angiography

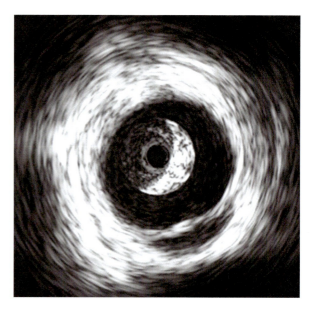

Fig. 4 Intravascular ultrasound (IVUS) demonstrating grade II BTAI

the need for the volume of intravascular contrast required by traditional angiography and decreases radiation exposure, it is predicated upon additional equipment, expertise, and placement of a slightly larger vascular sheath. This modality holds promise, as IVUS has demonstrated improved sensitivity over angiography [36, 37] for diagnosis of BTAI in several series.

Management: Medical

Immediate management of all BTAI injuries includes aggressive blood pressure control. Effective pharmacologic suppression of aortic pressure fluctuations is used to reduce impulse and stress on the injured aortic wall. This has been reported to decrease the risk of aortic rupture after BTAI from 12% to 1.5% [38]. SVS grade 1 injuries can be treated by medical management alone. For higher-grade injuries, SVS guidelines recommend medical management as a bridge to subsequent repair [15]. Some groups have reported successful nonoperative management of both grade I and grade II injuries finding that only 5% advanced [22]. Optimal blood pressure control regimen is not well established, with protocols varying by institution. Esmolol is often chosen due to its short half-life and titratability. For example, Fabian et al. reported the use of intravenous beta-blockers (esmolol or labetalol), titrated to a systolic blood pressure <100 mmHg and heart rate <100 bpm. Nitroprusside was added if adequate blood pressure control could not be obtained with beta-blockade alone [39].

Polytrauma patients with competing injury priorities may have contraindications to maintaining hemodynamics within these parameters. In the setting of traumatic brain and spinal cord injury, maximal neurologic recovery is predicated on maintenance of adequate vertebral and spinal cord perfusion pressures. This may necessitate use of vasopressors to maintain an elevated peripheral blood pressure, which is in direct contradistinction to medical management of BTAI. The heterogeneity of trauma patients and competing injury priorities requires close cooperation with trauma and neurosurgical providers in a multidisciplinary approach to determine if early endovascular repair for lower-grade BTAI is warranted.

Patients undergoing medical management of their BTAI must be closely monitored. Providers must be vigilant for the manifestation of obvious signs of malperfusion or possible early progression of injury among those selected for medical management of BTAI. With effective monitoring and in-patient imaging follow-up, however, progression of these injuries can be detected early and intervened upon safely. In the largest retrospective multicenter series of BTAI to date, the Aortic Trauma Foundation (ATF) reported that medical therapy alone was selected for 32.2% of BTAI patients. Only two in-hospital failures of medical therapy were noted in this population, both undergoing endovascular salvage without subsequent complication [16].

Upon diagnosis of BTAI, anti-impulse medications should be initiated in the absence of contraindication. Although SVS clinical practice guidelines recommend urgent (<24 h) repair [15], several large series suggest that delayed therapy is well tolerated and may be associated with improved outcomes. In one of the largest series on the topic, comparison of patients undergoing early endovascular (<24 h) and delayed endovascular (>24 h) repair showed a significantly lower mortality rate in the delayed group compared to those patients subjected to early repair (5.8% vs. 16.5%, $p = 0.034$) [19].

Open Repair

Early case reports of blunt traumatic aortic injury initially appeared in the literature in the 1960s. Early repairs were performed through left posterolateral thoracotomy with left atrium to femoral artery bypass [40] or via left posterolateral thoracotomy without bypass [41].

In the modern day, when open repair is required, a variety of approaches can be considered depending on the site and length of the descending thoracic aorta involved. A left posterolateral thoracotomy through the fourth interspace is usually the most expedient approach, as this provides excellent access to the area of the aortic isthmus where the majority of these injuries occur. This exposure is the most commonly described when employing the "clamp and sew" technique required by emergent repair or when extracorporeal support is not feasible or available. In the context of this approach, the chest is opened with the initial objective to rapidly acquire proximal and distal control around the area of injured thoracic aorta. The proximal clamp is typically applied between the left common carotid and left subclavian arteries, while the distal clamp is placed at some point on the distal descending thoracic aorta distal to the zone of injury.

While the clamp and sew technique has been demonstrated to be a safe method of operative management of BTAI [42], depending on the clinical scenario and patient condition, a distal aortic perfusion strategy should be employed to improve tolerance of proximal aortic clamping. The most expeditious technique for establishing distal aortic perfusion is "left-sided bypass," which can be performed through cannulation of the left inferior pulmonary vein and distal thoracic aorta. Rarely, the proximal clamp positioning is untenable. In this scenario, full cardiopulmonary bypass (CPB) is advisable, commonly through a femoral artery and a femoral vein cannulation. If total circulatory arrest is warranted, then careful venting of the left ventricle during times of cooling and rewarming is crucial.

In the setting of multiply injured trauma patient with competing injury priorities, the need for systemic anticoagulation with the use of bypass utilized in open repair is problematic. When left-sided bypass is performed, an activated clotting time >200 s is targeted; when full cardiopulmonary bypass is required, an activated clotting time >480 s is targeted [43]. Once the patient is on bypass and the perfusion circuit has appropriate flows, the periaortic hematoma is incised, the extent of injury is defined, and the aortic repair is undertaken. It is paramount that the aortic adventitia is incorporated into the subsequent suture lines, as this layer provides most of the tensile strength of the aorta. The patient is gradually rewarmed during the latter phase of the anastomosis to facilitate removal of the clamps at a moderate degree of hypothermia (32–34 °C). Once the clamps are off, the patient is weaned from bypass until adequate hemostasis is achieved and the wound is closed.

A significant consideration when undertaking open BTAI repair is spinal cord protection and the importance of distal aortic perfusion in minimizing the risk of postoperative paraplegia [44]. Several potential strategies to mitigate this risk have been described in the literature [45–49]. The most significant contributor to spinal cord ischemia as a result of aortic clamping is the occlusion of critical segmental spinal cord arterial branches originating from the distal thoracic aorta. Important factors in determining the incidence of immediate onset or delayed paraplegia following aortic repair include duration of cross-clamping, level and length of aortic segment excluded by clamping, duration of systemic hypotension, cerebrospinal fluid pressure, distal aortic pressure, and the number of intercostals ligated during repair [50]. Multiple adjuncts have helped lower the incidence of paraplegia following aortic repair for BTAI, including cerebrospinal fluid drainage, administration of steroids, generalized and localized hypothermia, and reimplantation of key intercostal arteries during the repair [47–50].

Management-Endovascular Repair

Endovascular repair has emerged as the mainstay of treatment of blunt thoracic aortic injuries. The first endovascular device, thoracic aortic graft (TAG) (W.L. Gore & Associates, Flagstaff, AZ), approved by the US Food and Drug Administration (FDA) for the treatment of thoracic aortic aneurysms was introduced in 2005. This device was utilized off-label for treatment of BTAI that same year [14]. The initial capabilities of this device limited TEVAR application to patients with a minimum aortic diameter of 23 mm. The subsequent approval of smaller diameter delivery systems, including the Talent (Medtronic, Santa Rosa, CA) and TX2 (Bloomington, IN) devices in 2008, made TEVAR feasible for a broader range of patients when employed in "off-label" fashion. The later introduction, and FDA approval for BTAI treatment, of two additional devices, CTAG (W.L. Gore, Flagstaff, AZ) and Valiant (Medtronic, Santa Rosa, CA), have further increased the tools available for definitive treatment of these injuries by effective endovascular means. In the largest multicenter retrospective BTAI examination to date conducted by the Aortic Trauma Foundation (ATF), TEVAR was utilized for 76.4% of the 382 BTAI patients studied, with only 23.6% requiring open repair during the study period [16].

A prospective, nonrandomized, multicenter trial utilizing Medtronic Valiant stents in 50 patients with blunt thoracic aortic injury (RESCUE trial) reported 100% successful device delivery and deployment, and 30-day all-cause mortality of 8.0%, which compares favorably to the previously reported 13% [51]. A recent American College of Surgeons National Trauma Databank review demonstrated a 196.8% increase in diagnosis of BTAI over the reviewed decade with a marked increase in TEVAR repair of BTAI, following FDA approval of capable endovascular devices (0.0 vs. 94.9% $p < 0.001$) overall [52].

The patient is prepped and draped such that both groins can be accessed and that the chest and abdomen may be rapidly entered if the procedure must convert to open. Femoral access is obtained and an arch aortogram is performed to confirm the location and characteristics of the injury. The cerebrovascular anatomy is evaluated with attention paid to determine if the take-off of the left subclavian artery will need to be covered in order to obtain an adequate proximal seal. IVUS can be utilized selectively based on the discretion of the attending surgeon and institutional capabilities to provide similar actionable information. Depending on the chosen device, most require femoral access with a sheath ranging in size from 20 to 24 F (6.67–8 mm) although lower profile devices (16 Fr) are now emerging on the market. These large-caliber devices can be challenging to place in the relatively small iliofemoral arteries of young trauma patients. The diameter of conduit vessels in this population is often less than 7 mm. Small iliac artery size has been demonstrated to be an independent risk factor for development of iliofemoral complications including dissection, rupture, and hematoma formation following TEVAR [53].

Heparin is administered using a weight-based protocol if there are no contraindications. In some situations a smaller dose of heparin (3000–5000 units) may be utilized. On occasion, as in patients with concomitant severe brain injury, anticoagulation use may represent a prohibitive risk. In these situations, thoughtful discussion with the other stakeholders of trauma patient care—including trauma surgeons and neurosurgical team members—must be undertaken in order to realistically balance the risk of thromboembolic complications for the limb that will occur without anticoagulation against the bleeding risk in the specific patient.

The thoracic device to be utilized for repair is selected, using CTA or angiographic images according to the manufacturer's sizing recommendations. Most commonly measurements are made based on two-dimensional, thin-cut axial CT scans with IV contrast. Once selected, the device is delivered and deployed using standard techniques without any pharmacological adjunct; extension pieces may be deployed as indicated but are not routinely required for these injuries (Fig. 5). Aggressive distal extension of the TEVAR device is likely to significantly increase the risk for subsequent spinal cord ischemia.

The subclavian artery may be covered as needed to obtain a proximal landing zone or gain better apposition with the lesser curvature of the aortic arch. Although this coverage does represent a theoretical increase in risk for malperfusion of the arm and vertebrobasilar steal postoperatively, a wealth of data suggests that BTAI patients will routinely tolerate LSCA coverage [54]. Post-deployment balloon angioplasty is performed only very selectively when there is significant incomplete apposition of the graft at the proximal landing zone noted. Heparin is then reversed with protamine at the surgeon's discretion. Postoperatively, patients are returned to the surgical-trauma intensive care unit and discharged following stabilization of their other injuries.

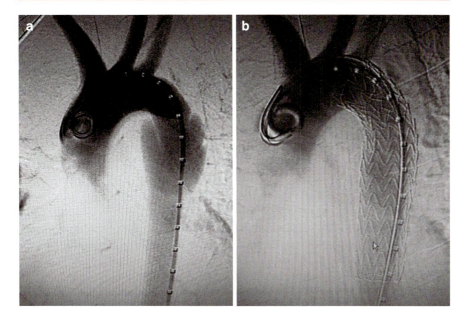

Fig. 5 (**a**) Grade IV BTAI prior to intervention. (**b**) Grade IV BTAI after TEVAR

When Is Open Repair Indicated in the Age of TEVAR?

Clinical Practice Guidelines from the Society for Vascular Surgery state that "endovascular repair be performed preferentially over open surgical repair or nonoperative management" [15].

A surgical repair is required if endovascular capabilities are unavailable or if a patient's anatomy is unsuitable for TEVAR. In the modern era, open repair is indicated when the patient shows signs of hemodynamic compromise and the need for emergent intervention when at a facility that does not have the capability to mobilize endovascular resources in an expedient fashion; local factors such as hybrid rooms, equipment, and surgical expertise come into play. A critical determinant of the need for open repair is the absence of an adequate proximal landing zone to allow for proper "seal" of the site of injury by the device. Arch aortogram is generally performed at the beginning of the procedure to delineate cerebrovascular anatomy. As outlined, left subclavian coverage is a frequently employed maneuver in TEVAR for BTAI, required in approximately 40% of patients [16]. Left arm claudication and vertebrobasilar insufficiency are potential sequelae of left subclavian artery coverage that must be assessed postoperatively. Data suggests, however, that the majority of patients requiring left subclavian artery coverage will have good short- and mid-term outcomes with regard to physical and mental health, without the need for subsequent bypass [16, 54]. Hybrid approaches utilizing planned carotid-carotid or carotid-subclavian bypasses may be utilized to provide for even more proximal coverage when the anatomy of injury treatment requires it. Within the last several years, more advanced thoracic branched endoprosthetics have begun to be utilized for treatment of aortic arch aneurysms [55]. As the vascular community becomes more familiar with these novel devices, even more patients with BTAIs will become safe candidates for endovascular-alone management of more proximal lesions.

Current data suggest that in comparison to open repair, TEVAR reduces early death, paraplegia, renal insufficiency, transfusions, reoperation for bleeding, cardiac complications, pneumonia, and length of hospital stay [19, 20]. The common concerns for paralysis and stroke that have been associated with open repair appear to be mitigated with the use of TEVAR. In the Aortic Trauma Foundation multicenter study of 382 BTAI patients, only 1 paralysis following TEVAR was noted, occurring in an 81-year-old male requiring 20 cm device coverage of the thoracic aorta. Likewise, stroke was a very rare occurrence, identified in only 2 patients, ages 62 and 85. Both required coverage of the left subclavian artery to facilitate TEVAR. These findings support the safety profile for TEVAR in the setting of BTAI, but suggest that older patients with possible native atherosclerotic disease and BTAI patterns requiring more extensive endograft coverage may have increased risk for these ischemic complications [16].

Access- and device-related complications also appear to be rare sequelae of TEVAR in contemporary practice. This improvement in safety profile has emerged as a benefit of increased experience and improvements in device technology. In the older 2008 report of the AAST BTAI study group, the investigators noted a significant rate of specific TEVAR-related complications. Demetriades and his group found that 18.4% of patients undergoing TEVAR had some form of stent graft-specific complication, most notably endoleak at 13.6% [20]. However, the Aortic Trauma Foundation study group has more recently reported a significantly lower rate of TEVAR-related complications. Of 382 BTAI patients, 6 malpositions of endograft at initial TEVAR occurred (3.0%) with a 2.5% post-TEVAR endoleak rate. Only one delayed stent migration was noted. Additionally, only two access site complications (one pseudoaneurysm, one bleeding requiring intervention) were identified. Among the six defined TEVAR treatment failures encountered in this large series, all underwent subsequent salvage with reintervention (two repeat TEVAR, four open repair).

The ATF study group identified only one patient treated with repeat TEVAR who suffered aortic-related mortality. No other mortalities were observed among the TEVAR failures [16]. Although increasingly rare in the modern era, it is important to note that complications during or after TEVAR remain possible in specific settings. Excessive oversizing or undersizing of endografts can lead to propagation of aortic injury or failure to achieve adequate seal. Patient-specific anatomical issues may also contribute, including the presence of a tight curvature of the aortic arch, native atherosclerotic disease, and the previously mentioned diameter limitations of iliac access vessels.

Is TEVAR the Answer for All Injuries?

The current SVS guidelines for BTAI management [15] published in 2011 were intended to provide an evidence-based, consensus-derived grading system and suggested course of treatment for BTAI. These guidelines still represent the most comprehensive effort in BTAI care optimization recommendations. The SVS guidelines do have some limitations and are specific to the aortic lesion alone. Under the SVS 2011 recommendations, grade I injuries are to be treated medically in patients without contraindication to the required anti-impulse blood pressure control. In a recent study by Osgood et al. [22], of 49 grade I and II injuries, investigators found that only 5% of these lesions advanced in grade on serial imaging. While there remains a need for additional studies to establish the relative risk of medical management verse TEVAR for these lower grade injuries, we have recently adopted a more selective approach to treatment of grade II injuries, managing some with medical therapy and serial imaging alone. In our present practice, grade II injuries deemed to require TEVAR and all grade III injuries are candidates for urgent repair via TEVAR. Grade IV injuries are transported expeditiously to the operating room for emergent repair, ideally by TEVAR [14].

Optimal management of patients with lower grade BTAI has recently emerged as a topic of considerable debate. Some group investigators have suggested that SVS grade I and II "minimal aortic injuries" do not universally require TEVAR [56–58]. The inclusion of SVS grade II injuries in this category conflicts with the present SVS clinical practice guidelines. In contrast, however, the findings from research conducted at several high-volume centers suggest that medical management with surveillance is a safe approach to BTAI treatment for patients in these categories [57, 58]. Ideal follow-up among patients selected for medical management and the natural history of SVS grade II injuries left untreated has not, however, been well established. Considering the small number of grade II injuries that present to each center on a yearly basis, properly addressing this issue will likely require a multi-institutional prospective study.

The ideal timing of BTAI treatment is another issue that requires further study. The results of the AAST Aortic Injury Study Group, reported in 2008, suggested that improved outcomes were associated with initial medical management including blood pressure and pulse pressure optimization. This group found that patients treated after a delayed (>24 h) period of optimization had improved survival compared to BTAI patients treated operatively within <24 h. However, there remains a need to adequately define whether there are specific risk factors associated with BTAI that represent a higher risk for early aortic rupture. If identified, these risk factors may inform considerations for more emergent timing of repair [19].

The long-term durability of these implanted endovascular devices for BTAI treatment also requires ongoing investigation. Improved conformability to aortic contour and various fixation element changes are attractive features of modern devices, but the impact of these design features on long-term integrity of the devices is not yet determined. Optimal graft sizing and graft utilization in patients with small aortic and iliac diameters are also inadequately studied issues. These challenges are exacerbated by the fact that optimal device indications and utilization have primarily been subjected only to industry-funded study, with associated inherent study bias potential. These issues require more objective investigation in a large, multicenter fashion.

The careful study of these issues also requires the foundation of a common vernacular to describe and categorize BTAI. The SVS grading system and associated guidelines for care are now widely utilized, but it is important to note that alternate algorithms have been proposed. Both the Vancouver simplified grading system [56] and the alternate classification scheme proposed by Starnes et al. [57, 58] have suggested that additional elements of imaging specific to BTAI may be of importance in guiding therapy. These groups have suggested that aortic lesion dimension measurements, which are not included in SVS criteria, are critical in determining the need for TEVAR. Initial work by investigators at the University of Maryland [23] has also demonstrated that associated secondary signs of injury are likely important for consideration. Specifically, this group has highlighted that the presence of extensive mediastinal hematoma and large left hemothorax may forecast impending aortic rupture. More recently, additional work by the Maryland group suggests that other markers of injury burden, including admission lactate, may also be predictive of early aortic adverse events [25].

A recent review of prospective trauma registry data suggests that limited aortic injury (grade I and II) may successfully be managed medically with observed complete resolution in approximately 8 weeks [59]. The routine employment of the SVS algorithm which prescribes liberal TEVAR for treatment of grade II injuries [15] may, subsequently, contribute to the overtreatment a significant number of injuries.

Conclusion

The future challenge for additional study of BTAI is to determine the ability to reconcile alternative viewpoints with those of the existing SVS BTAI grading system and treatment guidelines. The development and implementation of a consensus grading system and treatment algorithm for the management of BTAI patients is a challenging enterprise given the relative rarity of the disease process and the complexity and heterogeneity of the patient population. It will require a multi-institutional cohort of professionals and improved data on the diagnosis, management, and long-term outcomes of BTAI. In the interim, the data suggests that initial medical management is appropriate for most lower-grade injuries and that, among those requiring repair, delayed TEVAR should be the intervention of choice.

References

1. Arthurs ZM, Starnes BW, Sohn VY, Singh N, Martin MJ, Andersen CA. Functional and survival outcomes in traumatic blunt thoracic aortic injuries: an analysis of the National Trauma Databank. J Vasc Surg. 2009;49(4):988–94.

2. Smith RS, Chang FC. Traumatic rupture of the aorta: still a lethal injury. Am J Surg. 1986;152(6):660–3.
3. Clancy TV, Gary Maxwell J, Covington DL, Brinker CC, Blackman D. A statewide analysis of level I and II trauma centers for patients with major injuries. J Trauma. 2001;51(2):346–51.
4. Richens D, Field M, Neale M, Oakley C. The mechanism of injury in blunt traumatic rupture of the aorta. Eur J Cardiothorac Surg. 2002;21(2):288–93.
5. Teixeira PG, Inaba K, Barmparas G, Georgiou C, Toms C, Noguchi TT, et al. Blunt thoracic aortic injuries: an autopsy study. J Trauma. 2011;70(1):197–202.
6. Parmley LF, Mattingly TW, Manion WC, Jahnke EJ Jr. Nonpenetrating traumatic injury of the aorta. Circulation. 1958;17(6):1086–101.
7. Estrera AL, Miller CC 3rd, Guajardo-Salinas G, Coogan S, Charlton-Ouw K, Safi HJ, et al. Update on blunt thoracic aortic injury: fifteen-year single-institution experience. J Thorac Cardiovasc Surg. 2013;145(3 Suppl):S154–8.
8. Fabian TC, Richardson JD, Croce MA, Smith JS Jr, Rodman G Jr, Kearney PA, et al. Prospective study of blunt aortic injury: multicenter trial of the American Association for the Surgery of Trauma. J Trauma. 1997;42(3):374–80; discussion 80–3.
9. Neschis DG, Scalea TM, Flinn WR, Griffith BP. Blunt aortic injury. N Engl J Med. 2008;359(16):1708–16.
10. Feczko JD, Lynch L, Pless JE, Clark MA, McClain J, Hawley DA. An autopsy case review of 142 nonpenetrating (blunt) injuries of the aorta. J Trauma. 1992;33(6):846–9.
11. Arajarvi E, Santavirta S, Tolonen J. Aortic ruptures in seat belt wearers. J Thorac Cardiovasc Surg. 1989;98(3):355–61.
12. Burkhart HM, Gomez GA, Jacobson LE, Pless JE, Broadie TA. Fatal blunt aortic injuries: a review of 242 autopsy cases. J Trauma. 2001;50(1):113–5.
13. Moore EE, Malangoni MA, Cogbill TH, Shackford SR, Champion HR, Jurkovich GJ, et al. Organ injury scaling. IV: thoracic vascular, lung, cardiac, and diaphragm. J Trauma. 1994;36(3):299–300.
14. Azizzadeh A, Keyhani K, Miller CC 3rd, Coogan SM, Safi HJ, Estrera AL. Blunt traumatic aortic injury: initial experience with endovascular repair. J Vasc Surg. 2009;49(6):1403–8.
15. Lee WA, Matsumura JS, Mitchell RS, Farber MA, Greenberg RK, Azizzadeh A, et al. Endovascular repair of traumatic thoracic aortic injury: clinical practice guidelines of the Society for Vascular Surgery. J Vasc Surg. 2011;53(1):187–92.
16. DuBose JJ, Leake SS, Brenner M, Pasley J, O'Callaghan T, Luo-Owen X, et al. Contemporary management and outcomes of blunt thoracic aortic injury: a multicenter retrospective study. J Trauma Acute Care Surg. 2015;78(2):360–9.
17. Murphy SL, Kochanek KD, Xu J, Heron M. Deaths: final data for 2012. National vital statistics reports: from the Centers for Disease Control and Prevention, National Center for Health Statistics, National Vital Statistics System. 2015;63(9):1–117.
18. Azizzadeh A, Charlton-Ouw KM, Chen Z, Rahbar MH, Estrera AL, Amer H, et al. An outcome analysis of endovascular versus open repair of blunt traumatic aortic injuries. J Vasc Surg. 2013;57(1):108–14; discussion 15.
19. Demetriades D, Velmahos GC, Scalea TM, Jurkovich GJ, Karmy-Jones R, Teixeira PG, et al. Blunt traumatic thoracic aortic injuries: early or delayed repair—results of an American Association for the Surgery of Trauma prospective study. J Trauma. 2009;66(4):967–73.
20. Demetriades D, Velmahos GC, Scalea TM, Jurkovich GJ, Karmy-Jones R, Teixeira PG, et al. Operative repair or endovascular stent graft in blunt traumatic thoracic aortic injuries: results of an American Association for the Surgery of Trauma multicenter study. J Trauma. 2008;64(3):561–70; discussion 70–1.
21. Azizzadeh A, Ray HM, Dubose JJ, Charlton-Ouw KM, Miller CC, Coogan SM, et al. Outcomes of endovascular repair for patients with blunt traumatic aortic injury. J Trauma Acute Care Surg. 2014;76(2):510–6.
22. Osgood MJ, Heck JM, Rellinger EJ, Doran SL, Garrard CL 3rd, Guzman RJ, et al. Natural history of grade I-II blunt traumatic aortic injury. J Vasc Surg. 2014;59(2):334–41.
23. Rabin J, DuBose J, Sliker CW, O'Connor JV, Scalea TM, Griffith BP. Parameters for successful nonoperative management of traumatic aortic injury. J Thorac Cardiovasc Surg. 2014;147(1):143–9.

24. Martinelli O, Malaj A, Gossetti B, Bertoletti G, Bresadola L, Irace L. Outcomes in the emergency endovascular repair of blunt thoracic aortic injuries. J Vasc Surg. 2013;58(3):832–5.
25. Harris DG, Rabin J, Kufera JA, Taylor BS, Sarkar R, O'Connor JV, et al. A new aortic injury score predicts early rupture more accurately than clinical assessment. J Vasc Surg. 2015;61(2):332–8.
26. Hoffer EK, Karmy-Jones R, Bloch RD, Meissner MH, Borsa JJ, Nicholls SC, et al. Treatment of acute thoracic aortic injury with commercially available abdominal aortic stent-grafts. J Vasc Interv Radiol. 2002;13(10):1037–41.
27. Tang GL, Tehrani HY, Usman A, Katariya K, Otero C, Perez E, et al. Reduced mortality, paraplegia, and stroke with stent graft repair of blunt aortic transections: a modern meta-analysis. J Vasc Surg. 2008;47(3):671–5.
28. Xenos ES, Abedi NN, Davenport DL, Minion DJ, Hamdallah O, Sorial EE, et al. Meta-analysis of endovascular vs open repair for traumatic descending thoracic aortic rupture. J Vasc Surg. 2008;48(5):1343–51.
29. O'Conor CE. Diagnosing traumatic rupture of the thoracic aorta in the emergency department. Emerg Med J. 2004;21(4):414–9.
30. Woodring JH. The normal mediastinum in blunt traumatic rupture of the thoracic aorta and brachiocephalic arteries. J Emerg Med. 1990;8(4):467–76.
31. Mirvis SE, Bidwell JK, Buddemeyer EU, Diaconis JN, Pais SO, Whitley JE, et al. Value of chest radiography in excluding traumatic aortic rupture. Radiology. 1987;163(2):487–93.
32. Gutierrez A, Inaba K, Siboni S, Effron Z, Haltmeier T, Jaffray P, et al. The utility of chest X-ray as a screening tool for blunt thoracic aortic injury. Injury. 2016;47(1):32–6.
33. Gavant ML, Menke PG, Fabian T, Flick PA, Graney MJ, Gold RE. Blunt traumatic aortic rupture: detection with helical CT of the chest. Radiology. 1995;197(1):125–33.
34. Wicky S, Capasso P, Meuli R, Fischer A, von Segesser L, Schnyder P. Spiral CT aortography: an efficient technique for the diagnosis of traumatic aortic injury. Eur Radiol. 1998;8(5):828–33.
35. Bruckner BA, DiBardino DJ, Cumbie TC, Trinh C, Blackmon SH, Fisher RG, et al. Critical evaluation of chest computed tomography scans for blunt descending thoracic aortic injury. Ann Thorac Surg. 2006;81(4):1339–46.
36. Patel NH, Hahn D, Comess KA. Blunt chest trauma victims: role of intravascular ultrasound and transesophageal echocardiography in cases of abnormal thoracic aortogram. J Trauma. 2003;55(2):330–7.
37. Azizzadeh A, Valdes J, Miller CC 3rd, Nguyen LL, Estrera AL, Charlton-Ouw K, et al. The utility of intravascular ultrasound compared to angiography in the diagnosis of blunt traumatic aortic injury. J Vasc Surg. 2011;53(3):608–14.
38. Hemmila MR, Arbabi S, Rowe SA, Brandt MM, Wang SC, Taheri PA, et al. Delayed repair for blunt thoracic aortic injury: is it really equivalent to early repair? J Trauma. 2004;56(1):13–23.
39. Fabian TC, Davis KA, Gavant ML, Croce MA, Melton SM, Patton JH Jr, et al. Prospective study of blunt aortic injury: helical CT is diagnostic and antihypertensive therapy reduces rupture. Ann Surg. 1998;227(5):666–76; discussion 76–7.
40. McKnight JT, Meyer JA, Neville JF Jr. Nonpenetrating traumatic rupture of the thoracic aorta. Ann Surg. 1964;160:1069–72.
41. DeMuth WE Jr, Roe H, Hobbie W. Immediate repair of traumatic rupture of thoracic aorta. Arch Surg. 1965;91(4):602–3.
42. Mattox KL, Holzman M, Pickard LR, Beall AC Jr, DeBakey ME. Clamp/repair: a safe technique for treatment of blunt injury to the descending thoracic aorta. Ann Thorac Surg. 1985;40(5):456–63.
43. DuBose J, Azizzadeh A. Thoracic vascular trauma. In: Sidawy A, Bruce A, editors. Rutherford's vascular surgery and endovascular therapy. 9th ed. Philadelphia, PA: Elsevier; 2019.
44. Moore WM Jr, Hollier LH. The influence of severity of spinal cord ischemia in the etiology of delayed-onset paraplegia. Ann Surg. 1991;213(5):427–31; discussion 31–2.
45. Adams HD, Van Geertruyden HH. Neurologic complications of aortic surgery. Ann Surg. 1956;144(4):574–610.

46. Gharagozloo F, Larson J, Dausmann MJ, Neville RF Jr, Gomes MN. Spinal cord protection during surgical procedures on the descending thoracic and thoracoabdominal aorta: review of current techniques. Chest. 1996;109(3):799–809.
47. Cambria RP, Davison JK, Zannetti S, L'Italien G, Brewster DC, Gertler JP, et al. Clinical experience with epidural cooling for spinal cord protection during thoracic and thoracoabdominal aneurysm repair. J Vasc Surg. 1997;25(2):234–41; discussion 41–3.
48. Kouchoukos NT, Daily BB, Rokkas CK, Murphy SF, Bauer S, Abboud N. Hypothermic bypass and circulatory arrest for operations on the descending thoracic and thoracoabdominal aorta. Ann Thorac Surg. 1995;60(1):67–76; discussion –7.
49. Fowl RJ, Patterson RB, Gewirtz RJ, Anderson DK. Protection against postischemic spinal cord injury using a new 21-aminosteroid. J Surg Res. 1990;48(6):597–600.
50. Safi HJ, Miller CC 3rd, Carr C, Iliopoulos DC, Dorsay DA, Baldwin JC. Importance of intercostal artery reattachment during thoracoabdominal aortic aneurysm repair. J Vasc Surg. 1998;27(1):58–66; discussion –8.
51. Demetriades D, Velmahos GC, Scalea TM, Jurkovich GJ, Karmy-Jones R, Teixeira PG, et al. Diagnosis and treatment of blunt thoracic aortic injuries: changing perspectives. J Trauma. 2008;64(6):1415–8; discussion 8–9.
52. Scalea TM, Feliciano DV, DuBose JJ, Ottochian M, O'Connor JV, Morrison JJ. Blunt thoracic aortic injury: endovascular repair is now the standard. J Am Coll Surg. 2019;228(4):605–10.
53. Vandy FC, Girotti M, Williams DM, Eliason JL, Dasika NL, Michael Deeb G, et al. Iliofemoral complications associated with thoracic endovascular aortic repair: frequency, risk factors, and early and late outcomes. J Thorac Cardiovasc Surg. 2014;147(3):960–5.
54. McBride CL, Dubose JJ, Miller CC 3rd, Perlick AP, Charlton-Ouw KM, Estrera AL, et al. Intentional left subclavian artery coverage during thoracic endovascular aortic repair for traumatic aortic injury. J Vasc Surg. 2015;61(1):73–9.
55. Patel HJ, Dake MD, Bavaria JE, Singh MJ, Filinger M, Fischbein MP, et al. Branched endovascular therapy of the distal aortic arch: preliminary results of the feasibility multicenter trial of the Gore thoracic branch endoprosthesis. Ann Thorac Surg. 2016;102(4):1190–8.
56. Lamarche Y, Berger FH, Nicolaou S, Bilawich AM, Louis L, Inacio JR, et al. Vancouver simplified grading system with computed tomographic angiography for blunt aortic injury. J Thorac Cardiovasc Surg. 2012;144(2):347–54.e1.
57. Gunn ML, Lehnert BE, Lungren RS, Narparla CB, Mitsumori L, Gross JA, et al. Minimal aortic injury of the thoracic aorta: imaging appearances and outcome. Emerg Radiol. 2014;21(3):227–33.
58. Starnes BW, Lundgren RS, Gunn M, Quade S, Hatsukami TS, Tran NT, et al. A new classification scheme for treating blunt aortic injury. J Vasc Surg. 2012;55(1):47–54.
59. Sandhu HK, Leonard SD, Perlick A, Saqib NU, Miller CC 3rd, Charlton-Ouw KM, et al. Determinants and outcomes of nonoperative management for blunt traumatic aortic injuries. J Vasc Surg. 2018;67(2):389–98.

Thoracic Vascular Trauma

Paul T. Albini, Megan L. Brenner, and Raul Coimbra

Introduction

Up to 90% of thoracic vascular injuries are due to penetrating mechanisms (Wall/Mattox Trauma). As with any vascular trauma, repair of injured thoracic vessels is guided by several key principles. First, with any hard signs of vascular injury, patients should go immediately to the operating room for exploration (Table 1). Second, for those presenting in extremis, a left anterolateral thoracotomy with or without extension through the right chest (clamshell thoracotomy) is the procedure of choice. Third, when pursuing open repair, it is imperative to obtain proximal and distal control of the injured vessel. Fourth, the principle of damage control also applies to chest vascular injuries; when complex arterial reconstruction may not be safely undertaken, temporary vessel shunting or packing the chest and temporarily closing with negative pressure therapy may be used while the patient is being resuscitated or other injuries are addressed first [1].

Table 1 Hard and soft signs of vascular injury [11]

Vascular injury	
Hard signs	Soft signs
Active pulsatile bleeding	Diminished pulses distal to the injury site
Absent pulses distal to injury site	Stable, small hematoma
Expanding or pulsatile hematoma	Proximity to major vessels
Bruit or thrill at injury site	Peripheral nerve deficit
Unexplained shock	History of hemorrhage at scene
	Suspicious pattern of fracture or dislocation

P. T. Albini · M. L. Brenner · R. Coimbra (✉)
Riverside University Health System Medical Center, Comparative Effectiveness and Clinical Outcomes Research Center - CECORC, Riverside, CA, USA

Loma Linda University School of Medicine, Loma Linda, CA, USA
e-mail: p.albini@ruhealth.org; m.brenner@ruhealth.org; r.coimbra@ruhealth.org

In this chapter we will briefly review the management of common vascular injuries in the chest, excluding the aorta. We will focus on open exposure and repair. However, it is worth noting that endovascular hemorrhage control by way of balloon occlusion as well as endovascular repair is increasingly utilized for these injuries and may have certain advantages such as decreased need for blood transfusion and improved mortality in certain patient groups [2].

Diagnosis

All patients presenting to the hospital suspected of having thoracic injuries should be evaluated according to ATLS guidelines. A chest X-ray should be obtained to evaluate for signs of pneumothorax, or chest hemorrhage which include hemothorax, and widened mediastinum. In the case of a pneumothorax or hemothorax, a chest tube is inserted and monitored for blood output. If the patient is unstable or in extremis, a left anterolateral resuscitative thoracotomy is performed to evaluate for thoracic hemorrhage. This can be extended across the sternum and continued toward the right to complete a clamshell thoracotomy (Fig. 1). If the patient is stable, and 1500 cc of blood is immediately evacuated upon chest tube insertion, or the chest tube evacuates 200 cc of blood/h for 4 consecutive hours, then ipsilateral anterolateral thoracotomy should be performed in the OR. Stable patients without clear indication for anterolateral thoracotomy but with hard signs of vascular injury should proceed directly to the Operating or hybrid room where a formal angiogram can be performed with open repair. Stable patients with soft signs of vascular injury may undergo further evaluation with a CT angiogram (CTA) [3, 4].

Innominate Artery Injury

Injuries to the innominate artery, the first branch of the aortic arch heading toward the right side of the thoracic outlet (Fig. 2), are very rare and reportedly range from 0 to 3% of all civilian vascular injuries [5]. Innominate artery injuries are most frequently caused by penetrating trauma.

Fig. 1 Clamshell thoracotomy

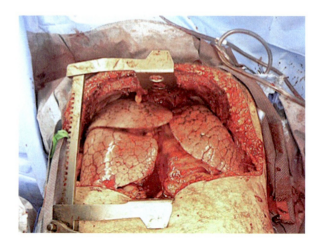

When these injuries occur, they have devastating consequences and 48%–71% of patients with innominate artery trauma die in the field prior to reaching a hospital.

A median sternotomy is the optimal exposure to access the injured innominate artery (Fig. 3). The innominate vein may be ligated to provide better exposure of the supra aortic branches and aortic arch. During repair of the innominate artery, consideration should be given to the need for adequate cerebral blood flow and utilization of an intraluminal shunt. Poor distal back bleeding, stump pressures in the carotid artery of less than 60 mmHg, or electroencephalogram changes during intraoperative monitoring suggest the need for shunt placement. Minor arterial injuries can be repaired primarily or with a patch graft. Large injuries, particularly those at

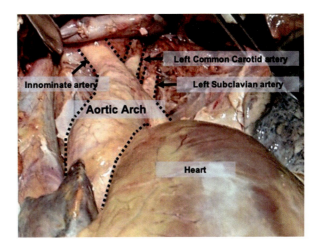

Fig. 2 Visualization of aortic arch branches, including the left subclavian artery. Note the superior displacement of the innominate vein to expose the takeoff of the right innominate artery

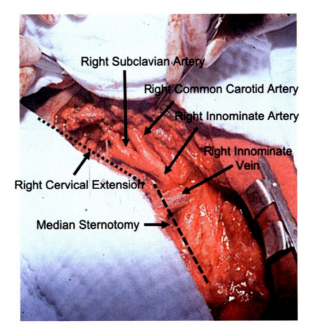

Fig. 3 Median sternotomy with right supraclavicular extension to expose the bifurcation of the innominate artery

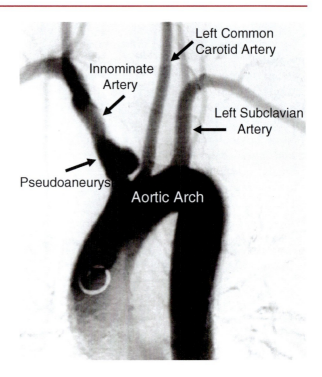

Fig. 4 Angiogram demonstrating an acute pseudoaneurysm of the innominate artery

the origin with the ascending aorta, may require bypass grafting between the proximal ascending aorta and the distal innominate artery, ligating and oversewing the injured section [3, 5, 6] (Fig. 4).

Isolated innominate vein injuries are rare and ligation is usually well tolerated.

Subclavian–Axillary Artery Injury

Subclavian and axillary arterial injuries are rare, affecting approximately 3% of all vascular injuries in multiple studies, and have a reported mortality rate between 10% and 34%. Difficulty in exposure may contribute to high lethality.

Most subclavian and axillary vascular injuries are caused by penetrating trauma. Overall, approximately 3% of all penetrating neck and chest injuries are associated with subclavian or axillary vascular injuries. In about 20% of patients, both the artery and vein are injured. Blunt trauma to these vessels is rare. Between 5% and 14% of first rib fractures are associated with these injuries. It is estimated that between 23% and 61% of patients sustaining subclavian–axillary artery injury die prior to hospital arrival [7–9].

The right subclavian is a branch of the innominate artery, the first great vessel branching from the aortic arch, after the takeoff of the right common carotid artery. The left subclavian artery is the third direct branch off of the aortic arch after the left common carotid artery (Fig. 2). The subclavian arteries extend toward the medial border of the anterior scalene muscle, then course posteriorly, and become the axillary artery at the lateral border of the first rib. The subclavian artery is itself divided into three different anatomic portions. The first portion extends from its origin in the aorta (left side) or innominate artery (right side), to the medial border of the scalene muscle. The second portion extends from the medial border of the scalene to the region where the artery crosses the clavicle posteriorly, and the third portion extends from the clavicle to the medial border of the pectoralis minor muscle [6].

Patients with subclavian injuries who are hemodynamically unstable require immediate operative intervention. Patients who are stable may be worked up with additional diagnostic tests such as CTA or conventional angiography. The advantages of CTA include its availability, speed, and less invasive nature. The advantages of conventional angiography include its dynamic nature and ability to perform definitive endovascular interventions.

It is recommended to consider conventional angiography in the OR or hybrid suite in stable patients presenting with hard signs of vascular injury. Most (60%) subclavian injuries are treated with an open surgical approach, followed by endovascular (17%), nonoperative (16%), and finally hybrid (6%) techniques [8].

The proximal right subclavian artery is exposed through a median sternotomy with optional right cervical or clavicular extension should these be necessary. The proximal left subclavian is exposed through a left lateral thoracotomy and supraclavicular incision or left anterolateral thoracotomy, full or partial sternotomy, and supraclavicular extension (trap door) (Fig. 2). It is a myth that the left subclavian artery cannot be controlled at its origin through a median sternotomy (Fig. 2). The second and third portions of the subclavian arteries are exposed via supraclavicular, infraclavicular or both (S-shaped) incisions. To expose the subclavian artery at the clavicular level, it may be necessary to disarticulate the clavicle from the sternum, resect the middle third of the clavicle, or divide the clavicle in half [6].

Endovascular repair is increasingly used in the management of subclavian–axillary artery injuries, particularly with proximal left subclavian injuries to avoid the morbidity of a median sternotomy. These endovascular repairs have reported success rates of 96.9% and long-term patency rates reported up to 84.4% [9] (Fig. 5).

Carotid Artery

The carotid artery is divided into three zones corresponding to that of the neck. Zone 1 extends from the sternal notch to the cricoid cartilage. Zone 2 extends from the cricoid cartilage to the angle of the mandible. Zone 3 extends from the angle of the mandible to the base of the skull. Cervicothoracic carotid injuries occurring from the aortic arch to the thoracic outlet are primarily Zone 1 injuries.

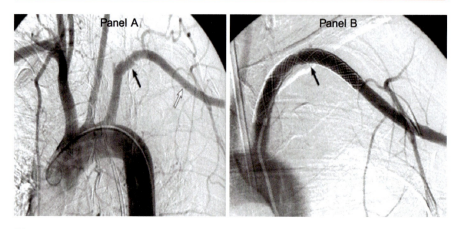

Fig. 5 (**Panel a**) Angiogram demonstrating an injury to the left subclavian artery (black arrow), starting at the takeoff of the left vertebral artery which is occluded. (**Panel b**) Stent graft placed to treat the left subclavian artery injury shown in **Panel a** (black arrow)

To obtain proximal control, it is often necessary to perform a median sternotomy. Distal control is obtained with an anterior sternocleidomastoid incision extension on the affected side. Dissecting deep to the anterior border of the sternocleidomastoid muscle reveals the carotid sheath. The vagus nerve lies in the posterior lateral position within the sheath and care is taken to identify it and protect it during the dissection.

In the mediastinum, the brachiocephalic veins are deep to the thymus. The left brachiocephalic vein can be retracted superiorly and medially to expose the aortic arch. Dissection along the arch will reveal the origin of innominate, left common carotid artery, and, posteriorly, the left subclavian artery. Proximal control of the left common carotid artery is obtained at this level [6, 10].

Internal Jugular Vein

Internal jugular venous injuries are caused almost exclusively by penetrating neck trauma. The low pressure venous system usually tamponades without major hemorrhage. When a jugular venous injury is encountered during neck exploration, the patient should be placed in Trendelenburg's position to prevent air embolism. Operative exploration to repair an isolated internal jugular vein is almost never performed, except for life-threatening hemorrhage. If known preoperatively from imaging, isolated penetrating injuries of the jugular vein can be safely managed nonoperatively. If encountered during a neck exploration, unilateral ligation of the jugular vein is well tolerated by patients. Minor injuries can be managed by a lateral suture repair; however there is a high incidence of thrombosis with venous repair. Rarely, when there are bilateral internal jugular vein injuries, one of the veins must be repaired to prevent cerebral venous congestion, which is associated with high mortality [10].

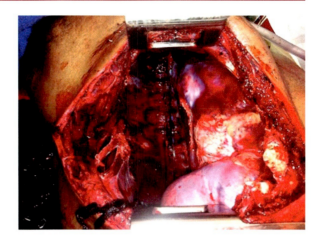

Fig. 6 Right pneumonectomy (Courtesy of Dennis Kim, MD, FACS)

Pulmonary Artery

Pulmonary artery injuries are rare, devastating, and associated with greater than 70% mortality. Intra-pericardial pulmonary arteries are approached via a median sternotomy. Minimal dissection is needed to expose the main and proximal left pulmonary arteries. Dissecting between the superior vena cava and ascending aorta exposes the right pulmonary artery. Anterior injuries to the pulmonary arteries can be repaired primarily. Posterior injuries may require cardiopulmonary bypass.

Distal pulmonary artery injuries present with massive hemothorax and are repaired through an ipsilateral posterolateral thoracotomy. When there is a major hilar injury, it may be necessary to perform a pneumonectomy [3] (Fig. 6).

Pulmonary Veins

Isolated pulmonary vein injuries are rare and associated with injuries to the heart, pulmonary artery, aorta, and esophagus. Injury to the pulmonary veins is difficult to manage through an anterior incision. With major hemorrhage, temporary occlusion of the entire hilum may be necessary (Fig. 7). When a pulmonary vein is ligated for hemorrhage control, the affected lobe of the lung should also be resected [3].

Venous Injury

Injuries to the superior vena cava (SVC) are rare, are highly lethal, should always be repaired, and may require temporary shunting to allow venous return to the heart. Eventually, injuries to the SVC may be repaired by simple lateral venorrhaphy. For complex injuries, a PTFE or Dacron interposition graft can be used and is favored over a more time-consuming saphenous vein graft tube reconstruction [3, 11].

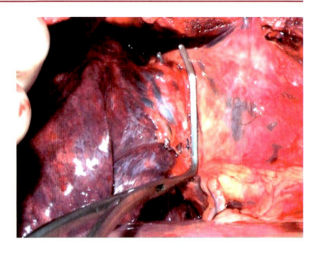

Fig. 7 Vascular clamp applied on the right pulmonary hilum

Repair of innominate vein injuries is desirable, although ligation is well tolerated in most cases. Both SVC and innominate vein injuries may be a source for air embolization. In the event of this complication, immediate direct aspiration of air from the pulmonary artery, right ventricle, atrium, and SVC is required. Subclavian venous injuries can be ligated with relative impunity [3].

Azygous vein injury is rare but may cause massive bleeding. Due to its posterior location, azygous vein injuries are difficult to diagnose and expose. They are often recognized when there is ongoing hemorrhage of dark blood from a posterior location in the right chest. The best approach to the azygous vein is through a right posterolateral thoracotomy. Most patients present with major bleeding through the chest tube requiring an emergent anterolateral thoracotomy. If azygous vein injury is suspected after the incision is made, it may be necessary to extend the incision posteriorly for adequate visualization of the injury and hemostasis through ligation [3, 6, 12].

Final Comments

Thoracic vascular injuries are rare; however they are life threatening due to the potential for exsanguinating hemorrhage and relative difficulty in accessing the structures anatomically. Mortality rates are high both in the pre-hospital and operative settings. Unstable patients and those with hard signs of vascular injuries should undergo emergent exploration and open repair. Those patients who are stable may undergo a diagnostic workup, including a chest tube and CT angiogram. The acute care surgeon should be familiar with basic chest exposures to expeditiously repair these injuries. Increasingly, certain populations of stable patients may be candidates for endovascular therapy including balloon occlusion and stent graft repair, particularly in those with proximal subclavian artery injuries. While applications for endovascular therapy continue to evolve, it is imperative the trauma surgeon understands open repair.

References

1. Weinberg JA, Moore AH, Magnotti LJ, Teague RJ, Ward TA, Wasmund JB, Lamb EMP, Schroeppel TJ, Savage SA, Minard G, Maish GO III, Croce MA, Fabian TC. Contemporary management of civilian penetrating cervicothoracic arterial injuries. J Trauma Acute Care Surg. 2016;81:302–6.
2. Faulconer ER, Branco BC, Loja MN, Grayson K, Sampson J, Fabian TC, Holcomb JB, Scalea T, Skarupa D, Inaba K, Poulin N, Rasmussen TE, Dubose JJ. Use of open and endovascular surgical techniques to manage vascular injuries in the trauma setting: a review of the American Association for the Surgery of Trauma PROspective observational vascular injury trial registry. J Trauma Acute Care Surg. 2018;84(3):411–7.
3. Wall MJ, Tsai PI, Mattox KL. Heart and thoracic vascular injuries. Chapter 26. In: Moore EE, Feliciano DV, Mattox KL, editors. Trauma. 8th ed. New York: McGraw-Hill Education; 2017.
4. Karmy-Jones R, Namias N, Coimbra R, Moore EE, Schriber M, McIntyre R, Croce M, Livingston DH, Sperry JL, Malhotra AK, Biffl WL. Western trauma association critical decisions in trauma: penetrating chest trauma. J Trauma Acute Care Surg. 2014;77(6):994–1002.
5. du Toit DF, Odendaal W, Lambrechts A, Warren BL. Surgical and endovascular Management of Penetrating Innominate Artery Injuries. Eur J Vasc Endovasc Surg. 2008;36:56–62.
6. Hoyt DB, Coimbra R, Potenza B, Rappold JF. Anatomic exposures for vascular injuries. Surg Clin N Am. 2001;81(6):1299–300.
7. Demetriades D, Asensio JA. Subclavian and axillary vascular injuries. Surg Clin N Am. 2001;81(6):1357–73.
8. Waller CJ, Cogbill TH, Kallies KJ, Ramirez LD, Cardenas JM, Todd SR, Chapman KJ, Beckman MA, Sperry JL, Anto VP, Eriksson EA, Leon SM, Anand RJ, Pearlstein M, Capano-Wehrle L, Cothren Burlew C, Fox CJ, Cullinane DC, Roberts JC, Harrison PB, Berg GM, Haan JM, Lightwine K. Contemporary management of subclavian and axillary artery injuries – a Western trauma association multicenter review. J Trauma Acute Care Surg. 2017;83(6):1023–31.
9. DuBose JJ, Rajani R, Gilani R, Arthurs ZA, Morrison JJ, Clouse WD, Rasmussen TE. Endovascular management of axillo-subclavian arterial injury: a review of published experience. Injury, int J. Care Injured. 2012;43:1785–92.
10. Kumar S, Weaver FA, Yellin AE. Cervical vascular injuries: carotid and jugular venous injuries. Surg Clin N Am. 2001;81(6):1331–44.
11. Dubose J, Teixeira PGR. Surgical Management of Vascular. Surgical Clinics North America. 2017;97:1133–55.
12. Wall MJ, Mattox KL, DeBakey ME. Injuries to the Azygous venous system. J Trauma. 2006;60:357–62.
13. Chang R, Fox EE, Greene TJ, Eastridge BJ, Gilani R, Chung KK, DeSantis SM, DuBose JJ, Tomasek JS, Fortuna GR, Sams VG, Todd SR, Podbielski JM, Wade CE, Holcomb JB, The NCTH Study Group. Multicenter retrospective study of noncompressible torso hemorrhage: anatomic locations of bleeding and comparison of endovascular versus open approach. J Tramua Acute Care Surg. 2017;83(1):11–8.
14. Kisat M, Morrison JJ, Hashmi ZG, Efron DT, Rasmussen TE, Haider AH. Epidemiology and outcomes of non-compressible torso hemorrhage. J Surg Res. 2013;184(1):414–21.
15. O'Connor JV, Scalea TM. Penetrating thoracic great vessel injury: impact of admission hemodynamics and preoperative imaging. J Trauma. 2010;68(4):834–7.

Diaphragm

Stefan W. Leichtle and Michel B. Aboutanos

Introduction

Diaphragm injuries can occur in the setting of blunt and penetrating trauma. They are more frequent in the latter but tend to be more severe in the former. They are often associated with injuries to heart, lungs, liver, or spleen, i.e., injuries that can be rapidly life-threatening and need to be addressed immediately [1–4]. The diaphragm rises to the level of the fourth and fifth intercostal spaces (nipple line) in full expiration, and iatrogenic diaphragm lacerations can be caused by inadvertent low chest tube placement or when the tube is placed erroneously below the sixth intercostal space.

In most cases, diaphragm injuries are small and per se asymptomatic. Therefore, a high index of suspicion is necessary based on trauma mechanism [3, 5, 6]. Missed diaphragm injuries can lead to severe short- and long-term complications such as chest infections and diaphragmatic hernias, respectively [5]. Herniation of abdominal contents through the diaphragm is more likely to occur in the setting of untreated left-sided injuries as the liver provides some protection to this complication on the right side. Right-sided diaphragm injuries, however, tend to be associated with a more severe injury burden and higher overall mortality. A solid understanding of gross anatomy of the diaphragm is helpful for the assessment and repair of diaphragm injuries.

Anatomy

The diaphragm is a dome-shaped muscle that separates the thoracic from the abdominal cavity. This location in the thoracoabdominal area (between fourth intercostal spaces/nipple line cranially and costal margin caudally) puts it at risk for

S. W. Leichtle · M. B. Aboutanos (✉)
Division of Acute Care Surgical Services, Department of Surgery,
Virginia Commonwealth University, Richmond, VA, USA
e-mail: Stefan.Leichtle@vcuhealth.org; michel.aboutanos@vcuhealth.org

© Springer Nature Switzerland AG 2021
J. M. Galante, R. Coimbra (eds.), *Thoracic Surgery for the Acute Care Surgeon*, Hot Topics in Acute Care Surgery and Trauma,
https://doi.org/10.1007/978-3-030-48493-4_18

damage particularly with penetrating trauma to lower chest, flank, and upper abdomen. The diaphragm consists of a central tendon and peripheral muscle, which attaches to ribs, sternum, and thoracic and lumbar vertebrae. It has three large openings for the aorta (accompanied by thoracic duct and azygos vein), esophagus (with the vagus nerve), and inferior vena cava (IVC). The phrenic arteries, the first branches off the aorta below the diaphragm, provide its main blood supply; venous drainage occurs into the IVC. On the right, the diaphragm covers the liver; on the left, it is in close proximity to the spleen and kidney, to which it is connected via the avascular phrenicosplenic and splenorenal ligaments, respectively. Heart and pericardium are located just cranial to the central tendon.

Innervation of the diaphragm occurs via the phrenic nerve, which originates from the cervical nerve roots C3, C4, and C5. The phrenic nerve reaches the diaphragm by coursing through the mediastinum along the pericardium and splits up to innervate left and right hemidiaphragm. As the primary respiratory muscle, diaphragmatic function is essential for effective respiration.

Diagnosis and Grading of Diaphragm Injuries

Trauma mechanisms that put patients at high risk for diaphragm injury are

– Penetrating thoracoabdominal trauma.
– Displaced lower rib fractures.
– Massive blunt force to the abdomen.

Initial workup for patients with possible diaphragm injury follows Advanced Trauma Life Support (ATLS) principles [7] to address immediately life-threatening injuries. Diagnostic imaging including chest X-ray (CXR) and computed tomography (CT) of chest and abdomen cannot reliably identify diaphragm injuries, particularly small ones [8]. Nonspecific findings associated with diaphragm injuries range from a small hemothorax or elevation of the diaphragm to a life-threatening (tension) pneumothorax or massive hemothorax (Figs. 1 and 2). Displacement of abdominal organs into the chest or coiling of a nasogastric tube in the chest are more specific for diaphragm injuries, but not sensitive. When concomitant injuries above and below the diaphragm are identified in the setting of penetrating trauma, e.g., left-sided hemothorax and a splenic laceration, diaphragm injury should be assumed until proven otherwise. While ultrasound has become an essential part of the ATLS algorithm with excellent sensitivity for the detection of hemo- and pneumothoraces, its role in the detection of diaphragm injuries is limited.

When left-sided diaphragm injury is suspected, but operative exploration for other injuries is not required, diagnostic laparoscopy should be considered [3, 6]. This is most commonly the case in hemodynamically stable patients with stab wounds to the thoracoabdominal area who have a benign abdominal exam. In their 2018 Practice Management Guideline using GRADE methodology, the Eastern Association for the Surgery of Trauma (EAST) provides a conditional recommendation (due to the availability of only very low grade evidence on the topic of

Fig. 1 Elevation of the right hemidiaphragm (arrow) in a patient with diaphragm injury from a gunshot wound to the right thoracoabdominal area

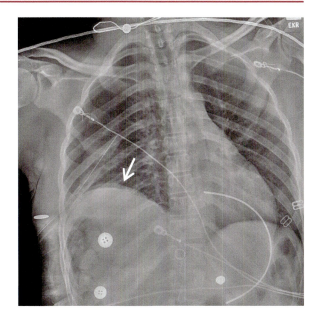

Fig. 2 Coronal views of a CT chest suggesting diaphragm injury (arrow) in a patient with a stab wound to the left thoracoabdominal area

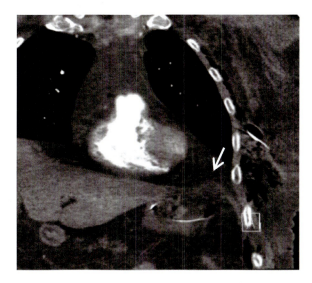

diaphragm injuries) for diagnostic laparoscopy as opposed to CT scan to identify diaphragm injuries in hemodynamically stable patients without peritonitis who sustained a left-sided thoracoabdominal stab wound [9]. For right-sided stab wounds in otherwise similar patients, EAST issued a conditional recommendation in favor of nonoperative management due to the lower risk of herniation on this side [9]. However, the risk for infectious complications and biliary spillage into the chest needs to be considered on a case-by-case basis, particularly if there is an associated ipsilateral hemo- or pneumothorax.

If a diaphragm injury is found, laparoscopic repair can be performed with minimal morbidity. In patients undergoing exploratory laparotomy, adequate mobilization of the liver and systematic examination of the diaphragm are necessary to detect small lacerations. A headlight is invaluable in these situations. Once a diaphragm injury has been identified, repair strategies depend on the extent of damage.

The American Association for the Surgery of Trauma (AAST) defines five grades of diaphragm injuries [10], shown in Table 1. This classification is best applied based on intraoperative findings and is helpful when choosing method of repair, in addition to allowing for a clear and universal description of this injury.

Table 1 AAST Grading System for Diaphragm Injuries (adapted from [10])

AAST Grade[a]	Description of injury
I	Contusion
II	Laceration, length ≤ 2 cm
III	Laceration, length 2 cm to 10 cm
IV	Laceration, length > 10 cm with tissue loss ≤25 cm^2 (Fig. 3)
V	Laceration with tissue loss >25 cm^2

[a]Add +1 to grade for bilateral injuries

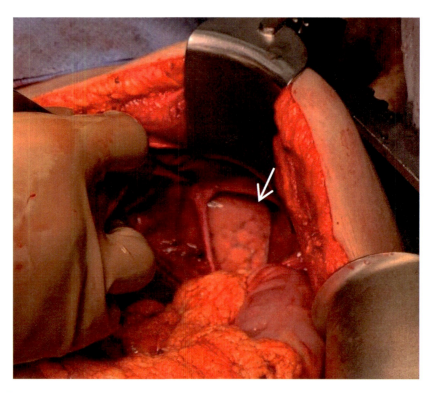

Fig. 3 Intraoperative image of an AAST grade 4 diaphragm injury (extensive tissue loss, less than 25 cm^2) in a patient with blunt abdominal trauma resulting in a grade V splenic injury (after splenectomy). The lower lobe of the left lung can be seen through the defect (arrow)

Surgical Repair

Repair During Exploratory Laparotomy

Good exposure is important and facilitated by the use of a Bookwalter retractor and adjustment of the table position as needed. To visualize the right diaphragm, the falciform ligament needs to be incised. On the left side, gentle traction needs to be applied to the spleen. Long Allis clamps are ideal to pull the edges of the diaphragmatic defect into view and approximate them (Fig. 4a, b). Most portions of the diaphragm are quite mobile. Clearly nonviable edges need to be debrided. Small diaphragmatic lacerations can be closed with vertical mattress sutures, while longer lacerations are most efficiently repaired using a running, interlocking suture. Suture material should be monofilament, non- or slowly absorbable, and heavy such as size 1 Prolene or PDS (Fig. 5a, b). If there was gross contamination of the abdomen,

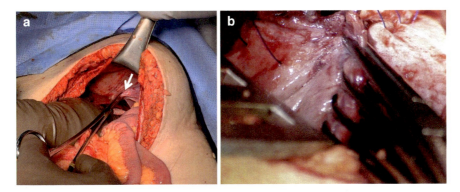

Fig. 4 (**a**) A long Allis clamp allows for retraction of the diaphragm into view (arrow) and approximation of the edges of a diaphragmatic laceration. This patient had undergone splenectomy resulting in excellent view of the left diaphragm. (**b**) Close-up view of the approximated edges of a diaphragmatic laceration

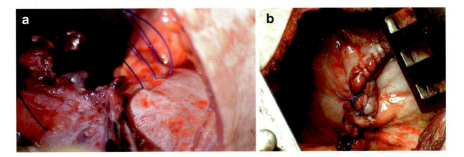

Fig. 5 (**a**) Repair of a diaphragmatic defect with size 1 Prolene suture. (**b**) Completed diaphragm repair

lavage of the ipsilateral thoracic cavity through the diaphragmatic defect should be performed prior to closure. An ipsilateral chest tube should be placed after most diaphragm repairs secondary to trauma, and more than one may be necessary depending on size of defect, degree of contamination, and associated pulmonary parenchymal injury. This is in contrast to elective diaphragm repair as seen in lower thoracic spine exposure, where the diaphragm can be taken down and repaired without the need for chest tube placement.

If incarcerated abdominal structures such as omentum (or solid organs and intestine in delayed repairs) need to be reduced, the diaphragmatic defect may need to be extended. The repair of larger and destructive diaphragm injuries is discussed below. In the setting of a damage-control laparotomy, the diaphragmatic defect does not necessarily need to be repaired during the initial operation, though destructive injuries that compromise respiratory function or result in herniation of abdominal organs into the chest do need to be addressed. Other reasons to repair these injuries during initial exploration, if reasonably possible, include prevention of abdominal bleeding or contamination to reach the thoracic cavity or the inability to provide effective packing in the setting of extensive liver injuries.

Laparoscopic Repair

Patients undergoing diagnostic laparoscopy for a suspected diaphragm injury need to be secured well on the operating room table. Steep Trendelenburg position with tilt to the side contralateral to the injury will facilitate view of and access to the site of injury. As in all laparoscopic operations, trocar placement can be adjusted to the individual patient as long as the principle of triangulation is observed. Hasson entry in supraumbilical position is a versatile option that works well in most situations. The subsequent placement of additional (usually two) trocars is based on location and extent of injury. Similar to open repair, a running, heavy, (non)absorbable suture is best to close diaphragm lacerations laparoscopically.

Throughout the operation, the patient needs to be observed closely for signs of a developing (tension) pneumothorax, which requires immediate placement of a chest tube. Washout of the thoracic cavity, as needed, and routine placement of an ipsilateral chest tube are performed in similar fashion as during open repair.

Thoracoscopic Repair

A thoracoscopic approach (video-assisted thoracoscopy, VATS) to the repair of diaphragmatic injuries can be considered for patients undergoing repair in the nonacute setting. This approach is particularly appealing in patients with multiple prior abdominal operations or other reasons to avoid laparoscopy or laparotomy. However, in the acute setting, an abdominal approach should be favored as it allows for the diagnosis of concomitant abdominal injuries. Strong data in favor of either approach does not exist [9].

Complex Diaphragm Injuries

Destructive diaphragm injuries with extensive loss of diaphragmatic muscle, chest, or abdominal wall are fortunately rare. Even larger tears can usually be approximated and repaired primarily (Fig. 5b), particularly in the acute setting. In delayed repair, larger defects may be encountered due to muscle contraction of the diaphragm. Permanent synthetic mesh allows for the reconstruction of larger defects in situations with no concern for contamination. Biologic or absorbable synthetic mesh allows for the closure of large defects in contaminated fields but is not well suited for a durable repair. For peripheral defects, the diaphragm can be attached to the ribs using horizontal mattress sutures around the ribs as anchoring stiches. For more extensive defects, various methods of reconstruction frequently used in congenital diaphragmatic abnormalities or after extensive oncologic resections exist, such as latissimus dorsi flaps [11].

Complications

Incidence and severity of acute complications in patients with diaphragm injury primarily depend on associated thoracic and abdominal injuries. Mortality rates of patients with diaphragm injuries are often reported to be 20% or higher [1, 2, 4]. Infectious complications, particularly in patients with bowel injury or other abdominal contamination include empyema and subphrenic abscess formation. Spillage of bile into the right thoracic cavity through an unrepaired right-sided diaphragmatic defect can also lead to bile pleuritis with associated severe systemic inflammatory reaction and potential infectious complications. These considerations should influence the decision whether to repair a right-sided diaphragm injury or not in patients with significant hepatic parenchymal damage.

The most severe long-term complication of missed diaphragm injuries is herniation of abdominal contents into the chest cavity, which can occur weeks and sometimes years after the initial trauma. Some patients may present with symptoms of a paraesophageal hernia or respiratory complications, while in other patients strangulation of stomach or intestine can lead to life-threatening complications [5].

Conclusion

Diaphragmatic lacerations are rare but important injuries. Hemodynamically stable patients with right-sided thoracoabdominal stab wounds and benign abdominal exam are at the highest risk for undetected diaphragm injuries and should be considered for diagnostic laparoscopy. Primary repair of diaphragm lacerations with a running size 1 Prolene or PDS suture is successful for most injuries. The outcomes of patients with diaphragm injuries are primarily dependent on associated injuries but a missed diaphragm injury is an important cause of long-term morbidity and mortality itself.

References

1. Zarour AM, El-Menyar A, Al-Thani H, Scalea TM, Chiu WC. Presentations and outcomes in patients with traumatic diaphragmatic injury: a 15-year experience. J Trauma Acute Care Surg. 2013;74(6):1392–8; quiz 1611.
2. Hanna WC, Ferri LE, Fata P, Razek T, Mulder DS. The current status of traumatic diaphragmatic injury: lessons learned from 105 patients over 13 years. Ann Thorac Surg. 2008;85(3):1044–8.
3. Powell BS, Magnotti LJ, Schroeppel TJ, Finnell CW, Savage SA, Fischer PE, et al. Diagnostic laparoscopy for the evaluation of occult diaphragmatic injury following penetrating thoracoabdominal trauma. Injury. 2008;39(5):530–4.
4. Fair KA, Gordon NT, Barbosa RR, Rowell SE, Watters JM, Schreiber MA. Traumatic diaphragmatic injury in the American College of Surgeons National Trauma Data Bank: a new examination of a rare diagnosis. Am J Surg. 2015;209(5):864–8; discussion 868–869.
5. Leppäniemi A, Haapiainen R. Occult diaphragmatic injuries caused by stab wounds. J Trauma. 2003;55(4):646–50.
6. Murray JA, Demetriades D, Asensio JA, Cornwell EE, Velmahos GC, Belzberg H, et al. Occult injuries to the diaphragm: prospective evaluation of laparoscopy in penetrating injuries to the left lower chest. J Am Coll Surg. 1998;187(6):626–30.
7. American College of Surgeons. Advanced Trauma Life Support® Student Course Manual [Internet]. 9th ed; 2012. http://web20.facs.org/MYATLS_RESOURCES/PDFDOCS_9TH/Student%20Manual.pdf. Accessed 16 Jan 2019.
8. Leung VA, Patlas MN, Reid S, Coates A, Nicolaou S. Imaging of traumatic diaphragmatic rupture: evaluation of diagnostic accuracy at a level 1 trauma centre. Can Assoc Radiol J. 2015;66(4):310–7.
9. McDonald AA, Robinson BRH, Alarcon L, Bosarge PL, Dorion H, Haut ER, et al. Evaluation and management of traumatic diaphragmatic injuries: a practice management guideline from the eastern Association for the Surgery of Trauma. J Trauma Acute Care Surg. 2018;85(1):198–207.
10. Moore EE, Malangoni MA, Cogbill TH, Shackford SR, Champion HR, Jurkovich GJ, et al. Organ injury scaling. IV: thoracic vascular, lung, cardiac, and diaphragm. J Trauma. 1994;36(3):299–300.
11. Bedini AV, Andreani SM, Muscolino G. Latissimus dorsi reverse flap to substitute the diaphragm after extrapleural pneumonectomy. Ann Thorac Surg. 2000;69(4):986–8.

Part III
Special Considerations

Acute Care Pediatric Thoracic Surgical Conditions

Julia Grabowski and L. R. Scherer III

Esophageal Rupture

Traumatic, non-iatrogenic, esophageal perforation is uncommon in children and accounts for less than 1% of thoracic injuries. Most are due to penetrating trauma. More commonly, esophageal perforation is an iatrogenic injury from nasogastric tube placement, endotracheal tube placement, or endoscopy. Newborns are specifically prone to esophageal perforation due to endotracheal intubation attempts or nasogastric tube placement. Young children are more prone to secondary perforation which occurs from ingestion of foreign bodies or chemicals (see next section). Most esophageal perforations occur in the hypopharynx or upper esophagus.

Presentation

Patients with pharyngeal perforations or injuries that are limited to the upper mediastinum most commonly present with respiratory distress, chest pain, neck pain, difficulty swallowing, excessive salivation, neck and upper chest emphysema, difficulty passing an orogastric or a nasogastric tube, fever, and tachycardia. Injuries that extend to the pleural space may present with respiratory distress, sepsis, and shock due to the flow of gastric and esophageal content into the mediastinum which initiates an inflammatory response and cytokine activations, leading to mediastinitis. Intraabdominal perforation may present with epigastric pain with or without peritonitis [1].

J. Grabowski (✉)
Division of Pediatric Surgery, Ann and Robert H. Lurie Children's Hospital, Northwestern University, Chicago, IL, USA

L. R. Scherer III
North Star Pediatric Surgery, Carmel, IN, USA

Diagnosis

When a patient is suspected of having an esophageal perforation, plain X-rays can assist in making the diagnosis. Radiographic findings will depend on the location of the injury. Air in the prevertebral facial plane may be noted on lateral films. Pneumomediastinum is the most common radiographic finding [2]. Mediastinal air can usually be noted within an hour of injury with pleural effusion and widening of the mediastinum occurring later. Hydropneumothorax can suggest the location of the perforation, with a right hydropneumothorax indicating a midesophageal injury and a left-sided hydropneumothorax indicating a more distal injury [2]. Esophagram is the standard study to diagnose an esophageal perforation. In general, a water-soluble agent is utilized and has a false-negative rate of about 10%. This may be followed up with a barium swallow study to increase sensitivity. More recently, chest CT with contrast has been utilized. Though flexible endoscopy has been shown to have a high sensitivity to identify esophageal perforations, the concern for the potential to worsen the injury has limited its routine use.

Treatment

Nonsurgical Treatment

Some patients, especially neonates, may be managed nonsurgically [3]. These patients must be clinically stable and have a well-contained leak with minimal contamination. They should be kept NPO, with fluid hydration and nutritional support and on broad-spectrum antibiotics. Antifungal medications are often utilized. Mediastinal and pleural fluid collections require drainage.

Surgical Intervention

Patients who have failed nonoperative treatments, with persistent sepsis or hemodynamic instability, require surgical intervention. The approach is determined by the location of the injury: the cervical esophagus is located in the left neck, the midesophagus is situated in the right side of the thorax, and the distal esophagus is in the left thorax.

The operative intervention for an esophageal perforation is similar to that of an adult (see Chap. 1). One notable caveat is that, though esophageal stenting has been used in adults with much success, the experience in children is limited and reports show a high rate of complications [4].

Caustic Ingestion

Acid- and alkali-containing substances are the agents that most commonly cause caustic injuries. These substances cause significant injuries in about 20% of cases. Button batteries are another cause of esophageal caustic injuries (see section "Esophageal Foreign Body"). Caustic ingestions occur in a bimodal fashion in the pediatric group; the first peak occurring in the 1–5-year-old age range. Children in this age group tend to ingest caustic substances accidentally. The second peak occurs later, in adolescents and young adults as a suicide attempt. The severity of the injury depends on the type, concentration, and amount of substance ingested [5].

Presentation

Patients may be asymptomatic, or they may have symptoms such as hoarseness, stridor, dysphagia, odynophagia, or abdominal pain. Patients who have a perforated viscus may present with sepsis and shock. Long-term sequelae of caustic ingestion may present with signs of stricture or gastric outlet obstruction.

Diagnosis and Initial Management

In a patient who is suspected to have swallowed a suspected caustic substance, initial management involves the fundamentals of ATLS by securing an airway, providing oxygenation and maintaining cardiovascular stability. No attempts should be made to neutralize or dilute the substance nor should attempts to elicit vomiting [5]. Direct visualization of the oral pharynx helps determine the extent of injury. In asymptomatic patients who have no signs of oral injury, a period of observation with a trial of oral intake may be adequate. Parents should be counseled to return if symptoms develop. Patients with symptoms or evidence of tissue injury require further evaluation. An initial chest X-ray is indicated as it may reveal evidence of a full-thickness injury if mediastinal emphysema or pneumothorax is identified.

In a symptomatic patient, endoscopy is the next step in diagnosing the presence and extent of esophageal injury and guides subsequent management. It should ideally occur within 12–24 h of the ingestion and should extend to the site of maximal esophageal injury. Contrast swallow studies are sometimes required after endoscopy to better identify the extent of grade 3 injuries and are also indicated in follow-up [5] (Table 1).

Table 1 Endoscopic grading schema of esophageal injury

Grade	Description
0	Normal
1	Edema and hyperemia of mucosa
2a	Friability: Hemorrhage, erosion, or blisters; superficial ulcers
2b	Conditions in 2a plus deep or circumferential ulcers
3a	Scattered areas of necrosis or brown/black/gray discoloration
3b	Extensive necrosis
4	Perforation

Nonsurgical Treatment, Including Alternative and Adjuvant Treatments

The acute care of a patient with a caustic esophageal injury often depends on the extent of injury. Proton-pump inhibitors and antibiotics are generally administered in patients with deep injuries. Systemic steroids are not currently recommended [6]. For patients with grade 1 or 2a injuries, limited in-hospital observation and diet advancement is recommended. Patients with grade 2b and higher injuries require longer hospital observation. These patients require monitoring for stricture formation (subacute and chronic) and longer-term follow-up is necessary. Stricture formation is common and often requires dilations, and there is concern for malignancies in the long term.

Patients with deep injuries may need a gastrostomy tube and NG left in place for feeding access and retrograde dilations.

Surgical Treatment

For the rare patients with full-thickness necrosis or perforation, urgent surgical intervention is needed. In the acute setting, the goal is to resect devitalized tissue and stabilize patient [7]. Just as in adults with necrosis of the esophagus or stomach, surgical intervention should involve a large incision (thoracotomy and laparotomy as needed) to best assess all tissue, with resection of all nonviable tissue. A cervical esophagoscopy and a feeding jejunostomy tube are often necessary in these urgent situations.

These patients should be referred to a tertiary care center with a plan for reconstruction after several months later using stomach, small intestine, or colon.

Tracheal Foreign and Esophageal Bodies

Airway Foreign Bodies

Diagnosis and Initial Management
Aspiration of a foreign body is common. Children younger than 4 years of age are most likely to aspirate foreign objects into the airway. The most common type of object aspirated is food with a peak incidence in children aged 1 to 2 years of age [8]. Though inhaled foreign bodies may have a benign course, severe complications or even death may develop if there is an acute and total obstruction of the larynx or trachea, and inhalation of a foreign body should be in the differential diagnosis in a child presenting with acute stridor or wheezing. Airway foreign bodies most frequently lodge in the main stem bronchus although they may also be located more distally. The right bronchial tree is more commonly involved than the left [8].

In a child with signs or symptoms consistent with airway obstruction (inability to phonate, cyanosis, stridor), the principles of ATLS apply and attention is paid immediately to stabilizing the airway. Direct laryngoscopy is used to evaluate for a foreign body in the oropharynx. A McGill forceps may be used to retrieve the object.

An emergent surgical airway is necessary if the foreign body obstructs the view of the vocal cords on direct laryngoscopy and prevents endotracheal intubation. Tracheostomy or needle cricothyroidotomy is preferred in children. Surgical cricothyroidotomy is not recommended in children younger than 8 years old [9]. If endotracheal intubation is not possible, an angiocatheter (14 or 12 gauge) placed directly into the trachea is recommended [10].

When a foreign body is suspected, chest X-ray with lateral view and expiratory films may be helpful, although there is a high rate of negative radiological findings [11, 12]. The lateral view, specifically, may help to further localize the object to the esophagus or airway. The observation of obstructive emphysema on chest radiography, a contralateral mediastinal shift, and ipsilateral paradox or restricted diaphragmatic motion during breathing support the diagnosis of air trapping with the ball-valve effect due to an endobronchial foreign body [13]. Bronchoscopy can both confirm the diagnosis and be therapeutic as a means to remove the foreign body.

Procedural Intervention

Rigid bronchoscopy under general anesthesia is the treatment of choice for aspirated foreign bodies. This is recommended as the instrumentation options are diverse, visualization is generally adequate, and ventilation is possible through the instrument [14, 15]. In older children and adolescents, however, flexible bronchoscopy through a laryngeal mask airway has been noted to be advantageous for small objects located in distal airways [14].

Post-Procedural Care

After bronchoscopic removal of an aspirated foreign body, a repeat chest X-ray should be obtained to prove successful retrieval. Repeat bronchoscopy is sometimes warranted. Patients should be monitored in the recovery room or higher level of care. Postoperative wheezing due to bronchospasm and/or laryngeal edema may be present after bronchoscopy and may be treated with both inhaled and systemic steroids [8].

Esophageal Foreign Bodies

Diagnosis and Initial Management

The esophagus is the site of 50 to 75% of pediatric gastrointestinal foreign body impactions and has the highest risk of complications in the alimentary tract [16]. Most esophageal foreign bodies become lodged at one of three areas of anatomical narrowing: the upper esophageal sphincter, the level of the aortic arch, and the lower esophageal sphincter. In patients with an esophageal stricture or previous esophageal surgery, such as those with a TEF repair, the foreign body often becomes impacted at the area of narrowing. The majority of esophageal foreign bodies either pass spontaneously or do not require an emergent intervention. There are, however, certain situations which require urgent intervention due to risk of high morbidity and even mortality [17]. According to the American Society for Gastrointestinal Endoscopy (ASGE), there are four broad scenarios that require prompt endoscopic or surgical management: patients with entrapped batteries (usually button batteries), high powered or multiple magnets or sharp objects (pins, needles, or glass), patients with complete obstruction leading to intolerance to liquids, those patients that present with objects trapped in upper third of the esophagus by the cricopharygneus muscle, and patient with objects that have been entrapped for longer than 24 h [18]. Symptoms for ingestion of a foreign body can vary from dysphagia, odynophagia, emesis, chest pain, drooling, or inability or refusal to eat. Airway and breathing are first priority. Plain posteroanterior (PA) and lateral X-rays of the neck and chest will identify most radiopaque objects. Two-view chest X-rays help to determine if the object is button battery (can be a surgical emergency—see below) as button batteries have a characteristic "double contour" sign. In patients with a non-diagnostic plain X-ray, a contrast esophagram may be helpful. CT scan is rarely necessary.

Nonoperative Management, Including Alternative and Adjuvant Treatments

In a child with a coin in the esophagus, coins can be removed on a semi-urgent basis, usually within 24 h; however those causing symptoms should be removed urgently. If patients are asymptomatic, consider glucagon to aid in passage of distal esophageal coins; however this has variable effectiveness [19]. Coins located in the stomach or beyond should be allowed to pass per rectum. It is suggested that a repeat X-ray should be performed at 2 weeks for retained coins, and endoscopic removal should be considered if the coin is retained in the stomach.

The most common sharp objects ingested are bones and toothpicks, and these require urgent or emergent removal, depending on symptoms. Other objects that require removal depend on symptoms or size. In infants, objects greater than 2 cm wide or 3 cm long are unlikely to pass through the pylorus and should be retrieved endoscopically. In older children and adolescents, objects greater than 2 cm thick or 5 cm long are unlikely to clear the duodenal c-sweep and, therefore, should be removed.

Procedural Intervention

Rigid esophagoscopy under general anesthesia is the gold standard to remove foreign bodies. For small lesions or those in the distal esophagus, flexible esophagoscopy is also often successful. Other techniques that have been described are bougienage and Foley extraction.

Bougienage entails a dilator being used to push the object from the esophagus into the stomach. It avoids general anesthesia and allows for the foreign body to pass through the gastrointestinal tract. This technique is also associated with lower hospital costs and length of stay [20]. Most centers that perform this technique for esophageal coins have specific criteria before attempting bougienage: only one coin on radiograph, the presentation within 24 h of ingestion, no previous esophageal abnormalities or surgery, the coin located between the clavicles and the diaphragm, and no respiratory distress or prior foreign bodies [21].

Some centers also perform removal of a smooth foreign body with a Foley catheter under fluoroscopy. In the fluoroscopy suite, without sedation, a Foley is inserted through the nares and passed below the level of the coin with the balloon deflated. With contrast injected to inflate the balloon, the catheter is gradually withdrawn to bring the coin into the oropharynx where it is coughed out by the patient or manually extracted. The coin is then manually removed or coughed out by the patient [22]. This technique should only be performed by experienced practitioners as there is the risk of aspiration after dislodgement [23].

Button Batteries

Button battery ingestion and impaction in the esophagus is somewhat unique to the pediatric population and constitutes a medical emergency. Typically, the batteries that get impacted are 20 mm in size with lithium batteries causing the most morbidity due to their higher voltage delivery. Disc batteries cause injury to the esophagus by generating and external current causing electrolysis of tissue fluids. Liquefactive necrosis can also occur due to leakage of alkaline electrolytes and tissue necrosis occurs from pressure phenomenon [24].

Disc battery removal is emergent as complications can occur in as little as 2 h or shorter [24]. Without prompt removal, erosive esophagitis, tracheoesophageal fistula, esophageal perforation, stricture, vocal cord paralysis, hemorrhage from aortoenteric fistula, or death can occur. Endoscopy, either rigid or flexible esophagoscopy using baskets is performed to remove the battery. Endoscopy allows inspection for mucosal injury. In order to inspect the airway, a bronchoscopy should be performed when the negative pole faces the trachea. Often, repeat endoscopy is warranted to assess for progressive damage.

A button battery in the stomach is not a surgical emergency. In most cases, the asymptomatic child with a button battery in the stomach may be discharged with follow-up in an outpatient setting. If the battery is not passed per rectum by 48 h (for batteries more than 20 mm) and in 10 to 14 days (for those less than 20 mm), an abdominal X-ray should be obtained. If the battery is identified at this time, or if symptoms develop, endoscopic retrieval should be performed.

Spontaneous Pneumothorax

Epidemiology and Presentation

The incidence of primary spontaneous pneumothorax PSP is estimated to be 7.4 to 18 per 100,000 in males and 1.2 to 6 per 100,000 in females. Though commonly reported to be significantly more common in males than in females, this difference

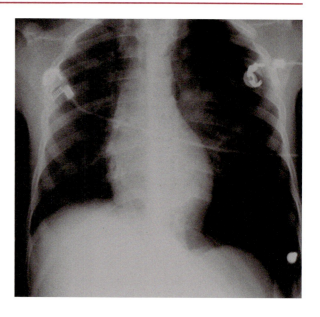

Fig. 1 Tension pneumothorax. The radiograph demonstrates the clinical findings of the shift of the heart to the right, right tracheal deviation, and depressed left diaphragm

may be less dramatic in younger pediatric patients. In pediatric series, the mean age at presentation ranges from 13.3 to 16.5 years old for PSP. The typical patient with PSP is tall and thin [25]. PSP is thought to have some significant differences in children compared to in adults; however much of the pediatric recommendations have been taken from adult data. PSP is distinguished from a secondary pneumothorax in that it occurs spontaneously in a patient without an underlying lung disease.

PSP usually presents with the acute onset of pleuritic chest pain characterized as a sharp pain (on the affected side) worsened by deep inspiration. There may also be shortness of breath. These symptoms frequently develop while at rest although they may be triggered by exertion or exercise.

These patients may only exhibit minimal tachycardia and slight dyspnea when there is only a small pneumothorax. In patients with a larger PSP, findings including decreased breath sounds; hyperresonant percussion and decreased vocal fremitus on the affected side [26]. Though rare, a large PSP can present as a tension pneumothorax (Fig. 1) with the additional findings of hypotension, cyanosis, jugular venous distention, and/or tracheal deviation [27].

Assessment

When working up a patient with a concern for a PSP, an upright posteroanterior (PA) plain chest radiograph (CXR) is standard and can often confirm the diagnosis. Often lateral films are also obtained. In addition to verifying the diagnosis, the CXR is to be used to determine the size of the pneumothorax (large vs. small) as this often helps determine a treatment plan. Though there are several methods to classify size of PSP in adults, these methods have not proven reliable in the pediatric population and are not routinely applied. Ultimately, a PSP is considered large when it is estimated to occupy greater than 15% of the thoracic volume [25].

The use of computerized tomography (CT scan for an initial, unilateral PSP) is not recommended based on available evidence. CT is indicated on the initial presentation only when bilateral PSPs are identified CXR or when underlying lung disease is suspected. If the patient experiences an ipsilateral recurrence or a new PSP on the contralateral side, chest CT may be indicated to guide subsequent surgical interventions [26].

Nonoperative Management

When a PSP has been diagnosed, initial noninvasive treatment begins with the administration of 100% oxygen via face mask, oxygen level, and cardiac monitoring [28]. High flow oxygen is used in order to aid reabsorption and is not titrated based on oxygen saturation [26]. If there is tension physiology, the chest should be emergently decompressed as for any other tension pneumothorax [25].

In asymptomatic patients with a small (classified as less than 15% thoracic volume) PSP, short term observation is all that is required. A stable X-ray 3–6 h later allows discharge if patients are given appropriate follow-up instructions and are able to return if symptoms arise [27].

There is considerable variation in practice patterns for pediatric patients with symptomatic or large PSPs. Both aspiration and tube thoracostomy have been studied and recommended in adult patients. No evidence-based consensus on treatment guidelines, however, has been possible in the pediatric population due to the lack of randomized controlled trials. Aspiration has been shown to be less invasive, more cost effective, and associated with fewer complications than tube thoracostomy [26]. Additionally, one study has shown that ambulatory management of large PSPs with a small-bore chest tube with a one-way Heimlich valve is effective in a majority of cases [29].

A PSP can most often be treated with a soft pigtail catheter (usually 8 French) that can be inserted under local anesthesia via the Seldinger technique. In some higher-risk patients, such as those with recurrence after bleb resection, a larger tube may be needed [27].

Whether aspiration or chest tube drainage is applied, if the initial PSP is completely evacuated within 3–4 days, the patient may be discharged home with follow-up instructions [27].

Operative Intervention

Though there is variation in the surgical treatment for PSP, in general, surgery is offered only to pediatric patients with a recurrent ipsilateral pneumothorax, contralateral pneumothorax, initial bilateral pneumothorax, persistent air leak (lasting more than 4 days), or spontaneous hemothorax [26, 30]. Surgical management of bleb disease often follows the first recurrence, though some authors encourage waiting for two recurrences in patients younger than 9 years old. There is ongoing debate about the role of surgery in an initial, uncomplicated PSP [27, 31].

The role of surgery is to identify and eliminate the cause of a continuous air leak and prevent recurrence. Blebs (cysts less than or equal to 2 cm) and bullae (greater than 2 cm) are most commonly noted in the apex of the lung. When identified, these lesions are typically treated with a nonanatomic apical wedge resection or *blebectomy* using a stapler [27]. While video-assisted thoracoscopic surgery (VATS) is the most common approach, open thoracotomy is also described. Many authors recommend an apical wedge resection even when blebs are not clearly visualized as they are thought to be present despite being elusive. Pleurodesis (mechanical and/or chemical) or pleurectomy is utilized to try to prevent recurrence [32]. Chemical pleurodesis refers to infusing a substance that induces inflammation into the pleural space [27]. Commonly studied substances include tetracycline, doxycycline, minocycline, and talc. No substance has proven superior. Mechanical pleurodesis refers to pleural abrasion. Pleurectomy refers to the removal of the entire parietal pleura. Regardless of technique, postoperative recurrence rates are higher than in adults and reported to vary from 16% to 28% [32].

Postoperative Considerations

With the high rate of recurrence, patients must be counseled to return to the hospital with any new symptoms. When a recurrence is identified, the options for a recurrent PSP after blebectomy include the same options for initial PSP management—observation, aspiration, chest tube placement, or repeat blebectomy with mechanical or chemical pleurodesis. There is a lack of evidence to guide this decision making. Computerized tomography scanning is often useful in these patients to identify the presence and location of new or previously overlooked blebs.

Parapneumonic Effusion and Empyema

Epidemiology and Presentation

Community-acquired pneumonia (CAP) is the leading cause of hospitalization in children in the United States with an incidence of 15 to 22 cases per 10,000 children younger than 18 years old [33]. It is also a leading cause of mortality globally. The incidence of empyema complicating CAP is between six and ten per 100,000 children younger than 18 years or approximately 5% of hospitalized CAP cases [33].

Children with parapneumonic effusion and empyema typically present with symptoms similar to those of children with uncomplicated community-acquired pneumonia. These symptoms may include fever, cough, malaise, tachypnea, and dyspnea. These patients often initially present as a typical CAP; however they often have persistent fever or no improvement in symptoms after 48–72 h of appropriate antibiotics [34].

The British Thoracic Society (BTS) guidelines for the management of pleural infection in children suggest many initial tests for pleural effusion. As there is limited evidence supporting the use of all of these investigations, investigations should be ordered based on clinical suspicion and availability of tests [34].

Initial investigations for suspected parapneumonic effusion:

- Chest radiograph.
- Ultrasound scan of chest.
- Blood culture.
- Antistreptolysin O titer.
- Complete blood count.
- Electrolytes (to detect inappropriate antidiuretic hormone syndrome).
- Serum albumin (often low; however, replacement is seldom required).
- C-reactive protein.
- Coagulation studies (in patients in whom a coagulation disorder is suspected).
- Tuberculosis testing.

Though chest CT is often not needed in the workup of children with pleural collections, it has a role in differentiating lung abscess or parenchymal disease from empyema. Additionally, it may demonstrate other serious clinical issues in immunocompromised children.

Medical Management

The mainstay of treatment in these patients is the treatment of the underlying pneumonia with the appropriate IV antibiotics. These patients should also be resuscitated with IV fluids, oxygen therapy (if $sPaO_2$ less than 92%), pain medication, and medications to reduce fever as needed. When these interventions have failed to improve symptoms and there is significant extrapleural fluid, an intervention (either tube thoracostomy with fibrinolysis as needed or a surgical debridement) is often warranted.

Surgical and Procedural Intervention

The aims of intervention for an empyema is to reduce the overall duration of symptoms, reduce hospital length of stay, and prevent long-term disability. Evacuating infected extrapleural fluid allows the underlying lung to expand thereby improving symptoms and facilitating treatment.

Early tube thoracostomy insertion may be helpful in children with a small effusion if there are severe symptoms (increased work of breathing, tachypnea, hypoxia) [35]. In general, however, interventions may be guided by the following algorithm (Fig. 2).

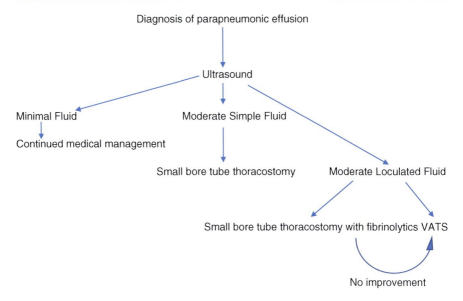

Fig. 2 Proposed algorithm for management of parapneumonic effusion (Original figure created by the author, Dr. Julia Grabowski)

The choice of tube thoracostomy with fibrinolysis versus VATS (video-assisted thoracoscopic surgery) has been the focus of much debate and study. Most available evidence suggest that, in the pediatric population, these two therapies have the same overall success rates. VATS has been shown to have increased costs and requires access to an operating room with thoracoscopic equipment and general anesthesia. Prior to the advent of VATS, thoracotomy was the surgical approach for these patients, but is rarely employed currently. VATS is indicated in patients in whom fibrinolysis is not effective or is contraindicated [35, 36].

Tube Thoracostomy

According to the BTS, placement of a chest tube is best performed (and has a lower associated risk of complications) by whichever service has access to the appropriate resources and the most experienced personnel. Unless there are known risk factors for a bleeding disorder, routine coagulation studies or platelet count is not needed. Ultrasound guidance, if available, can assist with placement of the tube [37].

When choosing the size of chest tube, the patient size should be taken into account. Several studies have shown that a larger tube does not confer an advantage; therefore tubes as small as 8 Fr can be used, though in larger children a size 12–14 Fr is often utilized [36]. These can be placed with the Seldinger technique [36, 38]. Though there are no evidence-based guidelines for chest tube removal, most authors suggest that tubes can be removed when there is no sign of air leakage and drainage output is less than 1 mL/kg per day [36].

In patients with loculated fluid, intrapleural *fibrinolytics* are used to break down the fibrin in these collections to improve drainage while avoiding systemic fibrinolysis [39]. Several fibrinolytic agents have been used, including urokinase and streptokinase, with tissue plasminogen activator (tPA) being the most commonly substance employed in children currently. A common technique is to instill the tPA by instilling the tPA solution (4 mg of tPA into 40 mL of sterile normal saline) directly into the tube with a dwell time of 1 h. The tPA solution is then re-instilled for two additional doses each given 24 h later to comprise three treatments in a 48-h span [36].

Surgical Cortical Debridement

When VATS is deemed necessary, either as initial approach or after failure of fibrinolytic therapy, it is usually performed with 2–3 incisions (1–2 5 mm ports and 1 10–12 ports). The procedure does not require single-lung ventilation. The camera can be placed through a 5 mm port and a large suction device and ringed forceps placed through the larger port. An attempt should be made to remove the fibrinous exudate and break up all loculations. In certain instances, the empyema is thick and organized precluding successful decortication with VATS and those patients require a thoracotomy [34].

Complications

Data suggest that children with failure of fibrinolysis should proceed to VATS and that children with failed VATS should be considered for trialing fibrinolysis, repeating VATS or performing a mini-thoracotomy [34]. One of the feared complications in the treatment of empyema is the formation of a bronchopleural fistula. A bronchopleural fistula is suspected when there is a persistent air leak or if a pneumothorax is noted after chest tube removal. The majority of bronchopleural fistulae are peripheral so most will resolve over time with continued tube thoracostomy which causes apposition of the visceral and parietal pleura. When persistent, further interventions may be needed. Surgical options include lung resection, decortication, and muscle flap formation. Bronchoscopy has also been reportedly successful in some instances [40, 41].

Pediatric Thoracic Trauma and Acute Surgical Care

Epidemiology
Blunt trauma represents 75% to 80% of thoracic injuries resulting in pediatric trauma admissions. In the urban setting, there is larger incidence of penetrating trauma. There are several characteristics to the injury patterns and children that are different from those in the adults [42]. Although thoracic injuries occur in less than 10% of injured children, one-quarter of fatal injuries include chest trauma. The

mechanisms of injury in children are well recognized and include pedestrian-motor vehicle, passenger-motor vehicle, and falls penetrating trauma. The largest group of children injured consists of those with pedestrian injuries (37%), second largest those involved in passenger-motor vehicle crashes (31%) [43].

In children with isolated thoracic trauma, the mortality rate is 5%. Children with abdominal injury in addition to their thoracic injury the mortality rate increases to 20%, and with an concomitant head injury, the mortality rate approaches 35%. Most of these deaths are due to the head injury.

In comparing the patterns of injury between adults and children, most adult deaths later in the bimodal distribution and result from pneumonia, adult respiratory distress syndrome, systemic inflammatory response syndrome, and multisystem organ failure, whereas most deaths in children occur in the acute phase of the injury. Although rib fractures in adults with blunt trauma to the chest occurring in 70% of patients, the incidence is only 30% in children. Conversely pulmonary contusions in children occur in as much as 50% vs. 30% of adults. Flail chest and aortic chair (rupture) rarely occur in children. Pneumothorax is common both groups, but the incidence of tension is much higher in children.

Anatomy and Physiology of the Pediatric Thorax

Physical factors creating injury are related to the mass (the victim and the colliding object), the velocity (the victim and the colliding object), the rate of change in the velocity, the area or volume of the body tissues involved in the transfer kinetic energy [42]. The degree of injury depends on the biomechanical features of the human tissue, including tensile strength, compliance, elasticity (soft tissue, muscle, cartilage), and compressive strength (bone). There are certain anatomic and physiologic characteristics to the thorax that are important to the biomechanics of injury [44]. The chest wall is very compliant because of the elastic nature of its tissues. The thoracic cage is mainly cartilage, minimal skeletal ossification. The pectoralis, intercostal, shoulder girdle, and paraspinal musculatures are often not fully developed. This creates a compliant chest wall that results in minimal damage to the thoracic cage transmission kinetic energy to the parenchyma [45].

The internal diameter of the trachea in a small child is often less than 6 mm, and therefore 1 to 2 mm of edema within the tracheal lumen may create a significant obstructed airway. Where similar edema in the adult may cause less than 50% narrowing of the airway, in the child this may result in a greater than 75% narrowing and critical airway obstruction. The length of the trachea in young children is as short as 5 cm in an infant and 10 cm and a school-aged child.

In children, there is no prominent point of fixation of the middle mediastinum to the posterior mediastinum. Therefore, the heart, thoracic great vessels, and the vena cava may freely shift within the chest cavity. With this lack of fixation, a pneumothorax with a tension component, the middle mediastinum may significantly impede venous return increasing cardiac output, leading to shock. Conversely, disruption of the descending thoracic aorta in children less than 10 years rarely occurs.

Cardiopulmonary physiology of the child provides significant buffer to the potential devastating consequences of trauma. The injured child often does not suffer from the comorbidity or underlying cardiac, renal, or hepatic illnesses.

Therefore, the unaltered organ physiology masks the hemodynamic effects of hypovolemia, hypoxia, and hypercarbia until late into the physiologic decline. Cardiac output of a child is maintained by a relatively fixed stroke-volume, and increases in cardiac output is determined by the increases in heart rate. Hypovolemic child cardiac output is similarly maintained by increases in heart rate and vasoconstriction. Tachycardia is an early sign of hypovolemia; other physical findings characteristic of hypovolemia include thready pulses, delayed capillary refill, and cool extremities. Because the child can maintain hemodynamic stability blood loss up to 30%, and late in complete decompensation occurs with blood loss in excess of 40%, clinician must be aware of the subtle hemodynamic changes of hypovolemia.

Pathophysiology of Thoracic Injuries

Blunt forces are the most common etiologies in children; 90% of injuries result from blunt force in young children, whereas penetrating trauma involves in 15 to 20% of injuries in adolescence [42]. The underlying pathophysiology of the injuries is often based on mechanism of injury. As described earlier, blunt forces may affect direct tissue damage by compression, crush, or shear forces or by rotational or decelerating-decelerating forces. The upper airway is particularly susceptible to direct forces to the trachea. The larynx is well protected by the mandible, therefore rarely injured. Injuries to the upper airway may present with airway obstruction, subcutaneous emphysema, or both. The airway obstruction may be caused by tracheal deviation, crush disruption, or mucosal edema. Deviation is most often the result of an associated vascular or intrathoracic injury causing a mass effect or shifting of the mediastinum. Direct blow to the trachea causing varying degrees of disruption results, and rapid airway compromise is due to mucosal edema and marked subcutaneous emphysema positive intra-airway pressure during expiration.

Because of its cartilaginous skeleton and thin musculature, the chest wall is very compliant in children. Therefore, kinetic energy is not absorbed by the thoracic cage as in the ossified ribs of the adult; it is transmitted to the pulmonary parenchyma and mediastinum. There can be severe pulmonary contusions in the absence of rib fractures, and unexplained hypoxemia without clinical or radiologic evidence of major chest wall injury [44]. Likewise, in the acute setting in the emergency department, almost all chest radiographs are obtained in supine position. Pre-fluid may be difficult to see in this position. Parenchymal hemorrhage and edema causing the hypoxemia resolved from loss of alveolar capillary integrity with immediate intrapulmonary shunting. The presence of a rib fracture increases the risk of life-threatening thoracic injury. The biomechanical of a rib fracture depending on the direct or indirect nature of transmission of the kinetic injury energy [43]. Direct blows to the chest result in the inward displacement of the rib and a fracture on the inner surface of the rib. The significant global forces of a crush injury bow the ribs outward either laterally or posteriorly, resulting in the fracture on the outer surface. Likewise, the direct forces from squeezing may result in a series of nerve fractures. Because of the significant kinetic energy necessary to cause rib fractures, resultant head and thoracic injuries are critical and the risk of death is much higher. In one study rib fractures were present in

25% of trauma-related deaths, and 42% of children with rib injury fracture with rib fractures die. Child abuse and motor vehicle crashes are frequent mechanisms of injury.

In the adult, if several rib fractures are noted, the examiner has a high index of suspicion for lung parenchymal injury such as a pulmonary contusion. The same index of suspicion is patient would hold for an aortic injury if there was a first rib fracture porch. Unfortunately, if no fractures are seen because of the relative compliance of the child's chest, the examiner may not be as attuned to the possibility of intrathoracic injury.

Biomechanically, traumatic hemothorax or pneumothorax from blunt forces to the chest can result from two different mechanisms [45]. Although infrequent in children, pulmonary parenchymal penetration from a rib fracture is well recognized as a cause of hemothorax and pneumothorax. Children, pneumothorax occurs more commonly when external compression produces a sudden, marked increase the intra-the internal pressure within the lung, resulting in rupture of distal bronchioles and leakage of air from the visceral pleura. Child inspires and closes the glottis, trapping air within the airway and a pneumothorax results.

Another injury related to the mobility of the mediastinum is a tear of the tracheobronchial tree. Partial or incomplete disruption caused by either shear forces that occur at a relatively thick head fix points, such as the carina of the segmental branches, or by severe crush injuries resulting in high intra-bronchial pressures with a closed glottis. Another mechanism involves the crush or impact that decreases the anteroposterior diameter of the chest, displacing and distracting the lung laterally from the main tracheobronchial structures.

Injury to the heart or great vessels requires traumatic events high velocity. The typical mechanism of injury is from blunt trauma and bolus rapid deceleration-acceleration in a motor vehicle crash as a passenger pedestrian or a fall from a great height. Because of the highly mobile mediastinum, aortic tearing or rupture is rare in children younger than 10 years of age. The tear results from the relatively fixed portion of the aorta at the ligamentum arteriosum sharing from the more mobile proximal aorta [43]. Survival (less than 25% from the scene) depends on the rupture being contained within the posterior mediastinum. Equally rare, cardiac rupture or papillary muscle tears are caused by rapid changes in speed or severe crush injury. Cardiac rupture most commonly involves the inferior or superior vena cava and the right atrium and decelerating injuries, and the right atrium when compressed during diastole. Papillary muscle disruption is thought to occur by the same mechanism. There is evidence that valvular insufficiency may be either acute or delayed after traumatic injury.

Life-Threatening Chest Injuries in the Unstable Patient

The unstable patient is categorized as having positive vital signs, but with an abnormal ventilatory pattern, poor skin perfusion, tachycardia, hypotension, altered sensorium, or decreased urine output. Patient requires immediate stabilization of the airway. Evaluating the patient for life-threatening thoracic injury, the surgeon must determine if the derangement results from a ventilatory or cardiac failure [46–48].

Injuries leading to ventilatory instability include tracheal injury, disruption of the tracheobronchial tree, and open pneumothorax flail chest. These injuries are recognized by subcutaneous, tracheal deviation, chest wall crepitus, and unilateral or bilateral impairment of ventilation. Flail chest is often presenting with paradoxical chest wall motion with inspiration [42]. Correction of ventilatory instability begins with establishment of a secure airway and positive pressure ventilation. The presence of a tracheal injury and emergency surgical airway may be necessary if endotracheal intubation is unsuccessful. Disruption of the major bronchial segments presents initially with inadequate ventilation, requiring endotracheal intubation and positive pressure ventilation. Simple pneumothorax is now converted into a tension pneumothorax [47]. Immediate decompression of the affected thorax is required by inserting catheter in the second intercostal space in the midclavicular line. This is followed by tube thoracostomy along the anterior axillary line 4th–sixth intercostal space. With significant bronchial injury, there is a persistent air leak from a chip from a tube thoracostomy, and a collapsed segment or low appears on chest radiograph [48].

Cardiac or pulmonary failure or both is seen in tension pneumothorax, hematoma thorax, and pericardial tamponade [42, 44, 48]. The pathophysiology of each of these injuries diminished venous return waiting to inadequate end-diastolic volume. Clinically this is apparent with hypotension distended neck veins and absent breath sounds (hemothorax-pneumothorax) or diminished heart tones and paradoxical pulses (pericardial tamponade not). Clinical features of pneumothorax-pneumothorax include decreased breath sounds, tracheal deviation hyperresonance (pneumothorax), or dullness (hemothorax) to percussion. Emergent care of these injuries requires placement of a large-diameter anterolateral thoracostomy for decompression. In children, size of the chest tube should be equal to the size of the child's thumb [46]. If the patient continues to have hemodynamically unstable stented neck veins (elevated central venous pressure) after placement of tube thoracostomy, the surgeon or emergency physician would suspect pericardial tamponade. If the patient is unstable, this condition requires needle pericardiocentesis. To evacuate the pericardial sac, the needle was inserted into the left sacral costal angle and directed posteriorly at a 45-degree angle toward the ipsilateral scapula. When the needle enters the pericardial space, there will be a return of nonclotting blood and there should be hemodynamic improvement in the child. This can occur with a return as little as 5 mL of blood in infants. This procedure only temporizes an unstable condition, and the patient still requires pericardial exploration.

Tension Pneumothorax
Due to the mobile middle mediastinum in the child, the mediastinum and trachea are displaced to the opposite side, decreasing venous return and compressing the opposite lung resulting in hemodynamic instability [49]. The most common causes of tension pneumothorax are mechanical ventilation with positive end-expiratory pressure, spontaneous pneumothorax with ruptured emphysematous bullae, and blunt chest trauma with a parenchymal lung injury. Occasionally traumatic defects in the chest wall may cause a tension pneumothorax. **Tension pneumothorax is a**

clinical diagnosis and should not be made radiologically [45]. A tension pneumothorax is characterized by respiratory distress, tachycardia, hypotension, tracheal deviation, unilateral absence of breath sounds, neck vein distention, and cyanosis as a late manifestation. Because of the similarity in their symptomatology, a tension pneumothorax initially may be confused with cardiac tamponade. Differentiation may be made by a hyper-resonant percussion noted over the ipsilateral chest. Tension pneumothorax requires **immediate decompression** and is managed initially by rapidly inserting a needle into the second intercostal space in the midclavicular line of the affected hemithorax. Definitive treatment usually requires only the insertion of a chest tube into the fifth intercostal space (nipple level), anterior to the midaxillary line.

Open Pneumothorax ("Sucking Chest Wound")
Large defects of the chest wall, which remain open, result in an open pneumothorax. or sucking chest wound. Equilibration between intrathoracic pressure and atmospheric pressure is immediate. If the opening in the chest wall is approximately two-thirds the diameter of the trachea, air passes preferentially through the chest defect with each respiratory effort, because air tends to follow the path of least resistance through the large chest-wall defect. Effective ventilation is thereby impaired, leading to hypoxia [43].

Manage an open pneumothorax by promptly closing the defect with a sterile occlusive dressing, large enough to overlap the wound's edges, and taped securely on three sides. Taping the occlusive dressing on three sides provides a flutter-type valve effect. As the patient inspires, the dressing occludes the wound, preventing air from entering. When the patient exhales, the open end of the dressing allows air to escape. A chest tube should be placed remote from the wound as soon as possible. Securely taping all edges of the dressing can cause air to accumulate in the thoracic cavity resulting in a tension pneumothorax unless a chest tube is in place. Any occlusive dressing (plastic wrap, petrolatum gauze, etc.) may be used as a stopgap so rapid assessment can continue. Definitive surgical closure of the defect is usually required.

Massive Hemothorax
Massive hemothorax results from a rapid accumulation of more than 20 mL/kg of blood in the chest cavity [46, 47]. It is commonly caused by a penetrating wound injuring great or hilar vessels. It may also be the result of blunt trauma. The blood loss is complicated by hypoxia. The neck veins may be flat secondary to severe hypovolemia or may be distended because of the mechanical effect of intrathoracic blood. This condition is discovered when shock is associated with the absence of breath sounds and/or dullness to percussion on one side of the chest. Massive hemothorax is initially managed by the simultaneous restoration of blood volume and decompression of the chest cavity. Large-caliber intravenous lines and rapid crystalloid infusion are begun, and type-specific blood is administered as soon as possible [50]. If an auto-transfusion device is available, it may be used. A single chest tube is inserted at the nipple level, anterior to the midaxillary line, and rapid restoration

of volume continues as decompression of the chest cavity is completed. When massive hemothorax is suspected, prepare for autotransfusion. If 20 mL/kg is immediately evacuated, it is highly likely that the patient will require an early thoracotomy. Some patients who have an initial volume output of less than 20 mL/kg, but continue to bleed, may require a thoracotomy. This decision is based on the rate of continuing blood loss (3–5 mL/h) [47]. During patient resuscitation, the volume of blood initially drained from the chest tube, and the rate of continuing blood loss must be factored into the amount of intravenous fluid replacement. The color of the blood (arterial or venous) is a poor indicator of the necessity for thoracotomy. Penetrating anterior chest wounds medial to the nipple line and posterior wounds medial to the scapula should alert the physician to the possible need for thoracotomy, because of possible damage to the great vessels, hilar structures, and the heart, with the associated.

potential for cardiac tamponade. **Thoracotomy is not indicated unless a surgeon is present, and the procedure is performed by a physician qualified by training and experience** [46, 51].

Flail Chest
A flail chest, uncommon in children, occurs when a segment of the chest wall does not have skeletal continuity with the rest of the thoracic cage. This condition usually results from trauma associated with multiple rib fractures. Due to the cartilaginous nature of a child's rib cage, ribs fractures are uncommon, but due to the force, injury to the underlying lung is significant, and serious hypoxia may result. Arterial blood gases, suggesting respiratory failure with hypoxia, also may aid in diagnosing a flail chest. Initial therapy includes adequate ventilation, administration of humidified oxygen, and fluid resuscitation. **In the absence of systemic hypotension,** the administration of crystalloid intravenous solutions should be carefully controlled to prevent overhydration. The injured lung in a flail chest is sensitive to both under resuscitation of shock and fluid overload. Specific measures to optimize fluid measurement must be taken for the patient with flail chest. The definitive treatment is to re-expand the lung, ensure oxygenation as completely as possible, administer fluids judiciously, and provide analgesia to improve ventilation. Some patients can be managed without the use of a ventilator. However, prevention of hypoxia is of paramount importance for the trauma patient, and a short period of intubation and ventilation may be necessary until the diagnosis of the entire injury pattern is complete. A careful assessment of the respiratory rate, arterial oxygen tension, and an estimate of the work of breathing will indicate appropriate timing for intubation and ventilation. Not all patients with a flail chest require immediate endotracheal intubation.

Cardiac Tamponade
Cardiac tamponade more commonly results from blunt injury causing the pericardium to fill with blood from the heart, great vessels, or pericardial vessels. The human pericardial sac is a fixed fibrous structure, and only a relatively small amount of blood is required to restrict cardiac activity and interfere with cardiac filling. Removal of small amounts of blood or fluid, often as little as 15 mL to 20 mL, by

pericardiocentesis may result in immediate hemodynamic improvement. The classic Beck's triad consists of venous pressure elevation, decline in arterial pressure, and muffled heart sounds. However, muffled heart tones are difficult to assess in the noisy emergency department. Distended neck veins caused by the elevated central venous pressure may be absent due to hypovolemia or the short child's neck. Pulsus paradoxus, a decrease in systolic pressure during inspiration in excess of 10 mmHg, also may be absent in some patients or difficult to detect in some emergency settings. In addition, tension pneumothorax—particularly on the left side—may mimic cardiac tamponade. Kussmaul's sign (a rise in venous pressure with inspiration when breathing spontaneously) is a true paradoxical venous pressure abnormality associated with tamponade. Electromechanical dissociation in the absence of hypovolemia and tension pneumothorax suggests cardiac tamponade [46, 51].

Pericardiocentesis is indicated for patients who do not respond to the usual measures of resuscitation for hemorrhagic shock and who have the potential for cardiac tamponade.

Insertion of a central venous line may aid diagnosis. Lifesaving pericardiocentesis should not be delayed for this diagnostic adjunct. A high index of suspicion coupled with a patient who is unresponsive to resuscitative efforts are all that is necessary to initiate pericardiocentesis by the subxyphoid method. Even though cardiac tamponade is strongly suspected, the initial administration of intravenous fluid will raise the venous pressure and improve cardiac output transiently while preparations are made for pericardiocentesis via the subxyphoid route. The use of a plastic-sheathed needle is preferable, but the urgent priority is to aspirate blood from the pericardial sac. Electrocardiographic monitoring may identify current of injury and needle-induced dysrhythmias. Because of the self-sealing qualities of the myocardium, aspiration of pericardial blood alone may relieve symptoms temporarily. However, all patients with positive pericardiocentesis due to trauma will require open thoracotomy and inspection of the heart. Pericardiocentesis may not be diagnostic or therapeutic because the blood in the pericardial sac is clotted. Preparations for transfer of these patients to the appropriate facility is necessary. Open pericardiotomy may be lifesaving but is indicated **only** when a qualified surgeon is available. Once these injuries and other immediate, life-threatening injuries have been treated, attention may be directed to the secondary survey and definitive care phase of potential, life-threatening thoracic injuries [43, 51].

Potentially Lethal Chest Injuries in the Stable Patient

The patient with stable vital signs usually can undergo more thorough evaluation for decisions about definitive treatment are undertaken. During the initial assessment, the surgeon should evaluate the patient as if they were potentially unstable and perform maneuvers to ensure an airway ventilation, oxygenation, trial of external bleeding, and securing intravenous access. Anteroposterior chest and lateral cervical spine radiograph should be obtained if the patient has any symptoms or signs of injury to the head neck, or torso [42–45].

The workup depends on the mechanism of injury and structures of the chest that may be at risk for injury. Evaluation of penetrating injury requires a diagnostic approach to identify injuries proximity to the penetrating wounds like the evaluation of such agents and trajectory as in adults. The child with a penetrating injury particularly gunshot wounds is the risk of injury to adjacent structures as the blast energy injury is more likely due to the close vicinity of vital structures. The tools esophagram, aerodigestive endoscopy, cardiac and thoracic ultrasound, and thoracic CT angiography are equally useful in children.

Evaluation of blunt injury to the thorax in a stable patient requires approach similar to penetrating injuries but the range of injuries is greater. In children younger than 10 years of age, transection of the thoracic aorta is extremely rare. In older children, this injury is often the result of pedestrian vs motor vehicle or side impact crashes. The incidence of aortic injury in young children is due to their mobile mediastinum without tethering of the distal aorta. Clinical signs and diagnostic evaluation are similar to adults. Tracheobronchial disruption (Fig. 3) is common in children exposed to high velocity blunt forces to the chest. Features of extra-pleural air and persistent air leak are similar to those seen in penetrating trauma.

Six potentially lethal injuries are considered herein:

1. Pulmonary contusion.
2. Myocardial contusion.
3. Aortic disruption.
4. Traumatic diaphragmatic rupture.
5. Tracheobronchial disruption.
6. Esophageal disruption.

Unlike immediately life-threatening conditions, these injuries are not obvious on

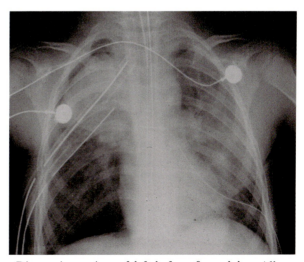

Fig. 3 Tracheobronchial disruption. The radiograph demonstrates incomplete expansion of the right lung and complete collapse of the right upper lobe. Despite 2 large chest tubes, there is a persistent air leak from the chest tubes. These are the clinical and radiographic features of proximal airway disruption, in this case of the take-off of the right upper lobe bronchus from the right mainstem

initial physical examination. Diagnosis requires a **high index of suspicion.** All are more often missed than diagnosed during the initial posttraumatic period. However, if these injuries are overlooked, lives may be lost.

Pulmonary Contusion With or Without Flail Chest

Pulmonary contusion is the most common chest injury seen in North America due to the use of CT imaging of the chest [52, 53]. The respiratory failure may be subtle and develops over time rather than occurring instantaneously. Therefore, careful monitoring and reevaluation of the patient is required in children with a supplemental oxygen requirement. Some patients with stable conditions may be managed selectively without endotracheal intubation or mechanical ventilation. Patients with significant hypoxia should be intubated and ventilated within the first hour after injury. Associated medical conditions, e.g., chronic pulmonary disease and renal failure, predispose to the need for early intubation and mechanical ventilation [54, 55]. If the patient cannot maintain satisfactory oxygenation or has any of the above complicating features, intubation and mechanical ventilation should be considered. Pulse oximetry, ABG determination, ECG monitoring, and appropriate ventilatory equipment are necessary for optimal management. Any patient with preexisting conditions and who is to be transferred should be intubated and ventilated.

Myocardial Contusion

Myocardial contusion, although difficult to diagnose, is another potentially lethal injury from blunt chest trauma. The patient's reported complaints of discomfort are often bypassed as being associated with chest wall contusion or fractures of the sternum and/or ribs. The diagnosis of myocardial contusion is established by abnormalities on the electrocardiogram, two-dimensional echocardiography, and associated history of injury. The electrocardiographic changes are variable and may even indicate frank myocardial infarction. Multiple premature ventricular contractions, unexplained sinus tachycardia, atrial fibrillation, bundle branch block (usually right), and ST segment changes are the most common electrocardiographic findings [56]. Elevated central venous pressure in the absence of obvious cause may indicate right ventricular dysfunction secondary to contusion. Patients with myocardial contusion are at risk for sudden dysrhythmias. They should be admitted to the critical care unit for close observation and cardiac monitoring.

Traumatic Aortic Rupture

As mentioned above, this injury is rarely seen in children less than 10 years of age, and present with similar clinical and radiographic findings [57, 58]. The evaluation and management are no different in children, but the use of endovascular techniques is limited in children and young adolescents. The treatment in the younger age population is either direct repair of the aorta or resection of the injured area and grafting. A qualified surgeon should surgically manage such a patient [59, 60].

Traumatic Diaphragmatic Rupture

A traumatic diaphragmatic rupture is more commonly diagnosed on the left side because the liver obliterates the defect on the right side, while the appearance of bowel, stomach, or nasogastric tube is more easily detected in the left chest. Blunt trauma produces large radial tears that lead to herniation. Penetrating trauma produces small perforations that often take some time, even years, to develop into diaphragmatic hernias [61]. These injuries are missed initially if the chest film is misinterpreted as showing an elevated left diaphragm, acute gastric dilatation, a loculated pneumohemothorax, or sub-pulmonary hematoma. If a laceration of the left diaphragm is suspected, a gastric tube should be inserted. When the gastric tube appears in the thoracic cavity on the chest film, the need for special contrast studies is eliminated. Occasionally, the diagnosis is not identified on the initial roentgenogram or after chest tube evacuation of the left thorax. An upper gastrointestinal contrast study should be performed if the diagnosis is not clear. Right diaphragmatic ruptures are rarely diagnosed in the early postinjury period. The liver often prevents herniation of other abdominal organs into the chest. The appearance of an elevated right diaphragm on chest roentgenogram may be the only finding. Operation for other abdominal injuries often reveals diaphragmatic tears. The treatment is direct repair.

Tracheobronchial Tree Injuries

Trachea

Direct trauma to the trachea, including the larynx, can be either penetrating or blunt [62–67]. Blunt injuries may be subtle, and history is all-important. Penetrating trauma is overt and requires immediate surgical repair [66, 68]. Penetrating injuries are often associated with esophageal, carotid artery, and jugular vein trauma. Because of the blast effect, penetrating injuries caused by missiles are often associated with extensive tissue destruction surrounding the area of penetration. Noisy breathing indicates partial airway obstruction that suddenly may become complete. Absence of breathing suggests that complete obstruction already exists. When the level of consciousness is depressed, detection of significant airway obstruction is more subtle. Observations of labored respiratory effort may be the only clue to airway obstruction and tracheobronchial injury. Endoscopic procedures and CT scanning aid in the diagnosis [44, 63].

Bronchus

Injury to a major bronchus is an unusual and fatal injury that is frequently overlooked.

Most of such injuries result from blunt trauma and occur within 20 mm of the carina [63, 64]. Although most patients with this injury die at the scene, those who reach the hospital alive have a 30% mortality, often due to associated injuries. If suspicion of a bronchial injury exists, immediate surgical consultation is warranted. A patient with a bronchial injury frequently presents with hemoptysis, subcutaneous emphysema, or tension pneumothorax with a mediastinal shift. A pneumothorax associated with a persistent large air leak after tube thoracotomy suggests a bronchial injury. More than one chest tube may be necessary to overcome a very large leak [68]. Bronchoscopy confirms the diagnosis of the injury. Treatment of tracheobronchial injuries may require only airway maintenance until the acute inflammatory and edema processes resolve [66]. Mediastinal deviation or compression of the trachea by extrinsic masses, i.e., hematomas, must be treated. Intubation frequently may be unsuccessful because of the anatomic distortion from paratracheal hematoma, major laryngotracheal injury, and associated injuries. For such patients, operative intervention is indicated. Patients surviving with bronchial injuries may require direct surgical intervention by thoracotomy [62, 65–68].

Esophageal Trauma

Esophageal trauma is commonly caused by mishaps of instrumentation (nasogastric tubes, endoscopes, dilators, etc.) [65]. The clinical picture is identical to that seen in adults. Esophageal injury should be considered for any patient who (1) has a left pneumothorax or hemothorax without a rib fracture, (2) has received a severe blow to the lower sternum or epigastrium and is in pain or shock out of proportion to the apparent injury, or (3) has particulate matter in their chest tube after the blood begins to clear. Presence of mediastinal air also suggests the diagnosis, which often can be confirmed by contrast studies and/or esophagoscopy [65, 67].

Wide drainage of the pleural space and mediastinum with direct repair of the injury via thoracotomy is the treatment if feasible. If the repair is tenuous or not feasible, esophageal diversion in the neck and gastrostomy of the lower and upper gastric segments usually is carried out, thereby avoiding continued soiling of the mediastinum and pleura by gastric and esophageal contents [67, 68].

Subcutaneous Emphysema

Subcutaneous emphysema may result from airway injury, lung injury, or, rarely, blast injury. Although it does not require treatment, the underlying injury must be addressed [65].

Crushing Injury to the Chest (Traumatic Asphyxia)

Findings associated with a crush injury to the chest include upper torso, facial, and arm plethora with petechiae secondary to superior vena cava compression. Massive swelling and even cerebral edema may be present. Underlying injuries must be treated [42, 43, 47].

References

1. Wu JT, Mattox KL, Wall MJ Jr. Esophageal perforations: new perspectives and treatment paradigms. J Trauma. 2007;63(5):1173–84.
2. Han SY, McElvein RB, Aldrete JS, Tishler JM. Perforation of the esophagus: correlation of site and cause with plain film findings. AJR Am J Roentgenol. 1985;145(3):537–40.
3. Johnson DE, Foker J, Munson DP, Nelson A, Athinarayanan P, Thompson TR. Management of esophageal and pharyngeal perforation in the newborn infant. Pediatrics. 1982;70(4):592–6.

4. Fallon BP, Overman RE, Geiger JD, Jarboe MD, Kunisaki SM. Efficacy and risk profile of self-expandable stents in the management of pediatric esophageal pathology. J Pediatr Surg. 2019;54(6):1233–8.
5. Millar AJ, Cox SG. Caustic injury of the oesophagus. Pediatr Surg Int. 2015;31(2):111–21.
6. Niedzielski A, Schwartz SG, Partycka-Pietrzyk K, Mielnik-Niedzielska G. Caustic agents ingestion in children: a 51-year retrospective cohort study. Ear Nose Throat J. 2019;99:52–7.
7. Ertekin C, Alimoglu O, Akyildiz H, Guloglu R, Taviloglu K. The results of caustic ingestions. Hepatogastroenterology. 2004;51(59):1397–400.
8. Cutrone C, Pedruzzi B, Tava G, Emanuelli E, Barion U, Fischetto D, et al. The complimentary role of diagnostic and therapeutic endoscopy in foreign body aspiration in children. Int J Pediatr Otorhinolaryngol. 2011;75(12):1481–5.
9. Melchiors J, Todsen T, Konge L, Charabi B, von Buchwald C. Cricothyroidotomy—the emergency surgical airway. Head Neck. 2016;38(7):1129–31.
10. Holm-Knudsen RJ, Rasmussen LS, Charabi B, Bottger M, Kristensen MS. Emergency airway access in children—transtracheal cannulas and tracheotomy assessed in a porcine model. Paediatr Anaesth. 2012;22(12):1159–65.
11. Silva AB, Muntz HR, Clary R. Utility of conventional radiography in the diagnosis and management of pediatric airway foreign bodies. Ann Otol Rhinol Laryngol. 1998;107(10 Pt 1):834–8.
12. Breysem L, Loyen S, Boets A, Proesmans M, De Boeck K, Smet MH. Pediatric emergencies: thoracic emergencies. Eur Radiol. 2002;12(12):2849–65.
13. Kenth J, Ng C. Foreign body airway obstruction causing a ball valve effect. JRSM Short Rep. 2013;4(6):2042533313482458.
14. Goyal R, Nayar S, Gogia P, Garg M. Extraction of tracheobronchial foreign bodies in children and adults with rigid and flexible bronchoscopy. J Bronchology Interv Pulmonol. 2012;19(1):35–43.
15. Soyer T. The role bronchoscopy in the diagnosis of airway disease in children. J Thorac Dis. 2016;8(11):3420–6.
16. Mosca S, Manes G, Martino R, Amitrano L, Bottino V, Bove A, et al. Endoscopic management of foreign bodies in the upper gastrointestinal tract: report on a series of 414 adult patients. Endoscopy. 2001;33(8):692–6.
17. Jayachandra S, Eslick GD. A systematic review of paediatric foreign body ingestion: presentation, complications, and management. Int J Pediatr Otorhinolaryngol. 2013;77(3):311–7.
18. Committee ASoP, Ikenberry SO, Jue TL, Anderson MA, Appalaneni V, Banerjee S, et al. Management of ingested foreign bodies and food impactions. Gastrointest Endosc. 2011;73(6):1085–91.
19. Peksa GD, DeMott JM, Slocum GW, Burkins J, Gottlieb M. Glucagon for relief of acute esophageal foreign bodies and food impactions: a systematic review and meta-analysis. Pharmacotherapy. 2019;39(4):463–72.
20. Arms JL, Mackenberg-Mohn MD, Bowen MV, Chamberlain MC, Skrypek TM, Madhok M, et al. Safety and efficacy of a protocol using bougienage or endoscopy for the management of coins acutely lodged in the esophagus: a large case series. Ann Emerg Med. 2008;51(4):367–72.
21. Heinzerling NP, Christensen MA, Swedler R, Cassidy LD, Calkins CM, Sato TT. Safe and effective management of esophageal coins in children with bougienage. Surgery. 2015;158(4):1065–70; discussion 71-2.
22. Harned RK 2nd, Strain JD, Hay TC, Douglas MR. Esophageal foreign bodies: safety and efficacy of Foley catheter extraction of coins. AJR Am J Roentgenol. 1997;168(2):443–6.
23. Burgos A, Rabago L, Triana P. Western view of the management of gastroesophageal foreign bodies. World J Gastrointest Endosc. 2016;8(9):378–84.
24. Kramer RE, Lerner DG, Lin T, Manfredi M, Shah M, Stephen TC, et al. Management of ingested foreign bodies in children: a clinical report of the NASPGHAN endoscopy Committee. J Pediatr Gastroenterol Nutr. 2015;60(4):562–74.
25. Dotson K, Johnson LH. Pediatric spontaneous pneumothorax. Pediatr Emerg Care. 2012;28(7):715–20; quiz 21-3.

26. Robinson PD, Cooper P, Ranganathan SC. Evidence-based management of paediatric primary spontaneous pneumothorax. Paediatr Respir Rev. 2009;10(3):110–7; quiz 7.
27. Lesher AP, et al. Spontaneous pneumothorax. In: Association APS, ed. Pediatric surgery NaT: APSA Webapp; 2018.
28. Harris M, Rocker J. Pneumothorax in pediatric patients: management strategies to improve patient outcomes. Pediatr Emerg Med Pract. 2017;14(3):1–28.
29. Voisin F, Sohier L, Rochas Y, Kerjouan M, Ricordel C, Belleguic C, et al. Ambulatory management of large spontaneous pneumothorax with pigtail catheters. Ann Emerg Med. 2014;64(3):222–8.
30. Williams K, Baumann L, Grabowski J, Lautz TB. Current practice in the management of spontaneous pneumothorax in children. J Laparoendosc Adv Surg Tech A. 2019;29(4):551–6.
31. Qureshi FG, Sandulache VC, Richardson W, Ergun O, Ford HR, Hackam DJ. Primary vs delayed surgery for spontaneous pneumothorax in children: which is better? J Pediatr Surg. 2005;40(1):166–9.
32. Yeung F, Chung PHY, Hung ELY, Yuen CS, Tam PKH, Wong KKY. Surgical intervention for primary spontaneous pneumothorax in pediatric population: when and why? J Laparoendosc Adv Surg Tech A. 2017;27(8):841–4.
33. Lee GE, Lorch SA, Sheffler-Collins S, Kronman MP, Shah SS. National hospitalization trends for pediatric pneumonia and associated complications. Pediatrics. 2010;126(2):204–13.
34. Balfour-Lynn IM, Abrahamson E, Cohen G, Hartley J, King S, Parikh D, et al. BTS guidelines for the management of pleural infection in children. Thorax. 2005;60(Suppl 1):i1–21.
35. Islam S, Calkins CM, Goldin AB, Chen C, Downard CD, Huang EY, et al. The diagnosis and management of empyema in children: a comprehensive review from the APSA Outcomes and Clinical Trials Committee. J Pediatr Surg. 2012;47(11):2101–10.
36. St Peter SD, Tsao K, Spilde TL, Keckler SJ, Harrison C, Jackson MA, et al. Thoracoscopic decortication vs tube thoracostomy with fibrinolysis for empyema in children: a prospective, randomized trial. J Pediatr Surg. 2009;44(1):106–11; discussion 11.
37. Laws D, Neville E, Duffy J, Pleural Diseases Group SoCCBTS. BTS guidelines for the insertion of a chest drain. Thorax. 2003;58(Suppl 2):ii53–9.
38. Thomson AH, Hull J, Kumar MR, Wallis C, Balfour Lynn IM. Randomised trial of intrapleural urokinase in the treatment of childhood empyema. Thorax. 2002;57(4):343–7.
39. Davies RJ, Traill ZC, Gleeson FV. Randomised controlled trial of intrapleural streptokinase in community acquired pleural infection. Thorax. 1997;52(5):416–21.
40. Boudaya MS, Smadhi H, Zribi H, Mohamed J, Ammar J, Mestiri T, et al. Conservative management of postoperative bronchopleural fistulas. J Thorac Cardiovasc Surg. 2013;146(3):575–9.
41. Jester I, Nijran A, Singh M, Parikh DH. Surgical management of bronchopleural fistula in pediatric empyema and necrotizing pneumonia: efficacy of the serratus anterior muscle digitation flap. J Pediatr Surg. 2012;47(7):1358–62.
42. Pearson EG, Fitzgerald CA, Santore MT. Pediatric thoracic trauma: current trends. Semin Pediatr Surg. 2017;26(1):36–42.
43. Bliss D, Silen M. Pediatric thoracic trauma. Crit Care Med. 2002;30(11 Suppl):S409–15.
44. Piccolo CL, Ianniello S, Trinci M, Galluzzo M, Tonerini M, Zeccolini M, Guglielmi G, Miele V. Diagnostic imaging in pediatric thoracic trauma. Radiol Med. 2017;122(11):850–65.
45. Pauzé DR, Pauzé DK. Emergency management of blunt chest trauma in children: an evidence-based approach. Pediatr Emerg Med Pract. 2013;10(11):1–22.
46. Leidel BA, Kanz KG. Cardiopulmonary resuscitation in cardiac arrest following trauma. Med Klin Intensivmed Notfmed. 2016;111(8):695–702.
47. Skinner DL, den Hollander D, Laing GL, Rodseth RN, Muckart DJ. Severe blunt thoracic trauma: differences between adults and children in a level I trauma centre. S Afr Med J. 2015;105(1):47–51.
48. Pandian TK, Hamner C. Surgical management for complications of pediatric lung injury. Semin Pediatr Surg. 2015;24(1):50–8.

49. Vasquez DG, Berg GM, Srour SG, Ali K. Lung ultrasound for detecting pneumothorax in injured children: preliminary experience at a community-based Level II pediatric trauma center. Pediatr Radiol. 2020;50(3):329–37.
50. Choi PM, Farmakis S, Desmarais TJ, Keller MS. Management and outcomes of traumatic hemothorax in children. J Emerg Trauma Shock. 2015;8(2):83–7.
51. Hunt PA, Greaves I, Owens WA. Emergency thoracotomy in thoracic trauma—a review. Injury. 2006;37(1):1–19. Epub 2005 Apr 20.
52. Medar SS, Villacres S, Kaushik S, Eisenberg R, Stone ME Jr. Pediatric acute respiratory distress syndrome (PARDS) in children with pulmonary contusion. J Intensive Care Med. 2019:885066619887666.
53. Chaari A, Chelly H, Fourati H, Mnif Z, Chtara K, Baccouche N, Bahloul M, Bouaziz M. factors predicting lung contusions in critically ill trauma children: a multivariate analysis of 330 cases. Pediatr Emerg Care. 2018;34(3):198–201.
54. Goedeke J, Boehm R, Dietz HG. Multiply trauma in children: pulmonary contusion does not necessarily lead to a worsening of the treatment success. Eur J Pediatr Surg. 2014;24(6):508–13.
55. Tovar JA. The lung and pediatric trauma. Semin Pediatr Surg. 2008;17(1):53–9.
56. Pediatric blunt cardiac injury: epidemiology, clinical features, and diagnosis. Pediatric Emergency Medicine Collaborative Research Committee: Working Group on Blunt Cardiac Injury.
57. Hiremath G, Morgan G, Kenny D, Batlivala SP, Bartakian S. Balloon expandable covered stents as primary therapy for hemodynamically stable traumatic aortic injuries in children. Catheter Cardiovasc Interv. 2020;95(3):477–83.
58. Erben Y, Trejo G, Brownstein AJ, Jean RA, Ziganshin BA, Carino D, Elefteriades JA, Maung AA. Endovascular thoracic aortic transection repair has equivalent survival to open repair after blunt thoracic aortic injury. Int Angiol. 2018;37(2):155–9.
59. Gandhi SS, Blas JV, Lee S, Eidt JF, Carsten CG III. Nonoperative management of grade III blunt thoracic aortic injuries. J Vasc Surg. 2016;64(6):1580–6.
60. Malgor RD, Bilfinger TV, McCormack J, Tassiopoulos AK. Outcomes of blunt thoracic aortic injury in adolescents. Ann Vasc Surg. 2015;29(3):502–10.
61. Marzona F, Parri N, Nocerino A, Giacalone M, Valentini E, Masi S, Bussolin L. Traumatic diaphragmatic rupture in pediatric age: review of the literature. Eur J Trauma Emerg Surg. 2019;45(1):49–58.
62. Wada D, Hayakawa K, Maruyama S, Saito F, Kaneda H, Nakamori Y, Kuwagata Y. A paediatric case of severe tracheobronchial injury successfully treated surgically after early CT diagnosis and ECMO safely performed in the hybrid emergency room. Scand J Trauma Resusc Emerg Med. 2019;27(1):49.
63. Shemmeri E, Vallières E. Blunt tracheobronchial trauma. Thorac Surg Clin. 2018;28(3):429–34.
64. Hamilton EC, Lazar D, Tsao K, Cox C, Austin MT. Pediatric tracheobronchial injury after blunt trauma. J Trauma Acute Care Surg. 2017;83(3):554–6.
65. Pryor SD, Lee LK. Clinical outcomes and diagnostic imaging of pediatric patients with pneumomediastinum secondary to blunt trauma to the chest. J Trauma. 2011;71(4):904–8.
66. Gabor S, Renner H, Pinter H, Sankin O, Maier A, Tomaselli F, Smolle Jüttner FM. Indications for surgery in tracheobronchial ruptures. Eur J Cardiothorac Surg. 2001;20(2):399–404.
67. Xu AA, Breeze JL, Jackson CA, Paulus JK, Bugaev N. Comparative analysis of traumatic esophageal injury in pediatric and adult populations. Pediatr Surg Int. 2019;35(7):793–801.
68. Grant WJ, Meyers RL, Jaffe RL, Johnson DG. Tracheobronchial injuries after blunt chest trauma in children—hidden pathology. J Pediatr Surg. 1998;33(11):1707–11.

Surgical Consideration of Bacteria, Fungi, and Parasites

Massimo Sartelli

Introduction

Since the introduction of pharmaceutical treatment, the mortality of pulmonary infections caused by bacteria, fungi, and parasites has declined, yet they still constitute serious illnesses and in certain situations they may require a surgical intervention.

This chapter will be broken down into three categories: lung abscesses, which are often polymicrobial and are caused by bacteria, fungus, or parasites, invasive pulmonary aspergillosis (IPV), and hydatidosis.

Lung Abscess

Background

A lung abscess or intrapulmonary abscess is a parenchymal necrosis with confined cavitation that results from a pulmonary infection. Traditionally intrapulmonary abscesses been managed by antibiotics or placement of a drainage. In patients who do not respond to antibiotics and have septic shock related to their intrapulmonary abscess, surgery may be necessary.

A lung abscess develops when a bacterial infection causes necrosis and produces cavities in the lung parenchyma. A primary lung abscess occurs when one or two cavities with air-fluid levels form in the lung parenchyma as the result of an aspiration of pathogen-laden secretion. A secondary lung abscess develops from predisposing conditions, such as congenital lung abnormalities, obstructing neoplasm, a foreign body, and bronchiectasis. In necrotizing pneumonia, multiple small cavities (<2 cm in diameter) develop in contiguous areas of the lung.

M. Sartelli (✉)
Department of Surgery, Macerata Hospital, Macerata, Italy

In most lung abscesses polymicrobial bacteria can be found [1]. Isolates often include anaerobic bacteria (Gram-negative *Bacteroides fragilis*, *Fusobacterium capsulatum* and *necrophorum*, Gram-positive *Peptostreptococcus* and *Microearophilic streptococci*) and aerobic bacteria (*Staphylococcus aureus* [including methicillin-resistant *Staphylococcus aureus* (MRSA)], *Streptococcus pyogenes* and pneumoniae, *Klebsiella pneumoniae*, *Pseudomonas aeruginosa*, *Haemophilus influenzae* (type B), *Acinetobacter* spp., *Escherichia coli*, and *Legionella*) [1–4]. Mycobacterium tuberculosis must also be considered when evaluating potential lung abscesses.

Fungal and parasitic pathogens for lung abscess include *Cryptococcus, Histoplasma, Blastomyces, Coccidioides, Entamoeba histolytica, Paragonimus westermani, Actinomyces* and *Nocardia asteroides*.

Diagnosis

Early signs and symptoms of lung abscess cannot be differentiated from pneumonia and include fever with shivering, cough, night sweats, dyspnea, weight loss and fatigue, chest pain and sometimes anemia. At the beginning cough is nonproductive, but when communication with bronchus appears, the productive cough (vomique) is the typical sign [5, 6]. Cough remains productive, sometimes followed by hemoptysis. In patients with chronic abscess, clubbing fingers can appear. Chest radiological show air-fluid or hydatid cysts in lung [7, 8].

Diagnostic bronchoscopy is a part of diagnostic protocol for taking the material for microbiological examination and to confirm intrabronchial cause of abscess-tumor or foreign body. CT imaging of the chest can further characterize the abscess and provide important information regarding underlying lung pathology. Pulmonary cystic lesions, such as intrapulmonary located bronchial cysts, sequestration or secondary infected emphysematous bullae can be difficult to differentiate, but localization of lesion and clinical signs can indicate the appropriate diagnosis. Localized pleural empyema can be distinguished by using CT scan [9].

Excavating bronchial carcinomas such as squamocellular or microcellular carcinoma are usually presented with thicker and irregular wall comparing to infectious lung abscess [10]. Absence of febricity, purulent sputum, and leukocytosis can indicate the carcinoma and not the infective disease.

Evaluation of intrathoracic lymph nodes is difficult given it would require a biopsy to determine if they were enlarged secondary to carcinoma or infection.

Treatment

Antibiotic therapy remains the mainstay for the treatment of lung abscess. Initial management of lung abscess is based on empirical therapy with broad-spectrum antibiotics, after taking into account the possible risk of multidrug-resistant causative bacteria. It is followed by antibiotic streamlining driven by microbiological documentation as resulted from cultures. Typical are known etiologic pathogens of lung abscess often requiring a long duration (6 months) of antibiotic therapy [11].

Percutaneous drainage of lung abscesses has been established as treatment of choice for patients who have failed to respond to antibiotic therapy. The percutaneous procedure is usually selected for lung abscesses with diameters greater than 4–8 cm and is performed under fluoroscopic, ultrasound or computed tomography guidance. Computed tomography is generally preferred due to additional information provided about location, content, and wall thickness of the abscess. In addition, it has been proven useful in differentiation between empyema and abscess and in exclusion of endobronchial lesions. Either the trocar or the Seldinger technique are used for abscess drainage, with no difference found when evaluating their respective therapeutic effectiveness.

Patients needing surgery are usually in septic or in septic shock due to abscesses and are not responding to pharmaceutical treatment either alone or combined with transcutaneous drainage. These patients usually present with extensive necrosis of lung parenchyma (abscess size >6 cm), bronchial obstruction due to a mass or a foreign body, empyema, bronchopleural fistula, or infection due to multidrug-resistant microorganisms. In most cases, emergency resection of lung parenchyma is necessary in order to control sepsis [12, 13]. When a lung abscess is complicated by massive hemoptysis due to rupture of a large blood vessel, emergency surgical resection is indicated [14].

The extent of surgical resection depends on the size of the underlying lesion. Lobectomy is the most common type of surgical resection required. Segmentectomies are performed in smaller abscesses (<2 cm), whereas a pneumonectomy should be performed at the presence of multiple abscesses or gangrene. The usual surgical approach is thoracotomy.

Surgical intervention due to failure of conservative treatment is required in only 10% of patients, with a success rate of up to 90% and postoperative mortality rates ranging between 0 and 33% [15].

Pulmonary Tuberculosis

Background

Pulmonary tuberculosis (TB) is the history of thoracic surgery. TB is mainly a medical disease. Surgery has been the unique therapeutic tool for a long time before the advent of specific antituberculous drugs, and the role of surgery was then confined to the treatment of the sequelae of tuberculosis and their complications [16].

However, nowadays, we are witnessing a resurgence of the role of surgery in managing TB due to the overall increase in global incidence, and the emergence of multidrug-resistant TB or extensive drug-resistant TB [17]. Moreover, there is a trend for an increasing incidence of TB in the western world due to migration from developing countries. Thoracic surgery may offer highly effective treatment of TB and its sequel with less operative trauma and postoperative morbidity than ever before. The advent of video-assisted thoracic surgery allowed a new approach to TB and the selected cases requiring lung resection can be performed through a mini-invasive approach.

Diagnosis

In preoperative evaluation, in addition to routine laboratory work and acid-fast bacilli sputum smears and cultures, an accurate assessment of TB lesions' localization should be done. Fiber-optic bronchoscopy has to be used to evaluate endo-bronchial tuberculosis, contralateral disease, and coexisting eventual malignant disease. Pulmonary-function tests are used to ensure adequate pulmonary reserve.

Treatment

Currently, the surgical indications in pulmonary TB are [17] the following: TB complications (e.g., hemoptysis, empyema, cavity formation associated with aspergilloma, adenopathy with fistula); cases displaying an inappropriate healing response to medication, in which clinical and radiological pictures remain unchanged or indicate progression (e.g., cavity, tuberculoma); acid-fast bacilli sputum smears positivity after 3-month treatment period, with a circumscribed radiological lesion or a destroyed lung; and previous relapse(s) in patients with histories of TB and proper drug regimen [17].

Invasive Pulmonary Aspergillosis

Background

Aspergillus is a fungus is common in the air. Individuals who are immunocompromised have allergies, or lung injury is susceptible to *Aspergillus* infections. Aspergillosis refers to a spectrum of disease caused by *Aspergillus* species. In immunocompromised and critically ill patients, invasive pulmonary aspergillosis (IPA) is relatively common and may be fatal [18, 19]. In non-immunocompromised patients, chronic pulmonary aspergillosis (CPA) may occur in those who have suffered a pulmonary insult such as tuberculosis and sarcoidosis [18, 20]. The older term chronic necrotizing pulmonary aspergillosis mostly refers to those with subacute IPA. The increase incidence of this infection is related to growing numbers of patients with impaired immune state associated with the management of malignancy, organ transplantation, and autoimmune and inflammatory conditions.

Diagnosis

Symptoms of IPA are nonspecific and usually mimic bronchopneumonia: fever unresponsive to antibiotics, cough, sputum production, and dyspnea. Patients may also present with pleuritic chest pain (due to vascular invasion leading to thromboses that cause small pulmonary infarcts) and hemoptysis, which is usually mild, but can be severe. IPA is one of the most common causes of hemoptysis in neutropenic patients and may be associated with cavitation that occurs with neutrophil recovery [21].

Chest radiography is not useful in the early stages of disease because the incidence of nonspecific changes is high. Usual findings include rounded densities, pleural-based infiltrates suggestive of pulmonary infarctions, and cavitations. Pleural effusions are uncommon. Chest computed tomography (CT), especially when combined with high-resolution images (HRCT), is much more useful. The routine use of HRCT of the chest early in the course of IPA leads to earlier diagnosis and improved outcomes [22].

Bronchoscopy with bronchoalveolar lavage is generally helpful in the diagnosis of IPA, especially in patients with diffuse lung involvement. The significance of bronchoscopic isolation of *Aspergillus* spp. in sputum samples depends on the immune status of the host. In immunocompetent patients, it generally represents a colonization. On the contrary isolation of an *Aspergillus* species from sputum is highly predictive of invasive disease in immunocompromised patients.

Treatment

Voriconazole has been used as the initial treatment of invasive aspergillosis and is currently considered the treatment of choice in many patients with IPA. Echinocandin derivatives such as caspofungin, micafungin and anidulafungin are also effective agents in the treatment of IPA refractory to standard treatment, or if the patient cannot tolerate first-line agents.

The surgical management of both IPA and CPA has been debated because of potential high mortality and morbidity. Surgery has been reserved for patients with unilateral, localized disease where curative resection is possible, as well as in patients with infection abutting the main pulmonary vessels to avoid fatal hemoptysis.

An aspergilloma is a fungus ball composed of *Aspergillus* hyphae, fibrin, mucus, and cellular debris found within a pulmonary cavity. Aspergillomas arise in preexisting pulmonary cavities that have become colonized with *Aspergillus* spp. or develop in chronic cavitary pulmonary aspergillosis [23].

Although data regarding the treatment of a simple aspergilloma are limited to case reports, surgical treatment is the mainstay of management for patients with simple aspergilloma. Surgical results are good [24–26].

Antifungal therapy provides limited benefit for the treatment of a simple aspergilloma. Antifungal therapy for a single aspergilloma is reserved for patients who are unable to undergo surgery but require therapy for symptoms or radiologic progression or because they are immunocompromised. The choice of antifungal agent is similar to that for chronic cavitary pulmonary aspergillosis.

Recurrent infection, inability to take azole therapy, azole resistance, and concurrent infection or tumor represent additional indications for surgical resection but carry greater risk.

Pre- and postoperative antifungal therapy is appropriate to minimize the risk of postoperative pleural aspergillosis, in case the cavity is opened inadvertently during surgery, leading to spillage [27].

Hydatidosis

Background

Hydatid disease is caused by larvae of *Echinococcus* tapeworm species, the definite hosts of which are members of the *Canidae* family (dogs and foxes). Although most cysts form in the liver, 20–30% form in the lung [28].

Diagnosis

Primary infection is asymptomatic, and patients may remain asymptomatic for years, during which time lung lesions may be discovered incidentally on a chest X-ray [29].

Cysts may cause symptoms by compression of adjacent structures, and lung cysts may present with chest pain, cough, hemoptysis, or pneumothorax. Symptoms may also occur if antigenic material is released from the cyst, causing a hypersensitivity reaction with fever, wheeze, and urticaria and, rarely, anaphylaxis. Cysts may become secondarily infected causing empyema or lung abscess formation.

Cysts can be seen as single or multiple well-defined homogenous lesions surrounded by otherwise normal lung parenchyma on a plain chest X-ray. A CT scan of the chest may reveal further diagnostic features including collapse of the laminated membrane from the surrounding host tissue, the presence of daughter cysts, and the presence of cyst rupture.

Peripheral blood eosinophilia may be found in no more than 50% of cases. A substantial rise in eosinophil count is often associated with a leakage of antigenic material from the cyst. Serological tests to support the initial diagnosis are available at reference laboratories but are less sensitive for the diagnosis of lung disease than for hepatic disease [30].

Treatment

In a small number of cases, hydatid cysts can resolve spontaneously; however in the majority of cases, the treatment of choice is surgical excision of cysts to preserve as much lung parenchyma as possible [31].

Albendazole should be avoided preoperatively as it may soften the cyst wall and increase the chance of rupture. It may be given as adjunctive therapy once the cyst has been removed. When surgery is contraindicated or not feasible in patients with multiorgan involvement, medical treatment with albendazole with or without praziquantel is recommended.

Conclusion

The mainstay of treatment for pulmonary infections remains appropriate pharmaceutical treatment regardless of underlying pathology. In certain situations, surgical interventions may be required.

References

1. Kuhajda I, Zarogoulidis K, Tsirgogianni K, et al. Lung abscess-etiology, diagnostic and treatment options. Ann Transl Med. 2015;3(13):183. https://doi.org/10.3978/j.issn.2305-5839.2015.07.08.
2. Stock CT, Ho VP, Towe C, et al. Lung abscess. Surg Infect (Larchmt). 2013;14:335–611.
3. Bartlett JG. Anaerobic bacterial infection of the lung. Anaerobe. 2012;18:235–9.
4. Takayanagi N, Kagiyama N, Ishiguro T, et al. Etiology and outcome of community-acquired lung abscess. Respiration. 2010;80:98–105.
5. Yen CC, Tang RB, Chen SJ, et al. Pediatric lung abscess: a retrospective review of 23 cases. J Microbiol Immunol Infect. 2004;37:45–9. [PubMed] [Google Scholar].
6. Chan PC, Huang LM, Wu PS, et al. Clinical management and outcome of childhood lung abscess: a 16-year experience. J Microbiol Immunol Infect. 2005;38:183–8. [PubMed] [Google Scholar].
7. Toleti S, Subbarao M, Dwarabu P. Hydatid disease of the lung presenting with hemoptysis and simulating a lung abscess. Tropenmed Parasitol. 2012;2:69–70. [PMC free article] [PubMed] [Google Scholar].
8. Schiza S, Siafakas NM. Clinical presentation and management of empyema, lung abscess and pleural effusion. Curr Opin Pulm Med. 2006;12:205–11. [PubMed] [Google Scholar].
9. Lin FC, Chou CW, Chang SC. Differentiating pyopneumothorax and peripheral lung abscess: chest ultrasonography. Am J Med Sci. 2004;327:330–5. [PubMed] [Google Scholar].
10. Dursunoğlu N, Başer S, Evyapan F, et al. A squamous cell lung carcinoma with abscess-like distant metastasis. Tuberk Toraks. 2007;55:99–102. [PubMed] [Google Scholar].
11. Yildiz O, Doganay M. Actinomycoses and Nocardia pulmonary infections. Curr Opin Pulm Med. 2006;12:228–34.
12. Refaely Y, Weissberg D. Gangrene of the lung: treatment in two stages. Ann Thorac Surg. 1997;64:970–3; discussion 973–4.
13. Chen C-H, Huang W-C, Chen T-Y, Hung T-T, Liu H-C, Chen C-H. Massive necrotizing pneumonia with pulmonary gangrene. Ann Thorac Surg. 2009;87:310–1.

14. Philpott NJ, Woodhead MA, Wilson AG, Millard FJ. Lung abscess: a neglected cause of life threatening haemoptysis. Thorax. 1993;48:674–5.
15. Marra A, Hillejan L, Ukena D. Management of lung abscess. Zentralbl Chir. 2015;140(Suppl 1):S47–53.
16. Kilani T, Boudaya MS, Zribi H, Ouerghi S, Marghli A, Mestiri T, Mezni F. Surgery for thoracic tuberculosis. Rev Pneumol Clin. 2015;71(2–3):140–58.
17. Bertolaccini L, Viti A, Di Perri G, Terzi A. Surgical treatment of pulmonary tuberculosis: the phoenix of thoracic surgery? J Thorac Dis. 2013;5(2):198–9. https://doi.org/10.3978/j.issn.2072-1439.2012.03.18.
18. Farid S, Mohamed S, Devbhandari M, et al. Results of surgery for chronic pulmonary Aspergillosis, optimal antifungal therapy and proposed high risk factors for recurrence—a National Centre's experience. J Cardiothorac Surg. 2013;8:180.
19. Brown GD, Denning DW, Gow NAR, Levitz SM, Netea MG, White TC. Hidden killers: human fungal infections. Sci Transl Med. 2012;4(165):165rv13.
20. Smith NL, Denning DW. Underlying conditions in chronic pulmonary aspergillosis including simple aspergilloma. Eur Respir J. 2011;37:865–72.
21. Albelda SM, Talbot GH, Gerson SL, et al. Pulmonary cavitation and massive hemoptysis in invasive pulmonary aspergillosis. Influence of bone marrow recovery in patients with acute leukemia. Am Rev Respir Dis. 1985;131:115–20.
22. Caillot D, Casasnovas O, Bernard A, et al. Improved management of invasive pulmonary aspergillosis in neutropenic patients using early thoracic computed tomographic scan and surgery. J Clin Oncol. 1997;15:139–47.
23. Denning DW, Riniotis K, Dobrashian R, Sambatakou H. Chronic cavitary and fibrosing pulmonary and pleural aspergillosis: case series, proposed nomenclature change, and review. Clin Infect Dis. 2003;37(Suppl 3):S265–80.
24. Massard G, Roeslin N, Wihlm JM, Dumont P, Witz JP, Morand G. Pleuropulmonary aspergilloma: clinical spectrum and results of surgical treatment. Ann Thorac Surg. 1992;54:1159–64.
25. Passera E, Rizzi A, Robustellini M, Rossi G, Pona Della C, Massera F, et al. Pulmonary aspergilloma: clinical aspects and surgical treatment outcome. Thorac Surg Clin. 2012;22(3):345–61.
26. Akbari JG, Varma PK, Neema PK, Menon MU, Neelakandhan KS. Clinical profile and surgical outcome for pulmonary aspergilloma: a single center experience. Ann Thorac Surg. 2005;80:1067–72.
27. Patterson TF, Thompson GR 3rd, Denning DW, Fishman JA, Hadley S, Herbrecht R, Kontoyiannis DP, Marr KA, Morrison VA, Nguyen MH, Segal BH, Steinbach WJ, Stevens DA, Walsh TJ, Wingard JR, Young JA, Bennett JE. Practice guidelines for the diagnosis and management of Aspergillosis: 2016 update by the Infectious Diseases Society of America. Clin Infect Dis. 2016;63(4):e1–e60.
28. Kunst H, Mack D, Kon OM, Banerjee AK, Chiodini P, Grant A. Parasitic infections of the lung: a guide for the respiratory physician. Thorax. 2011;66(6):528–36.
29. Gottstein B, Reichen J. Hydatid lung disease (echinococcosis/hydatidosis). Clin Chest Med. 2002;23:397–408, ix.
30. Erdem CZ, Erdem LO. Radiological characteristics of pulmonary hydatid disease in children: less common radiological appearances. Eur J Radiol. 2003;45:123–8.
31. Keshmiri M, Baharvahdat H, Fattahi SH, et al. A placebo controlled study of albendazole in the treatment of pulmonary echinococcosis. Eur Respir J. 1999;14:503–7.

Travel and Transport

Allison Berndtson and Jay Doucet

Physiology and Limitations of Air and Ground Transport

Confined Spaces

Space aboard ambulances and aircraft is limited; in some vehicles, access to parts of the patient's body may be difficult. Performing procedures such a thoracostomy may be impeded by the patient being placed alongside a cabin wall or due to overhanging cabinets and equipment or due to presence of multiple patients, sometimes in "stacked" arrangements. Detection or replacement of malfunctioning or dislodged tubes, lines, and drains can also be difficult. It is critical that the patient is well "packaged"— tubes, lines, and devices are well secured, such as by tape and sutures and cannot be easily dislodged. Patients who may become candidates for procedures such as endotracheal intubation or thoracostomy tube placement due to known or suspected conditions are safest if such procedures are performed under controlled conditions at the referring facility. Procedures done urgently in the cabin of an aircraft or ambulance during patient deterioration are more likely to fail. A handoff discussion between the referring facility and the transport team should include a discussion of contingencies that may occur *en route* and reconsideration made for any procedures that may be reasonably done before departure to ensure a safe trip for the patient.

A. Berndtson · J. Doucet (✉)
Division of Trauma, Surgical Critical Care, Burns and Acute Care Surgery, Department of Surgery, University of California San Diego, San Diego, CA, USA
e-mail: aberndtson@ucsd.edu; jdoucet@ucsd.edu

Lighting

Vehicles often use low intensity cabin lighting that may not be sufficiently intense or focused for patient assessment. Bright general cabin illumination may not be permitted to protect the night vision of pilots or drivers. Tactical environments may require the use of subdued or colored lighting such as red light, which makes assessment of the skin for pallor or cyanosis impossible. Blood may appear black rather than red on surfaces in such conditions and bleeding can be missed. Some military critical care helicopter transport teams may need to work under night vision goggle conditions with very low light conditions. Daytime may result in glare in cabins with windows without moveable shades. Vehicles and teams must be trained and equipped to work under a variety of lighting conditions.

Noise, Vibration, Turbulence, G-Loading

Vehicles in motion will generate noise and vibration. This may make some clinical assessments such as chest auscultation or percussion difficult or impossible. In some vehicles, detection of spontaneous respiration or even a palpable pulse may be difficult. In patients who are given paralytics or deep sedation, the only detectable patient signs of life on board the vehicle may be pupillary response and the vital signs detected by the monitors. Aircraft may experience turbulence and G-loads which can be uncomfortable for patients and providers. Motion sickness can occur in any vehicle; this risk is worsened when there are no nearby windows to provide an external visual horizon reference as is common in many medical evacuation vehicles.

Temperature

The outdoor environment frequently intrudes into the cabin of the vehicle—this may occur during prolonged loading or unloading of multiple patients on transport aircraft or by a tactical need to keep doors or windows open for defensive purposes. The patient must have adequate insulated coverings to maintain body warmth. Many critically ill or injured patients cannot maintain body temperature due to poor perfusion, vasodilation, burns, or heat losses from ventilators or insensible losses. Provision for equipment to maintain a stable thermal environment is required. Medications, intravenous fluids, and blood products also need thermostabilized storage.

Gas Laws

Aeromedical evacuation aircraft must fly at a sufficient altitude to avoid terrain, ensure communication with air traffic control, follow assigned airways and routes, and have enough fuel economy and speed to make the trip in a timely fashion.

Helicopters and piston aircraft are typically unpressurized, and the cabin altitude is the aircraft altitude. Most turboprop and jet aircraft have pressurized cabins; these aircraft usually do not allow the cabin altitude to exceed 8000 ft (2500 m) at cruising altitudes. The cabin pressure typically is not below 564 mmHg (75 kPa) or about 0.75 atmospheres [1]. This cabin pressure is well tolerated by most healthy persons, who will typically have a drop in peripheral oxygen saturation (SaO_2) of about 4% [2]. Cardiopulmonary patients requiring ventilation with a FiO_2 of 70% or greater may require ventilation with increased PEEP and FiO_2 [3]. Ventilated patients with ARDS with PaO_2/FiO_2 ratio of 100 or less may require advanced ARDS management techniques such as proning, inhaled nitric oxide or prostacyclin, or initiation of extracorporeal life support (ECLS) [4–6]. Decreased cabin pressure also means that trapped gasses in the body can expand, up to about 25% greater volume at a cabin pressure of 8000 ft as compared to sea level. This may increase the size or pressure of a pneumothorax, pneumomediastinum, or pneumopericardium. Generally, a known pneumothorax is managed by tube thoracostomy before flight. A symptomatic pneumothorax detected after ascent may be treated successfully with needle thoracostomy, although there is a significant failure rate. Finger or simple thoracostomy may be more reliable and is endorsed by the Advanced Trauma Life Support Course (ATLS) tenth edition. Tube thoracostomy may be required during transport of a cardiopulmonary patient and this is a required crew skill for critical care transport [7–9].

Available Monitoring and Equipment

The vehicle must be equipped to allow monitoring of patient vital signs during transport and provision of care up to critical care if needed. Monitors and associated equipment must be compatible with the power systems available on the vehicle and be resistant to shock, vibration, and impacts and provide displays and controls that can be used in a wide variety of lighting and temperatures. This equipment must not interfere with vehicle systems, such as aircraft controls, communications and navigation systems. In many jurisdictions, a regulatory authority must certify equipment for ground vehicle or aeromedical use. In the USA, some states, counties, or trauma systems have required equipment lists for ambulances. Aircraft including aeromedical helicopters are exempt from state, county, or city regulations under the Airline Deregulation Act [10]. Voluntary industry standards exist from the Commission on Accreditation of Medical Transport Systems (CAMTS), which has equipment lists for vehicles including aircraft at the Basic Life Support (BLS), Advanced Life Support (ALS), Emergency Critical Care and Intensive Critical Care levels, as well as specialty vehicles such as for Neonatal Intensive Critical Care (NICU) [11]. For example, CAMTS standards specify equipment for the Intensive Critical Care level vehicle should include cardiac monitoring (e.g., pacemaker/defibrillator), noninvasive monitoring (e.g., waveform capnography, pulse oximetry), multimodality ventilators capable of invasive ventilation (pressure, volume, ventilator appropriate to all age groups transported), and invasive hemodynamic monitoring (e.g., transvenous pacemakers, central venous pressure, arterial pressure) as well as an experienced aeromedical crew able to manage multiple infusions, perform transfusions, and perform procedures such as tube thoracostomy.

Imaging

The advent of handheld, portable ultrasound units now means that imaging is available during transport of the cardiopulmonary patient. Ultrasound can be diagnostic and can elucidate shock states, fluid responsiveness, hypovolemia, cardiac arrest, and cardiac failure including cor pulmonale and detect hemoperitoneum and pneumothorax [12–14]. It can also aid procedures such as central line insertion, simple, finger, Seldinger, or open tube thoracostomy and confirms correct placement of an endotracheal tube [15–17]. Aeromedical services in some locales have adopted ultrasound [18, 19].

Choice of Appropriate Transport Mode

Ground EMS

There are about 35,000 ground emergency medical services (EMS) ambulances in the USA, and more than half of these are BLS level ambulances. In many cases, the ALS ambulance may be faster than a helicopter as the ambulance is often closer to the scene or transferring facility and does not need to move long distances to pick up the patient. In most of the USA, the ALS EMS ground ambulance contains the first medical responders to arrive at the scene of a trauma patient, and the majority of thoracic trauma patients are transported by ground to their first medical facility. The ALS ambulance is typically staffed by two emergency medical technicians (EMTs) at least one of which is a paramedic. Dispatch of a helicopter direct to the scene either requires dispatch based on the assessment of a paramedic at the scene or automatic dispatch based on reports of law enforcement, witnesses, or remote sensing.

HEMS

EMS helicopters (HEMS) (Fig. 1) offer higher speeds than ground transport; in addition they are usually staffed with flight nurses and flight paramedics with a broader skill set than many paramedics. HEMS helicopters are usually capable of Emergency Critical Care or higher-level care. Altitudes encountered are usually less than 8000 ft, except in mountainous areas. Depending on helicopter prepositioning and utilization, HEMS is often not significantly faster than ground EMS. While HEMS may have advantages when traffic is heavy or ground routes are slow or impassible, most HEMS cannot be used when weather conditions are poor, such as

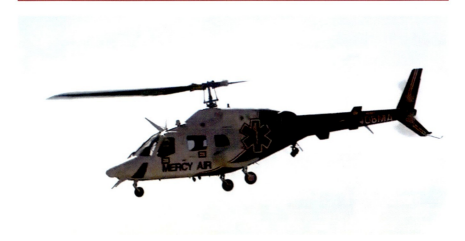

Fig. 1 This Bell 222B helicopter has a range of 434 miles (700 km) and cruises at 155 mph (250 kmh). It is unpressurized and typically carries a single patient, a flight nurse, and/or paramedic and a single pilot. (Photo Credit: Pat Choothesa 2012, with permission)

poor visibility, low cloud ceilings, high winds, or freezing precipitation. In some rural areas, insufficient ground EMS ambulances mandate the use of HEMS helicopters to avoid depleting local ambulance coverage.

HEMS operations had an accident rate in 2002 of 5 accidents per 100,000 flight hours; in 2017 it was 2.5 per 100,000 h, which still is significantly higher than the airline aviation accident rate of 0.16 per 100,000 h [20]. Inappropriate use of HEMS should be avoided to minimize excess risk to patients and crews. Retrospective analysis and meta-analysis of the benefits of HEMS over ground EMS are unclear, but are probably confined to those patients who are injured enough to benefit from the critical care on board and not due to any time saving by HEMS [21, 22]. The validated Air Medical Prehospital Triage (AMPT) score has shown that the prehospital trauma patients most likely to benefit from HEMS are those with Glasgow Coma Scale <14, a respiratory rate <10 or >29 breaths/min, unstable chest wall fractures, suspected hemothorax or pneumothorax, paralysis, multisystem trauma, or any one physiologic criterion plus any one anatomic criterion present from American College of Surgeons Committee on Trauma national field triage guidelines (Table 1) [23, 24]. The AMPT score may also be instructive for selection of patients for interfacility transport by HEMS.

Fixed Wing

Fixed wing aircraft require runways. Fixed wing aircraft may be a dedicated aeromedical vehicle at the BLS to ICU level or may only be a business aircraft with seats folded down to accommodate a stretcher with portable medical equipment and crew brought aboard for a single trip (Fig. 2). They may be capable of instrument flight

Table 1 Air Medical Prehospital Triage (AMPT) score

Criterion	Points
Glasgow coma scale <14	1
Respiratory rate <10 or >29 breaths/min	1
Unstable chest wall fractures[a]	1
Suspected hemothorax or pneumothorax[b]	1
Paralysis	1
Multisystem trauma[c]	1
PHY + ANA[d]	2

Consider helicopter transport if AMPT score ≥2 points

Brown JB, Gestring ML, Guyette FX, Rosengart MR, Stassen NA, Forsythe RM, et al. External validation of the Air Medical Prehospital Triage score for identifying trauma patients likely to benefit from scene helicopter transport. J Trauma Acute Care Surg. 2017;82(2):270–9

[a]Any chest wall instability or deformity including flail chest or multiple ribs fractures on physical exam
[b]Absence of breath sounds on affected hemithorax PLUS objective signs of respiratory distress (cyanosis, SpO_2 <92%, signs of tension physiology)
[c]3 or more anatomic body regions injured
[d]Any 1 physiologic criterion plus any 1 anatomic criterion present from American College of Surgeons Committee on Trauma national field triage guidelines

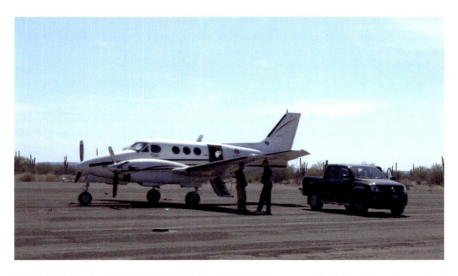

Fig. 2 This Beechcraft King Air C-90 turboprop fixed wing pressurized aircraft awaits a patient near Mulegé, Mexico. This type of aircraft has range up to 1000 miles (1609 km) and cruises at 245 mph (394 kph). (Photo Credit: Jay Doucet, 2012)

rules trips in poor visibility or low ceilings if the aircraft, crew, and operation is so certified. Depending on runway locations, they may be nearly equivalent in speed to HEMS, but require an ambulance transport on each end, with the additional discomfort and risk of moving the patient between vehicles. Piston fixed wing aircraft typically are unpressurized but rarely exceed 8000 ft except in mountainous areas. These aircraft may be more spacious than HEMS. Turboprop and jet aircraft

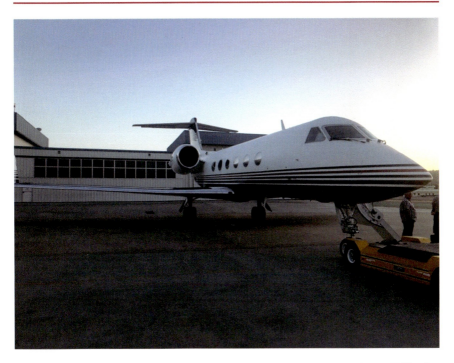

Fig. 3 This Gulfstream IV air ambulance is a pressurized jet with a range of over 4800 miles (8000 km) and cruises at 552 mph (888 kph). It can perform transoceanic air evacuations. (Photo Credit; Jay Doucet, 2019)

typically have pressurized cabins that do not exceed 8000 ft despite cruising at higher altitudes (Fig. 3). These aircraft are the most comfortable with less noise and turbulence and have the most space on board. Some jet aeromedical aircraft are capable of transoceanic flights.

Critical Care Air Transport Team

There are examples of military critical care air transport teams (CCATS) (Figs. 4 and 5) that provide critical care during flight including long distance flights, multiple patients, and advanced organ failure support including Extracorporeal Life Support (ECLS). These teams are usually composed of flight nurses, but may be accompanied by technicians and a flight surgeon or anesthesiologist. Typically they are embarked on a military transport aircraft. Normally the patient is stabilized at the referring facility before transport, but in some case, patients still undergoing resuscitation after damage control surgery, including those with an open chest or abdomen, can be transported. Specialized Medical Emergency Response Teams (MERTs) are anesthesiologist or intensivist-led teams aboard medium military helicopters that travel in conflict areas to the wounded patient

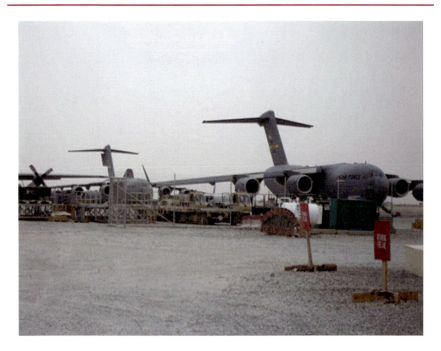

Fig. 4 US Air Force C-17 Globemaster III Transport aircraft stand by on the flight line at Kandahar Airfield, Afghanistan, to take Critical Care Air Transport Teams (CCAT) and their patients to Landstuhl, Germany. The C-17 has a range of 6456 mi (10,390 km) and cruises at 516 mph (830 kph). It can carry up to 36 litter and 54 ambulatory patients. (Photo Credit: Jay Doucet, 2006)

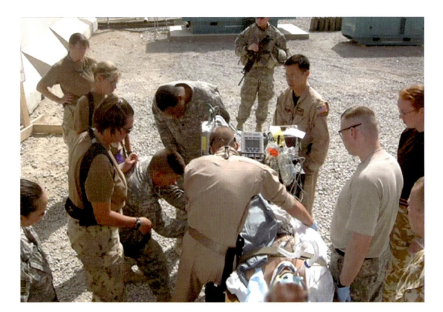

Fig. 5 US Air Force Critical Care Air Transport Team (CCAT) and 1st Canadian Field Hospital personnel make final preparations at Kandahar Airfield, Afghanistan, to place a ventilated patient aboard a military transport aircraft to Landstuhl, Germany. (Photo Credit: Jay Doucet, 2006)

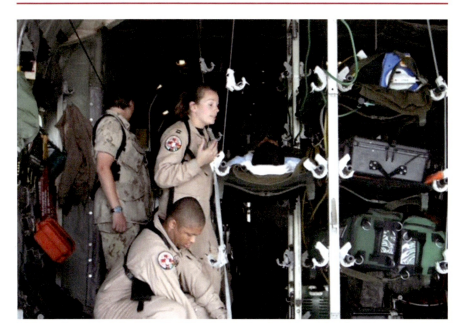

Fig. 6 US Air Force Critical Care Air Transport Team (CCAT) aboard a C-130 Hercules transport aircraft—an example of the "stacked" patient arrangement used on some military aircraft. (Photo Credit: Jay Doucet, 2006)

and perform initial resuscitation and stabilization *en route* to a field hospital. The experience of the CCAT and MERT teams provide examples on how initial stabilization and damage control surgery could be performed prior to the cardiopulmonary patient arrival at the major medical center, given appropriate transport resources (Fig. 6). There are a handful of civilian HEMS services that provide ECLS on board.

Commercial Airliner

Flying aboard a commercial passenger aircraft during scheduled airline service is not advisable for patients recovering from thoracic surgery or trauma until the risk of complications of transport has passed. Physiologic deterioration at altitude for such patients has considerable risks including lack of available skilled medical care, lack of sufficient medical equipment and medications, and the risk and expense to the other passengers and crew of diversion to an unplanned airport. Older recommendations for safe air travel following traumatic pneumothorax were to wait 2 to 3 weeks after radiographic resolution and were based on small experiences [25, 26]. Zonies et al. reported on 73 combat-injured patients who had a thoracostomy tube in place which had been removed a median of 2.5 days before subsequent flight without a pneumothorax recurrence. Those authors suggested that after a 72-h period of observation, air travel after tube thoracostomy removal appears to be safe for both mechanically ventilated and nonventilated patients [27]. Of course, to fly on a commercial aircraft, the patient will have to be ambulatory or be reasonably able to travel via wheelchair, which may be problematical in that a significant percentage of thoracic trauma patients have associated orthopedic trauma or other injuries [28].

Complications During Transport

Pneumothorax

A pneumothorax can be defined as free air within the pleural space. Traumatic pneumothoraces are due to injuries to the lung, trachea, or chest wall. Pneumothorax can also occur after chest surgery. Penetrating trauma can create a pneumothorax by exposing the relatively negative pressure of the pleural space to the atmospheric pressure, allowing air to enter—i.e., an open pneumothorax. Penetrating injury to the lung parenchyma or airways can also cause escape of air into the pleural space. Blunt trauma can cause rib fractures which then can lacerate lung parenchyma or airways, it can also cause focal rupture of the lung parenchyma or cause parenchymal tears of the lung. Postoperative causes include leakage from a resection margin of the lung or from a bronchial stump, repair, or anastomosis. The escaped free air within the plural space can create a simple pneumothorax, which means it does not have hemodynamic affects but can affect expansion of the lung within that hemithorax. Tension pneumothorax develops when the trapped air is under pressure, usually as a result of a one-way valve action of the injury to the bronchus, lung, or chest wall, which does not allow the escape of the trapped air. This increasing pressure of the trapped air will eventually cause collapse of the ipsilateral lung and increasing shift of the mediastinal structures. The increasing intrathoracic pressure can preclude spontaneous ventilation and halt venous blood return to the right heart; eventually progressing to complete cardiovascular collapse, arrest, and death. A simple pneumothorax can be converted into a tension pneumothorax by the initiation of positive pressure ventilation. Therefore, instability in a newly intubated patient may be due to tension pneumothorax. A previously asymptomatic pneumothorax may become symptomatic with increasing cabin altitude with increase in the simple pneumothorax size or by development of a tension pneumothorax. A high index of suspicion for worsening or tension pneumothorax should be maintained.

Hemothorax

The collection of blood within one or both hemithoraces may lead to respiratory failure as well as hemodynamic instability, shock, and circulatory collapse. The blood may emanate from postoperative bleeding or from trauma to chest wall structures, intercostal vessels, and mediastinal structures or from lung, heart, or great vessel injuries. Hemothorax if undetected can lead to rapid deterioration, circulatory collapse, and death. Each hemithorax and its pleural space is potentially large enough to contain enough blood to allow for lethal exsanguination. Unlike other body cavities, the thoracic cavity is large and compliant, and therefore significant bleeding can occur without any localized tamponade effect from adjacent structures. During transport, typical imaging such as chest X-ray is not available. Hemothorax must be picked up by careful clinical evaluation, a high level of suspicion and possibly by use of ultrasound. Massive hemothorax is usually defined as having more than 1500 mL of hemothorax in a typical sized adult. This amount of hemothorax will produce symptoms of hemodynamic shock and is an indication for emergency thoracotomy for evacuation and hemostasis. Ongoing blood loss of more than 500 mL per hour from a chest tube for more than 2 h is also an indication for emergency thoracotomy.

Chest Tube Management

Pneumothorax and hemothorax are typically managed by placement of a chest tube prior to transport. Unstable patients with suspected hemothorax or pneumothorax should not normally be transported until a chest tube is placed and the patient stabilized. During transport, the amount of chest tube output must be carefully monitored. Autotransfusion by reinfusing blood lost via chest tubes back into the patient intravenously can be accomplished if an autotransfusion chest drainage set or inline autotransfusion blood bags are available. During conflicts and mass disasters, patients who are hemodynamically stable with chest bleeding may sometimes be transported with a CCAT team equipped with transfusion and autotransfusion capabilities.

A complication that it can occur during transport is chest tube obstruction, typically with clotted blood. Signs of increasing hemodynamic instability with low chest tube output should raise suspicion for this problem. In such cases it is usually necessary to try to clear the clot from the tube by such techniques as "stripping" the tube, using a suction catheter within the tube, or by placing a new chest tube. Chest tubes should also be well secured and monitored to avoid accidental dislodgement.

Pneumomediastinum

Air leakage from the trachea, bronchi, esophagus, and major airways may track into the mediastinum rather than the pleura, resulting in pneumomediastinum or pneumopericardium. Subcutaneous emphysema is often detected at the neck and upper chest in significant cases. This may produce the sensation of "rice crispies" felt to be crunching below the skin when palpated. In severe cases subcutaneous air may track up into the face and cause distention of the face, including eyelid swelling and closure. This may have an alarming appearance but only rarely will lead to airway obstruction. In trauma patients pneumomediastinum should lead to investigations for presence of an airway injury or an esophageal leak. Small amounts of pneumomediastinum such as that detected only on CT scan are not a contraindication to aeromedical evacuation. Patients with large amounts of subcutaneous emphysema may be better transported by ground. Patients with large amounts of subcutaneous emphysema also have increased risk of pneumothorax and may need a chest tube during transport. Pneumopericardium may be asymptomatic on the ground but with expansion at altitude may produce tamponade physiology. If these patients must transported by air, a pericardial drain or xiphisternal pericardial window should be performed prior to aeromedical evacuation.

Tracheobronchial Bleeding

Significant bleeding into the airway can be life threatening and is associated with a high mortality rate. This may result from direct airway injury, penetrating or blunt lung injury. It can also be a complication of lung inflammation, infection, burns, pulmonary hypertension, malignancy, radiation, or presence of a pulmonary arterial catheter. It can also be a postoperative complication of tracheostomy and thoracic surgery. Immediate management requires intubation and administration of oxygen. If the bleeding side can be determined, this side is placed down as the patient is rolled into a decubitus position. If the bleeding is from the left lung, advancing the endotracheal tube into a right mainstem position may reduce entry of blood into the airway and allow single-lung ventilation. If a bronchoscope is available, a bronchial blocker balloon may be used to occlude the side with the bleeding bronchus. If the patient is coagulopathic, this should be corrected. Angiography or surgery is often required to control the bleeding vessels by embolization or ligation, respectively. Transport of the patient with tracheobronchial bleeding should be considered only after the correction of coagulopathy and establishment of single-lung ventilation as these can be very difficult to accomplish once on board a vehicle as bronchoscopy tools and blood banking are typically not available.

Cardiac Tamponade

Development of cardiac tamponade is usually the result of penetrating cardiac injury, although it can occur in rare cases of blunt chest trauma and occasionally as a result of post-pericardiotomy syndrome. The traditional diagnostic triad of medical cardiac effusions—"Beck's triad"—muffled heart sounds, hypotension, and distended neck veins, possibly with pulsus paradoxus is not useful in trauma and postsurgical patients aboard a vehicle. The best diagnostic tool is echocardiography, either transthoracic or transesophageal. Penetrating torso trauma requires a screening echocardiogram to rule of cardiac effusion or tamponade. When surgical capability to perform exploration and repair of the source of the pericardial bleeding is unavailable, the only temporizing measures are placement of a pericardial drain and/or administration of intravenous fluids to improve right heart preload with administration of pressors. Few ground EMS or HEMS crews have pericardiocentesis within their scope of practice, although there are a few case reports [29]. In patients undergoing interfacility transport with potentially symptomatic cardiac effusion, placement of a pericardial drain should be considered as it will be unlikely to be done *en route* if needed.

Loss of Airway

Patients with significant chest and torso trauma, large burns, traumatic brain injury, and potential postsurgical complications may suffer loss of airway events during transport. The loss of the airway may be due to dislodgement of an airway placed on the ground at the scene or at the referring facility. It may also be due to progressive swelling or airway obstruction leading to the need to immediately obtain an airway during transport. It may also result in worsening oxygenation and ventilation from clinical deterioration or due to complications of injuries or surgery. It is important that definitive airways placed prior to transport are very well secured and that patients are appropriately restrained or sedated as needed, to prevent dislodgment. Patient transported with a definitive airway should be accompanied by personnel who are capable of replacing the airway if dislodged. Successful surgical airways such as cricothyroidotomy performed on helicopters or ambulances are extremely rare, occurring in fewer than 0.57% of HEMS transports in a large trauma system [30].

Management of Specific Injuries During Transport

Flail Chest and Pulmonary Contusion

Flail chest is often defined as two or more adjacent ribs fractured in two or more places, such that a segment of the chest wall can move paradoxically than the rest of the chest wall during spontaneous respiration—as the patient inspires, the normal chest wall expands, but the flail segment retracts. Flail chest is usually the result of blunt trauma, but can occur in multiple or large penetrations or in blast injury. Flail chest is painful, which limits the patient's ability to fully inspire, and large flail segments may impair the effectiveness of spontaneous ventilation. Unless the patient has very brittle bone, flail chest is usually accompanied by pulmonary contusion underlying it. The lung parenchyma suffers alveolar hemorrhage and capillary rupture, leading to impaired ventilation, perfusion, and gas exchange. Flail chest may also be accompanied by atelectasis, pneumothorax, hemothorax, and pleural effusion. Significant pulmonary contusions can progress to acute respiratory distress syndrome (ARDS) and lung necrosis. Deterioration in pulmonary status can occur in the first 48 to 96 h and often requires intubation and mechanical ventilation. Optimal care requires attention to effective pain control, pulmonary toilet, incentive spirometry, bronchodilators, management of pneumothoraces, and possible chest tube placement. Transport of flail chest patients in the first 2–3 days after injury requires careful consideration of possible deterioration and contingencies *en route*; endotracheal intubation and placement of chest tubes before interfacility travel must be considered.

Tracheobronchial Injuries

Disruption of the intrathoracic airways—trachea and bronchi—is usually the result of penetrating trauma, but can occur after severe blunt trauma or blast injury. These injuries have a high prehospital mortality and even in tertiary referral centers may have a mortality of 13–30% [31, 32]. The patient may have simultaneous airway obstruction, tracheobronchial hemorrhage, large or tension pneumothorax, pneumomediastinum, hemothorax, pulmonary contusion, and flail chest. Surgery is usually required and specialized ventilation techniques may be necessary, such as dual lumen—dual- ventilator ventilation. Air leaks are common after surgical repair. Such patients are not good candidates for transport unless a critical care transport team is available. ECLS may be an option to provide oxygenation during transport and surgery [33].

Esophageal Injuries

Perforation of the esophagus may be the result of penetrating trauma, blunt trauma, caustic ingestion, and accidents during instrumentation or effort rupture of the esophagus (Boerhaave syndrome). Leakage of esophageal contents into the mediastinum and pleural spaces risks mediastinitis and sepsis. Prior to transport the patient usually has a nasogastric tube placed. Chest tubes may also be placed to drain the mediastinum. Broad-spectrum antibiotics are started and continued *en route*. Due to the risk of aspiration due to dysphagia and difficulty swallowing secretions, and possible clinical deterioration due to sepsis, precautionary intubation prior to transport may be warranted. Patients may require significant fluid resuscitation if septic shock develops.

Damage Control, the Open Chest

An extension of the damage control laparotomy to avoid abdominal compartment syndrome and shorten operative time is the temporary abdominal closure. Temporary chest closure has also been used in cases of damage control thoracotomy, mostly to avoid excess peak or plateau airway pressures or to accommodate intrathoracic packing [34–36]. Transport of such patients in the prehospital trauma environment has occurred after physician performed roadside thoracotomies with survival and low rates of infection [37]. Interfacility transport would require a critical care team, ventilation, and possibly critical care adjuncts such as vasopressors and transfusions.

Special Considerations During Transport

Pain Control

Effective pain control is required for cardiopulmonary patients during transport. Typically this has been accomplished by intermittent doses of opioids such as intravenous morphine or fentanyl. The fentanyl "lollypop" or stick lozenge has been used in field care and en route phase of combat casualties by the US Army. Non-opioid multimodal pain control is more commonly used which may include acetaminophen or non-steroidal anti-inflammatory drugs (NSAIDs) such as ketorolac, if there is no history of gastrointestinal ulcers, renal insufficiency, or coagulopathy. Regional techniques such as thoracic epidurals may provide good pain control, but must be monitored by the crew. Low-dose ketamine is increasingly being used in prehospital and inpatient care and can be added to a multimodal pain regimen [38].

Respiratory Therapy

Non-intubated patients after thoracic trauma or surgery are quickly started on a regimen of pain control, incentive spirometry, bronchodilators, secretion management, and chest physiotherapy. That regimen should be maintained during transport to avoid deterioration which can result from increased atelectasis, hypercarbia, and hypoxia and need for invasive pulmonary support including intubation.

Fluid Management

Cardiopulmonary trauma and emergency operations are frequently associated with hemorrhagic shock, massive transfusion, large intravascular and intracellular fluid shifts, and significant tissue edema. Excess crystalloid administration has been associated with tissue edema, pulmonary edema, increased ventilator and ICU days, and abdominal compartment syndrome. In the past, the pulmonary artery catheter was thought to aid management of fluid resuscitation of trauma patients, but this has nearly been abandoned due to lack of evidence of efficacy and increased complications, although it is sometimes used in cardiac injuries. The central venous catheter has not fared any better as a predictor of fluid responsiveness. The transport crew has no easy way to determine volume status or cardiac performance. Noninvasive and minimally invasive measures such as stroke volume variation (SVV) are commonly used in ICUs but are less suited in HEMS and ground ambulances which often produce too much motion artifact for good use. This leaves crews with no options other than to continue prior intravenous fluid orders or to attempt to increase or decrease intravenous fluid rates based on changing vital signs, though as ultrasound becomes more widely adopted in the prehospital setting it may have utility in assessing volume status.

ECMO/ECLS

Extracorporeal Life Support (ECLS), often called Extracorporeal Membrane Oxygenation (ECMO) (Fig. 7), is technology that uses a pump and oxygenator to increase blood oxygenation. Venovenous (VV) ECMO provides lung support only, so the patient's cardiac function must be intact. Two cannulas are placed into femoral and/or jugular veins or a dual-lumen venous catheter can be used. Venoarterial (VA) ECMO provides both oxygenation and cardiac support by bypassing a significant amount of blood from the patient's heart. This requires a venous and arterial catheter, typically femoral arterial and jugular venous catheters. Recently, more compact membrane oxygenators have made the ECMO machines less bulky and better suited for transport; these can be carried by one person. Worldwide, the number of ECMO centers has more than tripled from 2004 (120) to 2018 (381). ECMO centers often provide mobile teams that travel by ground or air to referring facilities, perform the cannulations, start ECMO, and transport the patient to the ECMO center. Most centers have adopted guidelines to identify suitable patients and prevent use of ECMO in patients with little chance of survival [39]. Since 1979, four randomized trials have studied the effectiveness of ECMO in ARDS and respiratory failure. The first three trials had

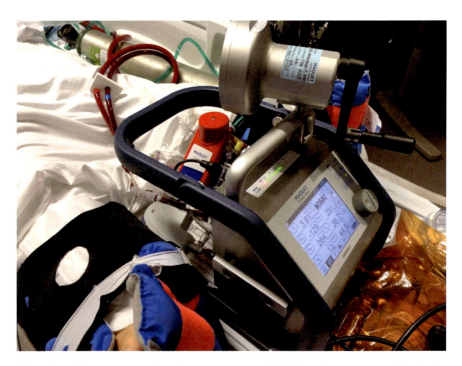

Fig. 7 Portable extracorporeal membrane oxygenator (ECMO) and pump system. This device weighs 10 kg and can be carried by one person onto an ambulance or helicopter. (Photo Credit—Jay Doucet, 2018)

significant selection and methodological issues. The EOLIA trial (ECMO to Rescue Lung Injury in Severe ARDS) was a multicenter randomized controlled trial published in 2018. The authors of the EOLIA trial concluded that in very severe ARDS, 60day mortality was not significantly lower with ECMO than with a strategy of conventional mechanical ventilation that included ECMO as rescue therapy. However, if the crossover rate is taken into account, and considering that the survival rate of the crossed-over patients without ECMO would have been between 0 and 33%, there was a significant increase in relative risk reduction with ECMO (from 0.74 to 0.62, $p < 0.001$ and $p = 0.045$, respectively) compared to the relative risk reduction of 0.76 ($p = 0.09$) described with the conventional intention-to-treat analysis [40]. It can be anticipated that the increasing use of ECMO for ARDS patients and their transport, will also increase its availability for transport of patients after thoracic trauma and emergency surgery and allow its further study.

Interfacility Transport

The ATLS course emphasizes the importance of proper interfacility transfers of trauma patients [9]. Transfer to definitive care should be considered whenever the patient's needs exceed the resources of the referring center. The course indicates that the referring doctor is responsible for:

- Diagnosing and treating immediate threats to life using the ATLS ABCs.
- Initiating transfer of the patient while resuscitative efforts are in progress.
- Selecting the mode of transportation and the level of care for the patient's treatment *en route*.
- Consulting with the receiving doctor and becoming familiar with the transporting agencies, their capabilities, and the arrangements for patient treatment during transport.
- Stabilizing the patient's condition before transfer to another facility and ensuring they are well "packaged"—(tubes, lines, devices are well secured and not easily dislodged).

Transfer should not be delayed for diagnostic tests that will not change management; however appropriate stabilization of the patient as above should be completed prior to transport. Physician-to-physician communication is a key component of interfacility transport and should occur before or while transportation is arranged; this ensures that the receiving physician is qualified and willing to accept the patient and allows them to assist the referring doctor in anticipating and preparing against potential transport pitfalls. Records and images from the referring facility should be sent with the patient whenever possible, to avoid unnecessary confusion or duplication of care at the receiving facility. Appropriate, timely, and prepared transport of patients with thoracic trauma provides physicians and transport crews with the best chance at excellent patient outcomes.

Safety of Transport

Safety during transport is always the first priority, and a decision to request HEMS, fixed wing, or ground transport should not require the acceptance of any unnecessary risks to the crew or patient. For example, there should never be second-guessing by referring providers after a HEMS crew refuses to fly due to operational limitations or safety issues should. So-called helicopter shopping is a fatally dangerous practice—contacting multiple HEMS operators to fly in weather conditions in which another HEMS operator has already refused to fly, especially without disclosing the first refusal to other operators [41]. Fatal accidents have occurred after such requests.

A "culture of safety" should exist within the trauma system for ground EMS, aeromedical services, hospitals, and trauma centers, including participation in safety management systems as appropriate [42]. Hospitals and trauma centers must ensure that their heliports are properly registered with FAA, state, and aviation databases. They must also ensure that safety and communications procedures, including radio, have been established and aligned with HEMS operators, including contingencies for multiple inbound helicopters. Referring and receiving facilities should have a coordinated air medical safety program with HEMS, which includes identification of safe landing sites, ingress and egress routes, proper loading and unloading procedures, and standardized communications with pilots and dispatchers. There should be safety procedures in proximity to an operating helicopter, including policies for "hot" (rotors turning) loading and unloading. The culture of safety must include referring and receiving physicians of thoracic trauma and surgery patients, so they will not cause the system and crews to exceed safe limitations and risk complications, injuries, and deaths to patients and crews.

References

1. Pressurized cabins, 14 C.F.R. § 25.841 (2006). 2006.
2. Muhm JM, Rock PB, McMullin DL, Jones SP, Lu IL, Eilers KD, et al. Effect of aircraft-cabin altitude on passenger discomfort. N Engl J Med. 2007;357(1):18–27.
3. Barnes SL, Branson R, Gallo LA, Beck G, Johannigman JA. En-route care in the air: snapshot of mechanical ventilation at 37,000 feet. J Trauma. 2008;64(2 Suppl):S129–34; discussion S34–5.
4. Cannon J, Pamplin J, Zonies D, Mason P, Sine C, Cancio L, et al. Acute respiratory failure. Mil Med. 2018;183(suppl_2):123–9.
5. Flabouris A, Schoettker P, Garner A. ARDS with severe hypoxia—aeromedical transportation during prone ventilation. Anaesth Intensive Care. 2003;31(6):675–8.
6. Reily DJ, Tollok E, Mallitz K, Hanson CW 3rd, Fuchs BD. Successful aeromedical transport using inhaled prostacyclin for a patient with life-threatening hypoxemia. Chest. 2004;125(4):1579–81.
7. Massarutti D, Trillo G, Berlot G, Tomasini A, Bacer B, D'Orlando L, et al. Simple thoracostomy in prehospital trauma management is safe and effective: a 2-year experience by helicopter emergency medical crews. Eur J Emerg Med. 2006;13(5):276–80.
8. Braude D, Tutera D, Tawil I, Pirkl G. Air transport of patients with pneumothorax: is tube thoracostomy required before flight? Air Med J. 2014;33(4):152–6.

9. Henry SM. Advanced trauma life support course student manual. 10th ed. Chicago, IL: American College of Surgeons; 2018.
10. Doucet J, Bulger E, Sanddal N, Fallat M, Bromberg W, Gestring M. Appropriate use of helicopter emergency medical services for transport of trauma patients: guidelines from the emergency medical system subcommittee, committee on trauma, American college of surgeons. J Trauma Acute Care Surg. 2013;75(4):734–41.
11. Systems CoAoMT. Accreditation Standards of the commission on accreditation of medical transport systems. Sandy Springs, SC; 2018.
12. Doucet J, Ferrada P, Murthi S, Nirula R, Edwards S, Cantrell E, et al. Ultrasonographic IVC diameter response to trauma resuscitation after one hour predicts 24 hour fluid requirement. J Trauma Acute Care Surg. 2020;88(1):70–9.
13. Dehqanzada ZA, Meisinger Q, Doucet J, Smith A, Casola G, Coimbra R. Complete ultrasonography of trauma in screening blunt abdominal trauma patients is equivalent to computed tomographic scanning while reducing radiation exposure and cost. J Trauma Acute Care Surg. 2015;79(2):199–205.
14. Press GM, Miller SK, Hassan IA, Alade KH, Camp E, Junco DD, et al. Prospective evaluation of prehospital trauma ultrasound during aeromedical transport. J Emerg Med. 2014;47(6):638–45.
15. Das SK, Choupoo NS, Haldar R, Lahkar A. Transtracheal ultrasound for verification of endotracheal tube placement: a systematic review and meta-analysis. Can J Anaesth. 2015;62(4):413–23.
16. Hanlin ER, Zelenak J, Barakat M, Anderson KL. Airway ultrasound for the confirmation of endotracheal tube placement in cadavers by military flight medic trainees—a pilot study. Am J Emerg Med. 2018;36(9):1711–4.
17. Mason R, Latimer A, Vrablik M, Utarnachitt R. Teaching flight nurses ultrasonographic evaluation of esophageal intubation and pneumothorax. Air Med J. 2019;38(3):195–7.
18. O'Dochartaigh D, Douma M, MacKenzie M. Five-year retrospective review of physician and non-physician performed ultrasound in a Canadian critical care helicopter emergency medical service. Prehosp Emerg Care. 2017;21(1):24–31.
19. Cover M, Tafoya C, Long B, Cranford J, Burkhardt J, Huang R, et al. Creation of a flight nurse critical care ultrasound program. Air Med J. 2019;38(4):266–72.
20. 1999–2018 Preliminary aviation statistics. Washington, DC: National Transportation Safety Board; 2019. https://www.ntsb.gov/investigations/data/Documents/AviationAccidentStatistics_1999-2018_20191101.xlsx. [cited 2018].
21. Galvagno SM Jr, Sikorski R, Hirshon JM, Floccare D, Stephens C, Beecher D, et al. Helicopter emergency medical services for adults with major trauma. Cochrane Database Syst Rev. 2015;12:CD009228.
22. Brown JB, Gestring ML, Guyette FX, Rosengart MR, Stassen NA, Forsythe RM, et al. Helicopter transport improves survival following injury in the absence of a time-saving advantage. Surgery. 2016;159(3):947–59.
23. Brown JB, Smith KJ, Gestring ML, Rosengart MR, Billiar TR, Peitzman AB, et al. Comparing the air medical Prehospital triage score with current practice for triage of injured patients to helicopter emergency medical services: a cost-effectiveness analysis. JAMA Surg. 2018;153(3):261–8.
24. Brown JB, Gestring ML, Guyette FX, Rosengart MR, Stassen NA, Forsythe RM, et al. External validation of the air medical Prehospital triage score for identifying trauma patients likely to benefit from scene helicopter transport. J Trauma Acute Care Surg. 2017;82(2):270–9.
25. Aerospace Medical Association Medical Guidelines Task F. Medical guidelines for airline travel, 2nd ed. Aviat Space Environ Med. 2003;74(5 Suppl):A1–19.
26. AMA Commission on Emergency Medical Services. Medical aspects of transportation aboard commercial aircraft. JAMA. 1982;247(7):1007–11.
27. Zonies D, Elterman J, Burns C, Paul V, Oh J, Cannon J. Trauma patients are safe to fly 72 hours after tube thoracostomy removal. J Trauma Acute Care Surg. 2018;85(3):491–4.

28. Cheatham ML, Safcsak K. Air travel following traumatic pneumothorax: when is it safe? Am Surg. 1999;65(12):1160–4.
29. Kaniecki DM. Pericardiocentesis in an ambulance: a case report and lessons learned. Air Med J. 2019;38(5):382–5.
30. High K, Brywczynski J, Han JH. Cricothyrotomy in helicopter emergency medical service transport. Air Med J. 2018;37(1):51–3.
31. Mahmodlou R, Sepehrvand N. Tracheobronchial injury due to blunt chest trauma. Int J Crit Illn Inj Sci. 2015;5(2):116–8.
32. Nishiumi N, Inokuchi S, Oiwa K, Masuda R, Iwazaki M, Inoue H. Diagnosis and treatment of deep pulmonary laceration with intrathoracic hemorrhage from blunt trauma. Ann Thorac Surg. 2010;89(1):232–8.
33. Hamilton EC, Lazar D, Tsao K, Cox C, Austin MT. Pediatric tracheobronchial injury after blunt trauma. J Trauma Acute Care Surg. 2017;83(3):554–6.
34. Lang JL, Gonzalez RP, Aldy KN, Carroll EA, Eastman AL, White CQ, et al. Does temporary chest wall closure with or without chest packing improve survival for trauma patients in shock after emergent thoracotomy? J Trauma Acute Care Surg. 2011;70(3):705–9.
35. Vargo DJ, Battistella FD. Abbreviated thoracotomy and temporary chest closure: an application of damage control after thoracic trauma. Arch Surg. 2001;136(1):21–4.
36. Garcia A, Martinez J, Rodriguez J, Millan M, Valderrama G, Ordoñez C, et al. Damage-control techniques in the management of severe lung trauma. J Trauma Acute Care Surg. 2015;78(1):45–51.
37. Lockey DJ, Brohi K. Pre-hospital thoracotomy and the evolution of pre-hospital critical care for victims of trauma. Injury. 2017;48(9):1863–4.
38. Laskowski K, Stirling A, McKay WP, Lim HJ. A systematic review of intravenous ketamine for postoperative analgesia. Can J Anesth. 2011;58(10):911.
39. Gutsche J, Vernick W, Miano TA, Penn LR. One-year experience with a mobile extracorporeal life support service. Ann Thorac Surg. 2017;104(5):1509–15.
40. Combes A, Hajage D, Capellier G, Demoule A, Lavoué S, Guervilly C, et al. Extracorporeal membrane oxygenation for severe acute respiratory distress syndrome. N Engl J Med. 2018;378(21):1965–75.
41. Gryniuk J, Leatham D. Helicopter shopping. EMS Mag. 2008;37(2):46–7.
42. American College of Emergency Physicians. A culture of safety in EMS systems. Policy statement. Ann Emerg Med. 2015;66(6):691.

Printed by Printforce, the Netherlands